AN UPDATE ON GLOMERULOPATHIES – ETIOLOGY AND PATHOGENESIS

Edited by **Sharma S. Prabhakar**

An Update on Glomerulopathies – Etiology and Pathogenesis
Edited by Sharma S. Prabhakar

Published by InTech

Janeza Trdine 9, 51000 Rijeka, Croatia

Publishing Process Manager Romina Krebel

Technical Editor Teodora Smiljanic

Cover Designer InTech Design Team

Additional hard copies can be obtained from orders@intechopen.com

An Update on Glomerulopathies – Etiology and Pathogenesis,
Edited by Sharma S. Prabhakar
p. cm.
ISBN 978-953-307-388-0

For EU product safety concerns:
IN TECH d.o.o., Prolaz Marije Krucifikse Kozulić 3, 51000 Rijeka, Croatia,
info@intechopen.com or visit our website at intechopen.com.

Meet the editor

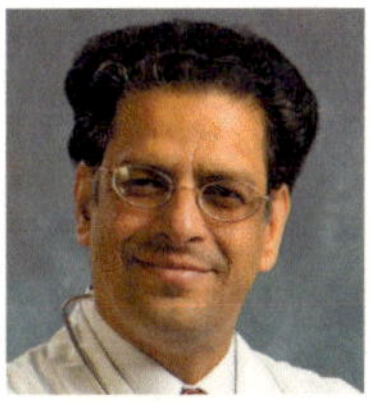

Dr. Sharma S. Prabhakar is a distinguished nephrologist currently at Texas Tech University Health Sciences Center, where he is a tenured professor in the Departments of Medicine and Cell Physiology and Molecular Biophysics, and the Chief of Nephrology Division and Vice Chairman, Department of Medicine. He is an established researcher examining pathophysiologic mechanisms of diabetic nephropathy and of insulin resistance in vitro and animal models. In the area of clinical research he initiated and is the principal investigator of a number of clinical studies. Dr. Prabhakar has over 100 publications including original articles, reviews, book chapters and published abstracts in prestigious journals, such as the American Journal of Physiology, Journal of American Society of Nephrology, and Kidney International. He has recently published a reference book entitled "Advances in the Pathogenesis of Diabetic Nephropathy". In recognition of his excellence in practice of medicine, Dr. Prabhakar was awarded an endowed chair by the University Medical Center. He is active in several professional societies and organizations and is the current President of American Federation for Medical Research.

Contents

Foreword

The past several decades have seen dramatic advances in understanding the etiopathogenesis of glomerulonephritis. The science of renal disease has progressed steadily from a discipline focused largely on whole organ physiology, through successive eras of cell and molecular biology, several omics (proteomics, genomics) and now into molecular mapping and personalized medicine. During that time, the processes which initiate and mediate glomerular inflammation have emerged with increasing clarity and complexity from early perceptions that they reflected largely immune complex driven processes involving exogenous antigens, antibodies and complement to today's recognition that most are autoimmune in nature. The role of both the innate and adaptive immune systems, the nature of the cellular responses to injury and their signalling pathways and the molecular events that produce the diseases seen by pathologists and clinicians have all become much more clearly defined.

This book is produced not as a comprehensive review of current understanding of the pathogenesis of glomerulonephritis but rather as a series of well selected individual update chapters that provide snapshots of the breadth and depth of renal science, as it exists today. Thus, chapters cover the dual roles of the innate immune system in mediating disease and initiating the immune response (Yahuan Lou), while others focus on both the humoral and cellular arms of the adaptive immune system (Tetsuhiro Tanaka et al., Mihály Józsi) and particularly the recent advances in understanding how auto-antibodies mediate membranous nephropathy (Gian Marco Ghiggeri et al., Chia-Chao Wu et al.). Considerable recent detail is provided on cytokines and signalling mechanisms which translate immune events into cellular pathology including prostaglandins (Andrey Sorokin), endoplasmic reticulum (Reiko Inagi), mTOR receptors (Lena Succar et al.), STAT3 signalling pathways (Fumio Tsuji et al.), TGF-ß (Hyun Soon Lee) and extracellular signal-regulated kinases (Maki Urushihara et al.). Animal models (Elena Goiman et al., Chia-Chao Wu et al., María Ángeles Jiménez et al.) and end results such as urinary biomarkers (Sophie Ohlsson) are updated as well.

The reader of "An Update on Glomerulopathies - Etiology and Pathogenesis" will find something of interest to all students and research investigators of glomerular disease in the assembled scientific reviews and updates that make up this book. As in all good stories, the best comes last when the material presented here is integrated into the clinical and treatment aspects of glomerular disease that are covered in the book "An Update on Glomerulopathies - Clinical and Treatment Aspects".

William G Couser, MD
Affiliate Professor of Medicine
University of Washington School of medicine
Woodinville, WA
USA

Preface

While various glomerular disorders account for the most cases of end stage renal failure, the etio-pathogenesis of these conditions intrigued many investigators for decades. A clear knowledge of the etiology and pathogenesis is crucial for developing novel strategies to prevent and to treat these disorders. Notwithstanding the continuous emergence of new discoveries, we still have a long way to get any closer to a thorough understanding of the mechanisms of glomerular injury. "An Update on Glomerulopathies - Etiology and Pathogenesis" is a monograph dedicated to compile recent advances in the experimental and clinical research that examined the etio-pathogenesis of various glomerular disorders. The book has fourteen chapters which are grouped under different sections for the purposes of convenience. The book is more of an update on several areas that are being very actively investigated, rather than comprehensive reviews of all the glomerular diseases.

The currently available treatment options for glomerular disorders are not optimal since most of them either respond only partially or poorly so that relapse and progression is often the rule. Inadequate understanding of the factors underlying the development and progression of glomerular injury in various clinical scenarios is primarily responsible for lack of ideal therapies. The section on immune system and glomerulonephritis has three chapters which basically cover some of the actively investigated areas. Tetsuhiro Tanaka et al. discuss adaptive immune responses, both humoral and cell mediated in the context of Glomerulonephritis. Gian Marco Ghiggeri et al. wrote an exhaustive review on the immunological aspects of membranous nephropathy. Finally, Mihály Józsi, in a very informative chapter reviewed the role of anti-compliment antibodies in membrano-proliferative glomerulonephritis and dense deposit disease.

An additional factor for lack of better therapeutic choices is the lack of suitable animal models to replicate human glomerular injury in order to develop and test novel treatment strategies. There are three detailed chapters that exemplify the recent advances in using animal models to explore the pathogenesis of glomerulonephritis. Immunopathogenic mechanisms in a murine model of membranous nephropathy are discussed by Chia-Chao Wu et al., while autoimmune glomerulonephritis complicating chronic graft versus host reaction was discussed by Elena Goiman et al.

An interesting comparative review on glomerular injury in domestic cats is described in a separate chapter by María Ángeles Jiménez et al.

Central to the development of glomerular inflammation and injury are alterations and abnormalities of various cytokines and signaling systems. There are four chapters in this book that deal with these aspects in the pathogenesis. The role of TGF-β in progressive glomerular disease is discussed in great detail in a chapter well written by Hyun Soon Lee, with particular reference to mesangial matrix accumulation, while the role of STAT3 activation in glomerulonephritis is elaborated in the well written chapter by Fumio Tsuji et al. There are two chapters that review the role of two signaling pathways in glomerular disorders – rennin angiotensin system and the mammalian target of rapamycin (mTOR). Finally, the significance of prostaglandin regulation in glomerulonephritis is well summarized in the chapter written by Andrey Sorokin.

Reiko Inagi reviewed very lucidly the role of endoplasmic reticulum in the stress of responses in glomeruli, while the pathogenic significance of dendritic cells in autoimmune glomerulonephritis is elaborated by Yahuan Lou. Finally, the relevance of urinary biomarkers in relation to pathogenesis of glomerulonephritis is put together in a concise chapter written by Sophie Ohlsson.

While the purpose of this volume is to serve as an update on recent advances in the etio-pathogenesis of glomerulopathies, the book offers the current and broad based knowledge in the field to readers of all levels in the nephrology community. The Editor expresses deep and sincere gratitude to all the authors for their valuable contributions which facilitated the prompt compilation of this invaluable resource.

Sharma S. Prabhakar, MD MBA FACP FASN
Texas Tech University Medical Center
USA

Part 1

Immune System and Glomerulonephritis

1

The Role of Humoral and Cell-Mediated Adaptive Immune Response

Tetsuhiro Tanaka[1], William G Couser[2] and Masaomi Nangaku[1]
[1]*Division of Nephrology and Endocrinology, University of Tokyo, Tokyo,*
[2]*Division of Nephrology, Department of Medicine, University of Washington, Washington,*
[1]*Japan*
[2]*USA*

1. Introduction

Glomerulonephritis is a major cause of chronic kidney disease worldwide and presents with various histological and clinical manifestations in terms of severity and duration, resulting in diverse clinical outcomes. Immune-mediated injury of the resident glomerular cells plays a critical role in many forms of glomerular injury and mounting evidence indicates that both humoral and cell-mediated mechanisms are involved.

2. The helper T cell paradigm

Studies in the past quarter of century have established a role for lymphocytes in the pathogenesis of immune-mediated glomerular diseases. CD4- expressing T helper cells are a subgroup of T lymphocytes that provide help for immunoglobulin production and direct cellular immune mechanisms through activation of effector cells, such as macrophages. The role of T helper cells is variable depending on the nature of disease, and differential activation of T helper cell subsets has been proposed as one of the plausible explanations for the diversity of injury in glomerular diseases.

The majority of T helper cells are naïve cells without specified patterns of cytokine production (Th0 cells). Upon stimulation by antigen-presenting cells, such as macrophages and dendritic cells (DC), they receive the signal via their α/β T cell receptor (TCR) and differentiate into either T helper 1 (Th1) or T helper 2 (Th2) cells. DC are specialized cells for uptake, transport, processing and presentation of antigens to T cells (Mellman and Steinman 2001), and subsets of DC have been identified that may influence Th1 and Th2 development (Moser and Murphy 2000). They facilitate Th1 differentiation when they are stimulated via toll-like receptors (TLRs), by secreting IL-12, while Th2 differentiation is mediated by IL-4. The cytokine milieu is a key factor in directing Th1 and Th2 polarization.

Differentiated Th1 and Th2 subclasses are functionally distinguished by their specific profiles of cytokine production and their ability to induce different types of effector responses. Th1 cells produce interferon (IFN)-γ, interleukin (IL)-2 and tumor necrosis factor (TNF)-α. They activate macrophages, induce delayed-type hypersensitivity responses, and stimulate B cells to produce complement-fixing antibody isotypes that mediate opsonization and phagocytosis. Th2 cells produce IL-4, IL-5, IL-10 and IL-13 and promote production of non-complement-fixing IgG isotypes and IgE. Therefore, Th1 cells are largely responsible for cell-mediated immunity, while Th2 cells play a central role in humoral immune response.

There is an interaction between the Th1 and the Th2 responses. They inhibit each other by several mechanisms. For example, IFN-γ produced in Th1 cells inhibit the expression of CD40 ligand (CD40L) on the surface of Th2 cells and suppress B cell activity. On the other hand, IL-4 and IL-10 from Th2 cells inhibit IFN-γ and IL-12 production in Th1 cells.

In the kidney, the Th2-mediated response is characterized by formation of immune complexes and deposition in the glomerulus, which is usually followed by complement activation. On the other hand, the Th1-mediated response is characterized by infiltration of circulating mononuclear cells and crescent formation. Both responses are capable of releasing mediators that are responsible for functional and structural changes as seen in primary glomerular diseases. Importantly, these apparently discrepant mechanisms of immune reactions, the Th1 and Th2 responses, are not always mutually exclusive and operate in a coordinated manner in glomerular injury, depending on etiology and pathological stages.

Recently, Th17 cells were identified as a new subset of T helper cells unrelated to Th1 or Th2 cells. They are a subset of T helper cells characterized by IL-17 production, differentiated from naïve T cells in the presence of both transforming growth factor (TGF)-β and IL-6 in mice, and are implicated in the pathogenesis of experimental allergic encephalomyelitis (EAE) and collagen-induced arthritis (CIA) (Langrish et al. 2005). Evidence suggests that the Th17 response may also pertain to inflammatory and autoimmune diseases in humans, such as rheumatoid arthritis, inflammatory bowel disease and psoriasis. Several cytokines such as IL-21 and IL-23 are involved in regulating activation and differentiation of Th17 cells. In the kidney, Th17 effector cells have been demonstrated in biopsy samples in human glomerulonephritis (Abdulahad et al. 2009) and may participate in the pathogenesis of proliferative glomerulonephritis via production of IL-17 and direct induction of renal inflammation (Kim et al. 2009; Miossec et al. 2009; Turner et al. 2010; Kitching and Holdsworth 2011). Recent studies utilizing genetically engineered mice showed that RORγt promotes the development of crescentic glomerulonephritis by directing nephritogenic Th17 responses (Steinmetz et al. 2011) . In contrast, the adaptive immune response by T cells is regulated by T regulatory cell (Treg)s (Jiang and Chess 2006). Treg cells are in charge of suppressing potentially deleterious activities of Th cells. Lyn-deficient mice, which increase titers of autoantibodies with age, develop immune complex-mediated glomerulonephritis, and Tregs are expanding in these mice in an effort to control the autoimmune disease, although they are simply overwhelmed by the disease process eventually (Tsantikos et al. 2009).

3. Humoral immune response

Many forms of glomerulonephritis are autoimmune in nature and loss of self-tolerance and exposure to etiologic agents lead to immune-complex formation, presumably by mechanisms of molecular mimicry and epitope spreading. Causative antigens include normal intrinsic structures of the glomerulus (eg. non-collagenous domain of the alpha-III chain of type IV collagen in Goodpasture's syndrome), non-renal self antigens (eg. DNA-nucleosome complex in systemic lupus erythematosus (Kalaaji et al. 2007)) or exogenous

agents (eg. HCV antigen-containing cryoglobulins in hepatitis C virus-associated membranoproliferative glomerulonephritis (MPGN) (Stehman-Breen and Johnson 1998)). Immune complexes are either formed in the systemic circulation and localize in the glomerulus through passive trapping (eg. serum sickness disease in rabbits) or are formed in situ and form immune deposits locally. In the latter case, an antibody either binds specific antigens intrinsic to the glomerulus, or soluble antigens that become localized due to charge interactions with the glomerular capillary wall or by nonspecific uptake by the mesangium.
Identification of responsible antigens in human glomerular diseases, however, is difficult, and multiple antigens and routes leading to immune complex formation appear to co-exist in a single disorder. In poststreptococcal glomerulonephritis (PSGN), for example, several candidate exogenous antigens, such as nephritis-associated plasmin receptor (NAPlr) and Streptococcal pyrogenic exotoxin B (SPE B) have been postulated. In systemic lupus erythematosus (SLE), circulating immune complexes composed of antibodies against double-stranded DNA and ribonucleoproteins are readily detectable, which correlate with disease activity (Izui et al. 1979), and anti-DNA and DNA immune complexes are enriched in kidney eluates (Koffler et al. 1967), leading to speculation that immune deposits are formed in circulation and accumulate in the kidney through passive trapping. However, immune complexes are formed in situ as well, via charge interactions between antibodies and DNA-histone complexes already deposited in the glomerulus (Schmiedeke et al. 1989; van Bruggen et al. 1997; Mortensen and Rekvig 2009; Crispin et al. 2010). Furthermore, some lupus autoantibodies appear to bind directly to intrinsic glomerular antigens.
Deposits are observed in subepithelial (eg. Heymann nephritis model in rats and human membranous nephropathy), subendothelial (eg. type 1 MPGN) and mesangial (eg. IgA nephropathy) spaces. In general, immune complexes formed in situ are more nephritogenic, because they are more capable of activating local complement response (Couser and Salant 1980), releasing vasoactive substances, reactive oxygen species, cytokines and procoagulants (Couser 1998). In fact, it is rather unusual that immunoglobulins themselves induce significant injury in the kidney, except for antibodies against components of the podocyte slit diaphragm (Holthofer 2007).
The complement system is an important mediator of tissue inflammation and injury. It is a family of more than 20 serum and cell-surface proteins and they operate as a cascade of reactions. The IgG immune complexes bind to complement factor C1q and activate the C1 complex, leading to the formation of C3 convertase and the enzymatic cleavage of the central complement component C3. C3 then releases the chemotactic factor C3a and the covalent C3b attaches to the host cells, which is an important step for continued activation of the terminal membrane attack complex, C5b-9, and for the amplification through the alternative pathway. C5b-9 is thought to be the key component responsible for the complement-mediated glomerular injury. It inserts in sublytic amounts into the glomerular membranes, triggers cell activation and mediates injury.
The complement cascade is tightly regulated by short half-lives of its components and a series of endogenous regulatory proteins. Complement regulatory proteins counteract the complement activity and protect glomerular cells from injury (Nangaku 1998). In vitro, overexpression of CD59 protected cultured glomerular cells from attack (Nangaku et al. 1996). In the rat Heymann nephritis model, simultaneous blockade of complement regulatory proteins by neutralizing antibodies was required to develop proteinuria following injection of anti-megalin antibody (Schiller et al. 1998). Furthermore, genetic ablation of decay-accelerating factor (DAF) and CD59 aggravated tissue injury in anti-GBM

nephritis (Sogabe et al. 2001), nephrotoxic nephritis (Lin et al. 2002) and ischemia-reperfusion (Yamada et al. 2004) models in mice. In humans, genetic abnormalities of factor H, a soluble complement regulatory protein at the hit point of C3b, compose approximately 15-30% of atypical HUS (Rougier et al. 1998; Warwicker et al. 1998; Noris et al. 1999), showing that failure to control intravascular complement activity can lead to endothelial injury, formation of thrombus, and eventually, HUS. Mice genetically deficient for Factor H, as well as pigs with congenital factor H deficiency develop type II MGPN (Pickering et al. 2002), again highlighting the critical relevance of complement regulation in maintaining normal glomerular structure.

3.1 Heymann nephritis model in the rat

The role of immune complexes formed in situ has been most extensively studied in the Heymann nephritis model in the rat, a human counterpart of membranous nephropathy (MN). This is a non-proliferative form of GN in which the humoral, Th2 responses play an important role. In human idiopathic MN, an increase in the percentage of IL-4 (Masutani et al. 2004) and IL-10 (Hirayama et al. 2002) was observed in peripheral blood T cells, which correlated with the amount of proteinuria.

Following induction of the disease, antibodies against gp330, megalin (Cavallo 1994; Ronco and Debiec 2005), are deposited at the subepithelial space of the glomerulus and trigger podocyte injury through activation of the complement system, particularly the membrane attack complex, C5b-9. C5b-9 inserts into the podocyte membrane and is then transported across the cell to be extruded into the urinary space, resulting in elevated levels of C5b-9 in the urine (Kerjaschki et al. 1989). C5b-9 is thought to be the major mediator of altered glomerular permeability function, although histologic changes are minimal by light microscopy (Nangaku et al. 2005). Depletion of complement complements using cobra venom factor greatly reduced the amount of proteinuria (Salant et al. 1980; Saran et al. 2003). At the cellular level, C5b-9 generates hydrogen peroxide (Shah 1988; Neale et al. 1993) triggers DNA damage (Pippin et al. 2003), causes reversible disruption of actin microfilaments (Topham et al. 1999), increases the expression of TGF-β and its receptors, leading to overproduction of extracellular matrix, GBM thickening and spike formation. It also induces apoptosis in podocytes, dissociation of nephrin from the actin cytoskeleton (Yuan et al. 2002), detachment and excretion in the urine (Cybulsky 2011). However, subepithelial deposits in general induce no inflammation, probably because they are located at a site inaccessible to circulating cells.

Several caveats exist in translating these findings in rats into human MN. First, the responsible antigen, megalin, shows a distinct pattern of spatial distribution among species. In rats, megalin is expressed both on the brush border of proximal tubules and the soles of podocyte foot processes at which immune complexes are initially formed. In humans, however, megalin is only expressed in proximal tubules and not in podocytes, excluding megalin from the list of responsible self-antigens in human MN. Nevertheless, findings obtained from the Heymann nephritis provide solid evidence that some components on the podocyte membrane serve as targets for immune complex formation in situ and trigger cascades of humoral immune responses that lead to massive proteinuria. Second, deposition of immunoglobulin in human MN is predominantly of the IgG4 subclass, which is theoretically incapable of triggering complement activation. This is in contrast to the fact that complements undoubtedly play an important role in the rat Heymann nephritis. It may be a relevant finding that C6-deficient PVG rats incapable of forming C5b-9 also develop massive proteinuria following injection of antisera, suggesting that complement-independent mechanisms may also exist in this model (Spicer et al. 2007).

To date, much effort has been made to identify podocyte antigens responsible for human MN, which are only beginning to be uncovered. Recent breakthrough studies revealed pathogenic antigens of human MN in podocytes; i.e. neutral endopeptidase (NEP) that causes neonatal MN and phospholipase A2 receptor (PLA2R) that causes adulthood MN.

The proposed mechanisms on the pathogenesis of anti-NEP antibody-mediated neonatal NM was as follows. A genetically NEP-deficient mother developed anti-NEP antibody during the first pregnancy, which was transferred to the second baby not deficient for NEP. As a result, antibody against NEP localized on the surface of podocytes, formed immune complex in situ and subepithelial immune deposits and eventually developed neonatal membranous nephropathy in the second baby (Debiec et al. 2002). Subsequently, families with truncating mutation in the MME gene (coding for NEP) were reported, in which cases second infants born from MME-mutated mothers developed neonatal MN, indicating that the MME gene product is a cause of alloimmunization during pregnancy (Debiec et al. 2004). Clearly, however, NEP is only responsible for a fraction of rare cases of neonatal MN and not likely a universal antigen.

In contrast, serum from approximately 70% of patients with idiopathic membranous nephropathy recognized a 185 kDa glycoprotein, which was identified as PLA2R by mass spectrometry. Anti-PLA2R antibodies in serum were mainly of IgG4 subclass, the predominant IgG subclass in glomerular deposits. PLA2R was expressed in podocytes of normal human glomeruli and colocalized with IgG4 in subepithelial immune deposits (Beck et al. 2009). These findings were recently supported by independent genomewide association studies of single-nucleotide polymorphisms (SNPs) in patients with idiopathic MN from three populations of white ancestry (Stanescu et al. 2011). The joint analysis of data from the 556 patients studied identified the gene encoding PLA2R as a risk allele of idiopathic MN.

3.2 Goodpasture's syndrome

Anti-GBM antibody disease (Goodpasture's syndrome) is a disorder in which circulating antibodies against an antigen intrinsic to the glomerular basement membrane (GBM) cause rapidly progressive glomerulonephritis (RPGN). Non-collagenous domain of the alpha-III chain of type IV collagen (α3IV-NCI) is likely a responsible antigen (Hudson et al. 2003; Hudson 2004), and eluates from patients contain antibodies against α5IV-NCI as well as α3IV-NCI. Of interest, the antigen requires certain quarternary structures to be recognized by the antibody, and the native cross-linked α345IV-NCI escapes recognition (Pedchenko et al. 2010). The disease is primarily initiated through autoantibody-mediated reactions, but an additional role of delayed hypersensitivity reactions is also suggested, because Th1 effector cytokines such as IL-12 and IFN-γ play important roles in this model (Kitching et al. 2004). Passive transfer of anti-GBM antibodies alone was not sufficient to induce disease in the absence of T cells (Kalluri et al. 1997) and T cells sensitized to the GBM antigen alone were sufficient to initiate injury (Wu et al. 2002). Furthermore, oral administration of α3IV-NCI ameliorated disease (Reynolds and Pusey 2001) and nasal application of this antigen protected from injury, which was associated with suppression of glomerular T cells and macrophages (Reynolds et al. 2005). These findings suggested the role of systemic suppression of T cell function in ameliorating disease. In this regard, the possible participation of Tregs is anticipated, but this remains to be proven.

Goodpasture's syndrome is clinically associated with alveolar hemorrhage. Because the α3IV-NCI is also expressed within the alveolar basement membrane, responsible antibodies recognize alveolar epithelium as well. Immune complexes then cause injury and subsequent effector responses, leading to pulmonary hemorrhage in affected patients.

3.3 Poststreptococcal glomerulonephritis

The major pathogenic mechanism of poststreptococcal glomerulonephritis (PSGN) is an in situ immune complex formation due to deposition of streptococcal nephritogenic antigens, such as nephritis-associated plasmin receptor (NAPlr) and Streptococcal pyrogenic exotoxin B (SPE B). Both are capable of activating the alternate pathway of the complement cascade and enhance the expression of adhesion molecules. SPE B also stimulates the production of chemotactic cytokines.

NAPlr was isolated from group A streptococcus and was shown to bind plasmin(ogen). In the original report, 92 percent of Japanese patients with the acute PSGN had anti-NAPlr antibodies, and about 80% of renal biopsy samples showed deposits of NaPlr, especially in the early stage of the disease, but the deposits did not colocalize with either C3 or IgG. NAPlr exhibits glyceraldehyde-3-phosphate dehydrogenase (GAPDH) activity in vitro. Mechanistically, it is speculated that NAPlr in the mesangium interacts with plasmin(ogen) and causes glomerular injury by degrading GBM through activation of metalloproteinase precursors. Then, circulating immune complexes move across damaged GBM and accumulate in the subepithelial space (Yamakami et al. 2000; Yoshizawa et al. 2004).

SPE B is a cationic cysteine proteinase and was found in 12 of 17 biopsies from patients in Latin America and Switzerland. SPE B deposits localized within the subepithelial electron dense deposits (humps) and colocalized with complement (Batsford et al. 2005). Antibodies to SPE B were detected in the convalescent sera in all patients tested.

To date, it is speculated that separate antigens may be responsible for PSGN in different parts of the world and among patients with distinct genetic backgrounds (Rodriguez-Iturbe and Batsford 2007; Rodriguez-Iturbe and Musser 2008).

3.4 Immune complex in the subendothelial space and the mesangium

Immune complexes can be formed and deposited in other compartments of the glomerulus as well. Deposition in the subendothelial space can be found in human type 1 MPGN and lupus nephritis (Class III and IV). They recruit circulating inflammatory cells, such as neutrophils, lymphocytes, macrophages and platelets (Adler and Brady 1999), activate effector responses and cause injury. Local chemotactic factors such as C5a and IL-8 recruit neutrophils to sites of inflammation. There, they phagocytose the immune complex aggregates, become activated and undergo a respiratory burst that generates reactive oxygen species. Macrophages are recruited through interaction with deposited immunoglobulins and by several chemokines, such as macrophage chemoattractant protein-1 (MCP-1) and RANTES. Lymphocyte-derived molecules such as macrophage inhibitory factor (MIF) and leukocyte adhesion molecules such as ICAM-1 and VCAM-1 also trigger their migration (Nikolic-Paterson and Atkins 2001). In contrast to neutrophils, they release tissue factors and TGF-β and facilitate extracellular matrix accumulation which eventually leads to glomerular sclerosis.

Immune deposits in the mesangium are a representative feature of human IgA nephropathy and lupus nephritis (Class I and II). Following deposit formation, these cells initiate a cascade of inflammatory processes, including complement activation, coagulation and release of cytokines and growth factors (Gomez-Guerrero et al. 2005). C5b-9-mediated mechanisms of complement activation are likely to be responsible for immunopathology in the mesangium, too. Furthermore, they undergo a dysregulated increase in proliferation and expansion that lead to glomerular hypercellularity, express markers of de-differentiation such as α-SMA and serve as a source of inflammatory cytokines and growth factors, such as transforming growth factor (TGF)-β and platelet-derived growth factor (PDGF) that contribute to glomerular sclerosis.

4. Cell-mediated immune response

In the kidney, T cell-mediated injury occurs primarily through effector responses, such as release of chemokines and recruitment of macrophages and is indispensable for glomerular immunopathology, and available data even suggest that a subset of Th17 cells have effector cell functions alone. On the other hand, some forms of glomerulonephritis do not require immune complexes to develop full-blown pathology. Crescentic glomerulonephritis was produced in a chicken with chemically blocked Bursa of Fabricius, indicating that the lesion was developed without antibody deposits (Bolton et al. 1984). Nephritis was also transferred to normal chickens using only T cells sensitized to GBM (Bolton et al. 1988), and to rats using lymphocytes sensitized to the Goodpasture antigen (Wu et al. 2002). These results indicate that T cells play important roles in the pathogenesis of certain forms of crescentic nephritis. Cell-mediated immune responses are also critical in several other types of glomerulonephritis, such as minimal change nephrotic syndrome (MCNS), focal and segmental glomerulosclerosis (FSGS), pauci-immune crescentic glomerulonephritis, and lupus (Class IV). Mononuclear cells such as lymphocytes and macrophages are recruited to the glomerulus and release tissue factors and TGF-β that initiate fibrin deposition and extracellular matrix accumulation, and there is speculation that T cells may be the source of permeability factors that contribute to proteinuria and noninflammatory glomerular injury.

4.1 Glomerular permeability factor(s)

The initial manifestations in MCNS and FSGS are dramatic increases in glomerular permeability, which are associated with little or no structural abnormality by light microscopy. In these disorders, the presence of non-immunoglobulin circulating permeability factors is postulated, for the following reasons. First, the rapid recurrence of MCNS and FSGS is clinically observed when normal kidneys are transplanted into patients with these disorders (Hoyer et al. 1972). Second, MCNS kidneys demonstrate rapid resolution when placed in a normal environment (Ali et al. 1994). Similarly, a market decrease in proteinuria is observed in some FSGS patients following plasma exchange. Third, serum from recurrent FSGS are able to increase the albumin reflection coefficient of isolated normal glomeruli in vitro (Savin et al. 1996) . However, the identity of these permeability factors is elusive and it remains unclear how non-immunoglobulin permeability factors increase glomerular permeability. One study implicated CLC1 as a candidate factor in recurrent FSGS (McCarthy et al. 2010). In contrast, up-regulation of the glomerular expression of angiopoietin-like-4 (Angptl4), a secreted glycoprotein, was shown in the serum and in podocytes in experimental models of MCNS and in the human disease (Clement et al. 2011). A pathogenic role of Angptl4 expression in podocytes was confirmed in genetically engineered animals.

4.2 Th1-mediated response in experimental crescentic nephritis

Severe crescentic injury in the glomerulus, regardless of its underlying cause, is regarded as the result of a Th1 predominant cellular response. It is presumably mediated by T cell- and macrophage- mediated, delayed hypersensitivity responses, which is suggested by the association of cellular immune mediators with local fibrin deposition (Tipping and Holdsworth 2006). Macrophages release ROS and inflammatory cytokines, cause injury in the Bowman's capsule and mediate crescent formation by facilitating compensatory cell growth and influx of inflammatory cells.

4.2.1 Nephrotoxic nephritis

Nephrotoxic nephritis is one of the most intensively studied models of experimental glomerulonephritis characterized by cellular proliferation and crescent formation. In this model, nephrotoxic serum is taken up and presented to naïve T helper cells by antigen-presenting cells, presumably DC. Naïve T cells then differentiate into Th1 effector cells (Schatzmann et al. 1999), which play a central role in the pathogenesis. The first evidence came from a study comparing histological features of injury in Th1 (C57BL6) - and Th2 (BALB/c) - dominant mice (Huang et al. 1997). Studies in Lewis and Brown Norway rats also demonstrated features of cell-mediated types of glomerular injury, which were accompanied by a Th1 polarized profile of cytokine production (Coelho et al. 1997). Analysis of cytokine profiles from biopsies of proliferative glomerulonephritis showed higher levels of IL-2 and IFN-γ, as compared to non-proliferative forms (Kim et al. 2001). In addition, studies in human anti-GBM glomerular disease supported a role for Th1 responses in injury, by demonstrating IFN-γ-predominant effector cell responses in active disease and IL-10 predominance in remission (Cairns et al. 2003).

Cytokines produced in response to Th1 polarization play an essential role for crescent formation. Glomerular T cell and macrophage accumulation was attenuated in mice with genetic deletion of Th1 cytokines, such as IL-12 (Kitching et al. 2000), IFN-γ (Kitching et al. 1999) and TNF (Timoshanko et al. 2003), which was associated with amelioration of crescentic injury. Conversely, administration of IL-12 augmented Th1 responses and crescentic nephritis (Kitching et al. 1999). On the other hand, Th2 cytokines attenuated proliferative and crescentic nephritis. Mice genetically deficient for IL-4 or IL-10 showed more pronounced Th1 responses and developed more severe crescentic nephritis (Kitching et al. 1998). Conversely, overexpression of IL-10 by gene transfer attenuated crescentic nephritis in Wistar Kyoto rats (Higuchi et al. 2003).

Not all Th1 predominant cytokines, however, behave in a similar way to augment injury, because discrepant results also exist for the role of IFN-γ, reporting ameliorating effect in nephrotoxic nephritis (Ring et al. 1999), and experimental anti-GBM nephritis (Kitching et al. 2004), suggesting the complex role of IFN-γ beyond the principle of simple Th1/Th2 predominancy. The cellular source and the co-producition of additional cytokines, such as IL-10, may determine whether IFN-γ is protective or harmful (Trinchieri 2007). Similarly, deficiency for IL-13, a Th2-associated cytokine, failed to aggravate nephrotoxic nephritis, despite augmented production of Th1-associated immunoglobulin subclasses (Kitching et al. 2004), leading to speculation that the pathogenic role of Th1-mediated delayed hypersensitivity reactions overweigh that of antibody-mediated immune responses.

DC are remarkably abundant in the tubulointerstitium in the normal kidney. However, DC form periglomerular infiltrates around inflamed glomeruli in nephrotoxic nephritis (Kruger et al. 2004), the rat anti-GBM model (Fujinaka et al. 2007) and some forms of human glomerular diseases, such as Wegener's granulomatosus and IgA nephropathy (Markovic-Lipkovski et al. 1990). Functionally, dendritic cells appear to have a protective role against injury, by interacting with Th1 cells locally and producing IL-10, thereby suppressing Th1 cell and macrophage functions. When DC were depleted, nephrotoxic nephritis was aggravated. (Scholz et al. 2008).

4.2.2 Other forms of crescentic glomerulopathies

A predominant role for Th1 responses has been described in other types of crescentic glomerular diseases as well. In ANCA-associated nephritis, T cells and macrophages accumulate in glomerular lesions (Cunningham et al. 1999) and glomerular biopsies show high IFN-γ and low IL-4 mRNA expression, suggesting a Th-1 predominant effector response. Peripheral blood T cells showed a high IFN-γ:IL-4 ratio as compared to non-proliferative forms (Masutani et al. 2003). There is also evidence suggesting the involvement of Th17 responses. Th17 cells promoted autoimmune anti-myeloperoxidase glomerulonephritis in mice (Gan et al. 2010) and patients with ANCA-associated vasculitis had elevated serum levels of IL-17 and IL-23 (Nogueira et al. 2010). It remains unclear, however, how the co-existing Th1 and Th17 responses cross-regulate each other. Available evidence suggests both synergism (O'Connor et al. 2008) and inhibition (Yi et al. 2008). In active Wegener's granulomatosis, peripheral blood T cells produced high levels of IFN-γ and monocytes produced high IL-12 regardless of disease activity (Ludviksson et al. 1998). Analysis of cytokine profiles in lesions from the nasal mucosa have yielded conflicting results, and both IL-2 and CCR5+ (Th1) and IL-4 and CCR3+ (Th2) cells were present in renal tissues (Balding et al. 2001).

Human lupus nephritis displays heterogenous patterns of Th1 and Th2 responses, which are probably associated with diverse histopathogolical presentations of this disease entity. In patients with WHO class IV crescentic disease, however, increases in peripheral blood T cell IFN-γ:IL-4 ratio, renal CD3+ cells and macrophages and IFN-γ positive cells were observed compared to patients with either WHO class V or mild glomerular lesions (Masutani et al. 2001). Th1 cytokine predominance was also shown in the urinary sediment of patients with active lupus nephritis (Chan et al. 2003). Murine models of lupus nephritis are also critically dependent on T helper cells, in addition to the almost certain dependency on B cells (Reininger et al. 1996; Chan et al. 1999). Depletion of CD4+ cells attenuated disease in MRL-lpr mice (Jabs et al. 1992), in New Zealand black/white (NZB/NZW) mice (Connolly et al. 1992) and in Y-chromosome-associated lupus mice (Lawson et al. 2001). In MRL/lpr mice, however, cytokine profiling showed conflicting results in terms of Th1 (Takahashi et al. 1996; Kikawada et al. 2003) and Th2 (Santiago et al. 1997) predominancy, again refleting the multifactorial nature of the disease.

A fraction of cases with IgA nephropathy also present with proliferative, crescentic lesions. In general, this is a disease with heterogeneity of Th responses. The onset may be related to factors favoring a Th2-predominnat environment that promotes dysregulated IgA production, but a severe proliferative disease is associated with Th1 predominant responses. This idea is supported by experimental observation that adoptive transfer of T helper cells alone was unable to initiate disease (Suzuki et al. 2007). Meanwhile, IL-12 induced glomerular crescents and macrophage accumulation in a ddY strain with high IgA, suggesting a role of Th1 subsets (Nogaki et al. 2000).

5. Conclusion

Immune-mediated mechanisms of injury are involved in a variety of primary glomerular diseases. In humoral immune injury, immune complexes against intrinsic renal antigens, exogenous agents and non-renal, self antigens are either formed in situ or are passively trapped in the glomerulus. Immune deposits then trigger injury by activating the complement cascade, releasing oxidants, cytokines and growth factors and recruiting effector cells. The membrane attack complex, C5b-9 plays a critical role in the majority of humoral responses in the kidney. On the other hand, proliferative, crescentic glomerulonephritis is almost always associated with cell-mediated immune responses, which are associated with effector cell activation such as macrophages and release of cytokines and growth factors, leading to delayed hypersensitivity response. Th1 cytokines, such as IFN-γ and IL-12 play important roles during the pathogenesis. The Th17 responses may also participate in cell-mediated injury in some forms of glomerulopathies, such as ANCA-associated nephritis. The humoral and cell-mediated mechanisms of injury are not necessarily exclusive, mutually, but play respective roles at each stage of a given disease category, depending on its nature. The critical, albeit complex, participation of both humoral and cell-mediated immune responses provides rationale for the current treatment strategies that target modulation of immunopathogenesis at multiple stages of glomerular injury.

6. References

Abdulahad, W. H., C. A. Stegeman, et al. (2009). "Review article: The role of CD4(+) T cells in ANCA-associated systemic vasculitis." Nephrology (Carlton) 14(1): 26-32.

Adler, S. and H. R. Brady (1999). "Cell adhesion molecules and the glomerulopathies." Am J Med 107(4): 371-86.

Ali, A. A., E. Wilson, et al. (1994). "Minimal-change glomerular nephritis. Normal kidneys in an abnormal environment?" Transplantation 58(7): 849-52.

Balding, C. E., A. J. Howie, et al. (2001). "Th2 dominance in nasal mucosa in patients with Wegener's granulomatosis." Clin Exp Immunol 125(2): 332-9.

Batsford, S. R., S. Mezzano, et al. (2005). "Is the nephritogenic antigen in post-streptococcal glomerulonephritis pyrogenic exotoxin B (SPE B) or GAPDH?" Kidney Int 68(3): 1120-9.

Beck, L. H., Jr., R. G. Bonegio, et al. (2009). "M-type phospholipase A2 receptor as target antigen in idiopathic membranous nephropathy." N Engl J Med 361(1): 11-21.

Bolton, W. K., M. Chandra, et al. (1988). "Transfer of experimental glomerulonephritis in chickens by mononuclear cells." Kidney Int 34(5): 598-610.

Bolton, W. K., F. L. Tucker, et al. (1984). "New avian model of experimental glomerulonephritis consistent with mediation by cellular immunity. Nonhumorally mediated glomerulonephritis in chickens." J Clin Invest 73(5): 1263-76.

Cairns, L. S., R. G. Phelps, et al. (2003). "The fine specificity and cytokine profile of T-helper cells responsive to the alpha3 chain of type IV collagen in Goodpasture's disease." J Am Soc Nephrol 14(11): 2801-12.

Cavallo, T. (1994). "Membranous nephropathy. Insights from Heymann nephritis." Am J Pathol 144(4): 651-8.

Chan, O. T., M. P. Madaio, et al. (1999). "B cells are required for lupus nephritis in the polygenic, Fas-intact MRL model of systemic autoimmunity." J Immunol 163(7): 3592-6.

Chan, R. W., L. S. Tam, et al. (2003). "Inflammatory cytokine gene expression in the urinary sediment of patients with lupus nephritis." Arthritis Rheum 48(5): 1326-31.

Clement, L. C., C. Avila-Casado, et al. (2011). "Podocyte-secreted angiopoietin-like-4 mediates proteinuria in glucocorticoid-sensitive nephrotic syndrome." Nat Med 17(1): 117-22.

Coelho, S. N., S. Saleem, et al. (1997). "Immunologic determinants of susceptibility to experimental glomerulonephritis: role of cellular immunity." Kidney Int 51(3): 646-52.

Connolly, K., J. R. Roubinian, et al. (1992). "Development of murine lupus in CD4-depleted NZB/NZW mice. Sustained inhibition of residual CD4+ T cells is required to suppress autoimmunity." J Immunol 149(9): 3083-8.

Couser, W. G. (1998). "Pathogenesis of glomerular damage in glomerulonephritis." Nephrol Dial Transplant 13 Suppl 1: 10-5.

Couser, W. G. and D. J. Salant (1980). "In situ immune complex formation and glomerular injury." Kidney Int 17(1): 1-13.

Crispin, J. C., S. N. Liossis, et al. (2010). "Pathogenesis of human systemic lupus erythematosus: recent advances." Trends Mol Med 16(2): 47-57.

Cunningham, M. A., X. R. Huang, et al. (1999). "Prominence of cell-mediated immunity effectors in "pauci-immune" glomerulonephritis." J Am Soc Nephrol 10(3): 499-506.

Cybulsky, A. V. (2011). "Membranous nephropathy." Contrib Nephrol 169: 107-25.

Debiec, H., V. Guigonis, et al. (2002). "Antenatal membranous glomerulonephritis due to anti-neutral endopeptidase antibodies." N Engl J Med 346(26): 2053-60.

Debiec, H., J. Nauta, et al. (2004). "Role of truncating mutations in MME gene in fetomaternal alloimmunisation and antenatal glomerulopathies." Lancet 364(9441): 1252-9.

Fujinaka, H., M. Nameta, et al. (2007). "Periglomerular accumulation of dendritic cells in rat crescentic glomerulonephritis." J Nephrol 20(3): 357-63.

Gan, P. Y., O. M. Steinmetz, et al. (2010). "Th17 cells promote autoimmune anti-myeloperoxidase glomerulonephritis." J Am Soc Nephrol 21(6): 925-31.

Gomez-Guerrero, C., P. Hernandez-Vargas, et al. (2005). "Mesangial cells and glomerular inflammation: from the pathogenesis to novel therapeutic approaches." Curr Drug Targets Inflamm Allergy 4(3): 341-51.

Higuchi, N., H. Maruyama, et al. (2003). "Hydrodynamics-based delivery of the viral interleukin-10 gene suppresses experimental crescentic glomerulonephritis in Wistar-Kyoto rats." Gene Ther 10(16): 1297-310.

Hirayama, K., I. Ebihara, et al. (2002). "Predominance of type-2 immune response in idiopathic membranous nephropathy. Cytoplasmic cytokine analysis." Nephron 91(2): 255-61.

Holthofer, H. (2007). "Molecular architecture of the glomerular slit diaphragm: lessons learnt for a better understanding of disease pathogenesis." Nephrol Dial Transplant 22(8): 2124-8.

Hoyer, J. R., R. L. Vernier, et al. (1972). "Recurrence of idiopathic nephrotic syndrome after renal transplantation." Lancet 2(7773): 343-8.

Huang, X. R., P. G. Tipping, et al. (1997). "Th1 responsiveness to nephritogenic antigens determines susceptibility to crescentic glomerulonephritis in mice." Kidney Int 51(1): 94-103.

Hudson, B. G. (2004). "The molecular basis of Goodpasture and Alport syndromes: beacons for the discovery of the collagen IV family." J Am Soc Nephrol 15(10): 2514-27.

Hudson, B. G., K. Tryggvason, et al. (2003). "Alport's syndrome, Goodpasture's syndrome, and type IV collagen." N Engl J Med 348(25): 2543-56.

Izui, S., P. J. McConahey, et al. (1979). "Association of circulating retroviral gp70-anti-gp70 immune complexes with murine systemic lupus erythematosus." J Exp Med 149(5): 1099-116.

Jabs, D. A., C. L. Burek, et al. (1992). "Anti-CD4 monoclonal antibody therapy suppresses autoimmune disease in MRL/Mp-lpr/lpr mice." Cell Immunol 141(2): 496-507.

Jiang, H. and L. Chess (2006). "Regulation of immune responses by T cells." N Engl J Med 354(11): 1166-76.

Kalaaji, M., K. A. Fenton, et al. (2007). "Glomerular apoptotic nucleosomes are central target structures for nephritogenic antibodies in human SLE nephritis." Kidney Int 71(7): 664-72.

Kalluri, R., T. M. Danoff, et al. (1997). "Susceptibility to anti-glomerular basement membrane disease and Goodpasture syndrome is linked to MHC class II genes and the emergence of T cell-mediated immunity in mice." J Clin Invest 100(9): 2263-75.

Kerjaschki, D., M. Schulze, et al. (1989). "Transcellular transport and membrane insertion of the C5b-9 membrane attack complex of complement by glomerular epithelial cells in experimental membranous nephropathy." J Immunol 143(2): 546-52.

Kikawada, E., D. M. Lenda, et al. (2003). "IL-12 deficiency in MRL-Fas(lpr) mice delays nephritis and intrarenal IFN-gamma expression, and diminishes systemic pathology." J Immunol 170(7): 3915-25.

Kim, A. H., M. A. Markiewicz, et al. (2009). "New roles revealed for T cells and DCs in glomerulonephritis." J Clin Invest 119(5): 1074-6.

Kim, Y. S., S. Zheng, et al. (2001). "Differential expression of various cytokine and chemokine genes between proliferative and non-proliferative glomerulonephritides." Clin Nephrol 56(3): 199-206.

Kitching, A. R. and S. R. Holdsworth (2011). "The emergence of TH17 cells as effectors of renal injury." J Am Soc Nephrol 22(2): 235-8.

Kitching, A. R., S. R. Holdsworth, et al. (1999). "IFN-gamma mediates crescent formation and cell-mediated immune injury in murine glomerulonephritis." J Am Soc Nephrol 10(4): 752-9.

Kitching, A. R., P. G. Tipping, et al. (1999). "IL-12 directs severe renal injury, crescent formation and Th1 responses in murine glomerulonephritis." Eur J Immunol 29(1): 1-10.

Kitching, A. R., P. G. Tipping, et al. (2000). "IL-18 has IL-12-independent effects in delayed-type hypersensitivity: studies in cell-mediated crescentic glomerulonephritis." J Immunol 165(8): 4649-57.

Kitching, A. R., P. G. Tipping, et al. (1998). "Interleukin-4 deficiency enhances Th1 responses and crescentic glomerulonephritis in mice." Kidney Int 53(1): 112-8.

Kitching, A. R., A. L. Turner, et al. (2004). "Experimental autoimmune anti-glomerular basement membrane glomerulonephritis: a protective role for IFN-gamma." J Am Soc Nephrol 15(7): 1764-74.

Kitching, A. R., A. L. Turner, et al. (2004). "Endogenous IL-13 limits humoral responses and injury in experimental glomerulonephritis but does not regulate Th1 cell-mediated crescentic glomerulonephritis." J Am Soc Nephrol 15(9): 2373-82.

Koffler, D., P. H. Schur, et al. (1967). "Immunological studies concerning the nephritis of systemic lupus erythematosus." J Exp Med 126(4): 607-24.

Kruger, T., D. Benke, et al. (2004). "Identification and functional characterization of dendritic cells in the healthy murine kidney and in experimental glomerulonephritis." J Am Soc Nephrol 15(3): 613-21.

Langrish, C. L., Y. Chen, et al. (2005). "IL-23 drives a pathogenic T cell population that induces autoimmune inflammation." J Exp Med 201(2): 233-40.

Lawson, B. R., S. I. Koundouris, et al. (2001). "The role of alpha beta+ T cells and homeostatic T cell proliferation in Y-chromosome-associated murine lupus." J Immunol 167(4): 2354-60.

Lin, F., S. N. Emancipator, et al. (2002). "Decay-accelerating factor confers protection against complement-mediated podocyte injury in acute nephrotoxic nephritis." Lab Invest 82(5): 563-9.

Ludviksson, B. R., M. C. Sneller, et al. (1998). "Active Wegener's granulomatosis is associated with HLA-DR+ CD4+ T cells exhibiting an unbalanced Th1-type T cell cytokine pattern: reversal with IL-10." J Immunol 160(7): 3602-9.

Markovic-Lipkovski, J., C. A. Muller, et al. (1990). "Association of glomerular and interstitial mononuclear leukocytes with different forms of glomerulonephritis." Nephrol Dial Transplant 5(1): 10-7.

Masutani, K., M. Akahoshi, et al. (2001). "Predominance of Th1 immune response in diffuse proliferative lupus nephritis." Arthritis Rheum 44(9): 2097-106.

Masutani, K., M. Taniguchi, et al. (2004). "Up-regulated interleukin-4 production by peripheral T-helper cells in idiopathic membranous nephropathy." Nephrol Dial Transplant 19(3): 580-6.

Masutani, K., M. Tokumoto, et al. (2003). "Strong polarization toward Th1 immune response in ANCA-associated glomerulonephritis." Clin Nephrol 59(6): 395-405.

McCarthy, E. T., M. Sharma, et al. (2010). "Circulating permeability factors in idiopathic nephrotic syndrome and focal segmental glomerulosclerosis." Clin J Am Soc Nephrol 5(11): 2115-21.

Mellman, I. and R. M. Steinman (2001). "Dendritic cells: specialized and regulated antigen processing machines." Cell 106(3): 255-8.

Miossec, P., T. Korn, et al. (2009). "Interleukin-17 and type 17 helper T cells." N Engl J Med 361(9): 888-98.

Mortensen, E. S. and O. P. Rekvig (2009). "Nephritogenic potential of anti-DNA antibodies against necrotic nucleosomes." J Am Soc Nephrol 20(4): 696-704.

Moser, M. and K. M. Murphy (2000). "Dendritic cell regulation of TH1-TH2 development." Nat Immunol 1(3): 199-205.

Nangaku, M. (1998). "Complement regulatory proteins in glomerular diseases." Kidney Int 54(5): 1419-28.

Nangaku, M., R. L. Meek, et al. (1996). "Transfected CD59 protects mesangial cells from injury induced by antibody and complement." Kidney Int 50(1): 257-66.

Nangaku, M., S. J. Shankland, et al. (2005). "Cellular response to injury in membranous nephropathy." J Am Soc Nephrol 16(5): 1195-204.

Neale, T. J., R. Ullrich, et al. (1993). "Reactive oxygen species and neutrophil respiratory burst cytochrome b558 are produced by kidney glomerular cells in passive Heymann nephritis." Proc Natl Acad Sci U S A 90(8): 3645-9.

Nikolic-Paterson, D. J. and R. C. Atkins (2001). "The role of macrophages in glomerulonephritis." Nephrol Dial Transplant 16 Suppl 5: 3-7.

Nogaki, F., E. Muso, et al. (2000). "Interleukin 12 induces crescentic glomerular lesions in a high IgA strain of ddY mice, independently of changes in IgA deposition." Nephrol Dial Transplant 15(8): 1146-54.

Nogueira, E., S. Hamour, et al. (2010). "Serum IL-17 and IL-23 levels and autoantigen-specific Th17 cells are elevated in patients with ANCA-associated vasculitis." Nephrol Dial Transplant 25(7): 2209-17.

Noris, M., P. Ruggenenti, et al. (1999). "Hypocomplementemia discloses genetic predisposition to hemolytic uremic syndrome and thrombotic thrombocytopenic purpura: role of factor H abnormalities. Italian Registry of Familial and Recurrent Hemolytic Uremic Syndrome/Thrombotic Thrombocytopenic Purpura." J Am Soc Nephrol 10(2): 281-93.

O'Connor, R. A., C. T. Prendergast, et al. (2008). "Cutting edge: Th1 cells facilitate the entry of Th17 cells to the central nervous system during experimental autoimmune encephalomyelitis." J Immunol 181(6): 3750-4.

Pedchenko, V., O. Bondar, et al. (2010). "Molecular architecture of the Goodpasture autoantigen in anti-GBM nephritis." N Engl J Med 363(4): 343-54.

Pickering, M. C., H. T. Cook, et al. (2002). "Uncontrolled C3 activation causes membranoproliferative glomerulonephritis in mice deficient in complement factor H." Nat Genet 31(4): 424-8.

Pippin, J. W., R. Durvasula, et al. (2003). "DNA damage is a novel response to sublytic complement C5b-9-induced injury in podocytes." J Clin Invest 111(6): 877-85.

Reininger, L., T. H. Winkler, et al. (1996). "Intrinsic B cell defects in NZB and NZW mice contribute to systemic lupus erythematosus in (NZB x NZW)F1 mice." J Exp Med 184(3): 853-61.

Reynolds, J., E. I. Prodromidi, et al. (2005). "Nasal administration of recombinant rat alpha3(IV)NC1 prevents the development of experimental autoimmune glomerulonephritis in the WKY rat." J Am Soc Nephrol 16(5): 1350-9.

Reynolds, J. and C. D. Pusey (2001). "Oral administration of glomerular basement membrane prevents the development of experimental autoimmune glomerulonephritis in the WKY rat." J Am Soc Nephrol 12(1): 61-70.

Ring, G. H., Z. Dai, et al. (1999). "Increased susceptibility to immunologically mediated glomerulonephritis in IFN-gamma-deficient mice." J Immunol 163(4): 2243-8.

Rodriguez-Iturbe, B. and S. Batsford (2007). "Pathogenesis of poststreptococcal glomerulonephritis a century after Clemens von Pirquet." Kidney Int 71(11): 1094-104.

Rodriguez-Iturbe, B. and J. M. Musser (2008). "The current state of poststreptococcal glomerulonephritis." J Am Soc Nephrol 19(10): 1855-64.

Ronco, P. and H. Debiec (2005). "Molecular pathomechanisms of membranous nephropathy: from Heymann nephritis to alloimmunization." J Am Soc Nephrol 16(5): 1205-13.

Rougier, N., M. D. Kazatchkine, et al. (1998). "Human complement factor H deficiency associated with hemolytic uremic syndrome." J Am Soc Nephrol 9(12): 2318-26.

Salant, D. J., S. Belok, et al. (1980). "A new role for complement in experimental membranous nephropathy in rats." J Clin Invest 66(6): 1339-50.

Santiago, M. L., L. Fossati, et al. (1997). "Interleukin-4 protects against a genetically linked lupus-like autoimmune syndrome." J Exp Med 185(1): 65-70.

Saran, A. M., H. Yuan, et al. (2003). "Complement mediates nephrin redistribution and actin dissociation in experimental membranous nephropathy." Kidney Int 64(6): 2072-8.

Savin, V. J., R. Sharma, et al. (1996). "Circulating factor associated with increased glomerular permeability to albumin in recurrent focal segmental glomerulosclerosis." N Engl J Med 334(14): 878-83.

Schatzmann, U., C. Haas, et al. (1999). "A Th1 response is essential for induction of crescentic glomerulonephritis in mice." Kidney Blood Press Res 22(3): 135-9.

Schiller, B., C. He, et al. (1998). "Inhibition of complement regulation is key to the pathogenesis of active Heymann nephritis." J Exp Med 188(7): 1353-8.

Schmiedeke, T. M., F. W. Stockl, et al. (1989). "Histones have high affinity for the glomerular basement membrane. Relevance for immune complex formation in lupus nephritis." J Exp Med 169(6): 1879-94.

Scholz, J., V. Lukacs-Kornek, et al. (2008). "Renal dendritic cells stimulate IL-10 production and attenuate nephrotoxic nephritis." J Am Soc Nephrol 19(3): 527-37.

Shah, S. V. (1988). "Evidence suggesting a role for hydroxyl radical in passive Heymann nephritis in rats." Am J Physiol 254(3 Pt 2): F337-44.

Sogabe, H., M. Nangaku, et al. (2001). "Increased susceptibility of decay-accelerating factor deficient mice to anti-glomerular basement membrane glomerulonephritis." J Immunol 167(5): 2791-7.

Spicer, S. T., G. T. Tran, et al. (2007). "Induction of passive Heymann nephritis in complement component 6-deficient PVG rats." J Immunol 179(1): 172-8.

Stanescu, H. C., M. Arcos-Burgos, et al. (2011). "Risk HLA-DQA1 and PLA(2)R1 alleles in idiopathic membranous nephropathy." N Engl J Med 364(7): 616-26.

Stehman-Breen, C. and R. J. Johnson (1998). "Hepatitis C virus-associated glomerulonephritis." Adv Intern Med 43: 79-97.

Steinmetz, O. M., S. A. Summers, et al. (2011). "The Th17-defining transcription factor RORgammat promotes glomerulonephritis." J Am Soc Nephrol 22(3): 472-83.

Suzuki, H., Y. Suzuki, et al. (2007). "Th1 polarization in murine IgA nephropathy directed by bone marrow-derived cells." Kidney Int 72(3): 319-27.

Takahashi, S., L. Fossati, et al. (1996). "Imbalance towards Th1 predominance is associated with acceleration of lupus-like autoimmune syndrome in MRL mice." J Clin Invest 97(7): 1597-604.

Timoshanko, J. R., J. D. Sedgwick, et al. (2003). "Intrinsic renal cells are the major source of tumor necrosis factor contributing to renal injury in murine crescentic glomerulonephritis." J Am Soc Nephrol 14(7): 1785-93.

Tipping, P. G. and S. R. Holdsworth (2006). "T cells in crescentic glomerulonephritis." J Am Soc Nephrol 17(5): 1253-63.

Topham, P. S., S. A. Haydar, et al. (1999). "Complement-mediated injury reversibly disrupts glomerular epithelial cell actin microfilaments and focal adhesions." Kidney Int 55(5): 1763-75.

Trinchieri, G. (2007). "Interleukin-10 production by effector T cells: Th1 cells show self control." J Exp Med 204(2): 239-43.

Tsantikos, E., C. Quilici, et al. (2009). "Perturbation of the CD4 T cell compartment and expansion of regulatory T cells in autoimmune-prone Lyn-deficient mice." J Immunol 183(4): 2484-94.

Turner, J. E., H. J. Paust, et al. (2010). "The Th17 immune response in renal inflammation." Kidney Int 77(12): 1070-5.

van Bruggen, M. C., C. Kramers, et al. (1997). "Nucleosomes and histones are present in glomerular deposits in human lupus nephritis." Nephrol Dial Transplant 12(1): 57-66.

Warwicker, P., T. H. Goodship, et al. (1998). "Genetic studies into inherited and sporadic hemolytic uremic syndrome." Kidney Int 53(4): 836-44.

Wu, J., J. Hicks, et al. (2002). "CD4(+) T cells specific to a glomerular basement membrane antigen mediate glomerulonephritis." J Clin Invest 109(4): 517-24.

Yamada, K., T. Miwa, et al. (2004). "Critical protection from renal ischemia reperfusion injury by CD55 and CD59." J Immunol 172(6): 3869-75.

Yamakami, K., N. Yoshizawa, et al. (2000). "The potential role for nephritis-associated plasmin receptor in acute poststreptococcal glomerulonephritis." Methods 21(2): 185-97.

Yi, T., D. Zhao, et al. (2008). "Absence of donor Th17 leads to augmented Th1 differentiation and exacerbated acute graft-versus-host disease." Blood 112(5): 2101-10.

Yoshizawa, N., K. Yamakami, et al. (2004). "Nephritis-associated plasmin receptor and acute poststreptococcal glomerulonephritis: characterization of the antigen and associated immune response." J Am Soc Nephrol 15(7): 1785-93.

Yuan, H., E. Takeuchi, et al. (2002). "Nephrin dissociates from actin, and its expression is reduced in early experimental membranous nephropathy." J Am Soc Nephrol 13(4): 946-56.

2

Immunological Basis of Membranous Glomerulonephritis

Gian Marco Ghiggeri[1] et al.*
[1]*Division of Nephrology and Laboratory on Pathophysiology of Uremia, G. Gaslini Children Hospital, Genoa Italy*

1. Introduction

Primary membranous glomerulonephritis (MGN) is a major glomerular disease causing proteinuria in humans (Jones, 1957). It is the prototype of an autoimmune disease (Couser, et al., 1978) characterized by sub-epithelial immune deposits within glomeruli. Its pathogenesis remains still unknown. Immune deposits are formed by IgG_4, their respective antigen and complement. The definition of the immune deposit architecture has been a main focus of the pathology research for years but advances were restricted, until recently, to animal models of the disease, in particular to Heymann nephritis (HN) (Heymann, et al., 1959; Heymann, et al., 1952; Van Damme, et al., 1978). Unfortunately, results from experimental HN cannot be readily exported to human MGN since the major antigen of immune deposits in rat is not present in human glomeruli. Therefore different podocyte antigens are involved in human MGN and their identification is a fundamental step in understanding human pathology. Technology problems, mainly concerning dissection of glomeruli and purification/characterization of glomerular antibodies from human biopsies, have limited the experimental approach in humans for years.

In the last 5 years, human MGN has become the topic of renewed nephrologic research. Debiec et al. (Debiec, et al., 2002, 2004) first showed that neutral endopeptidase (NEP) emerges as podocyte antigen in a rare form of congenital MGN due to maternal NEP deficiency and alloimmunization during pregnancy. More recently, the existence of three new glomerular auto-antigens, i.e. phospholipase A2 receptor (PLA2R), aldose reductase (AR) and superoxide dismutase 2 (SOD2) have been proposed by independent groups (Beck, et al., 2009; Prunotto, et al., 2010).

Technology evolution in the field of laser capture and proteomics allowed a direct experimental approach in humans, a crucial step for a direct analysis *'in vivo'*. It is now clear that IgG_4 eluted from glomeruli of MGN patients recognize a panel of podocyte proteins

---

* Corrado Murtas[1], Maria Luisa Carnevali[2], Giovanni Candiano[1], Maurizio Bruschi[1], Marco Prunotto[1], Riccardo Magistroni[3] and Landino Allegri[2].
1 Division of Nephrology and Laboratory on Pathophysiology of Uremia, G. Gaslini Children Hospital, Genoa, Italy,
2 Department of Clinical Medicine, Nephrology and Health Sciences, University of Parma, Parma, Italy,
3 Chair of Nephrology, University of Modena, Italy.

that have been only in part characterized and that represent good candidates for being involved in the pathogenesis of MGN as "auto-antigens".

The same approach might be extended to different renal auto-immune pathologies. However, before proceeding, the scientific community needs a consensus on criteria and technologies that should be utilized for recognizing and validating auto-antigens.

2. Animal models

Heymann nephritis (Heymann, et al., 1952, 1959) is the animal model most frequently used for studying mechanisms implicated in the process of deposition of antibodies within glomeruli. Passive Heymann nephritis is induced in susceptible rat strains by injection of heterologous antisera from sheep or rabbit immunized with a crude extract of rat proximal tubular antigens known as Fx1A. This model is highly similar to human MGN: renal pathology in HN is constantly charachterized by the presence of glomerular sub-epithelial immune deposits. Heymann nephritis is quite simple to be produced and has offered for years the unique chance to study the structure of immune deposits and the mechanisms involved in their formation. This goal has been completed many years ago. Several studies, between 1980 and 1990, demonstrated that megalin is the target antigen of sub-epithelial IgG. Complement factors, mainly C5b-9, and other ancillary proteins such as receptor associated protein (RAP) and anti-RAP IgG complete the structure of immune deposits (Couser, et al., 1978; Kerjaschki, 2004; Kerjaschki & Farquhar, 1982; Kerjaschki, et al., 1987, 1992; Saito, et al., 1994; Salant, et al., 1980a, 1980b; Van Damme, et al., 1978).

The presence of IgG directed against a podocyte antigen triggers the complement cascade that ends with the formation of C5b-9, the key mediator of podocyte damage in MGN. C5b-9 aggregation on the podocyte membrane causes the activation of the epithelial cell. The podocyte starts the production of a cascade of mediators with phosphorylation of PKC and formation of free oxygen radicals (Cybulsky, et al., 2000). The result is a rearrangement of the cytoskeleton and the consequent loss of cell junction that leads to a pathologic alteration of the glomerular filter and to the appearance of proteinuria.

Immune deposits also contain clusterin (Ghiggeri, et al., 2002; Rastaldi, et al., 2006), a natural binder of megalin, that probably represents an endogenous inhibitor of C5b-9.

The definition of pathology features and physiopathology events in Heymann nephritis represented a breakthrough in research of renal autoimmunity. Unfortunately, in spite some of the components above have been detected in human MGN (i.e. C5b-9, clusterin), Heymann nephritis could not be utilized as a direct model of human MGN because megalin is not present in human glomeruli. Moreover, many years later, it was described that megalin structural homolog, the LDL-receptor, is not recognized by circulating IgG_4 in human MGN (Bruschi, et al., 2009).

Diverse animal models of membranous nephropathy have been developed and different podocyte antigens have been identified such as neutral endopeptidase in rabbit, and dipeptidyl peptidase IV in mouse (Table 1) (Assmann, et al., 1992; Ronco, et al., 1989). These proteins are present in human glomeruli; however they were not identified in immune deposits and their involvement in idiopathic MGN was never proved (Allegri, 1997).

After all, animal models showed the heterogeneity of potential podocyte antigens in MGN and straightened the concept of 'in situ' formation of immune deposit. Problems related to the translation of the lesson from animal models to human beings slowed progression in understanding of mechanisms of human MGN. After twenty years, however, new insights were generated by the observation of familial models of MGN and from the characterization of antigens involved in their pathogenesis.

Animal Models		Ref.
Megalin	*rat*	Kerjaschki & Farquhar, 1982
Dipeptidyl peptidase IV	*rat, mouse, rabbit*	Assmann, et al., 1992
Neutral endopeptidase	*rabbit*	Ronco, et al., 1989
Neonatal MGN		
Neutral endopeptidase	*humans*	Debiec, et al., 2002
Idiopathic MGN		
Phospholipase A2 receptor	*humans*	Beck, et al., 2009
Aldose reductase	*humans*	Prunotto, et al., 2010
Mn-superoxide dismutase	*humans*	Prunotto, et al., 2010
Alpha enolase	*humans*	Bruschi, et al., 2011
Others	*humans*	Bruschi, et al., 2011

Table 1. Glomerular antigens in experimental models and in human MGN

3. Human MGN

3.1 Neonatal MGN

Seminal studies by Debiec and Ronco (Debiec, et al., 2002; Debiec, et al., 2004) represented a fundamental passage on the road of comprehension of human MGN many years after the definition of HN. These authors' contributions led to the definition of neutral endopeptidase as the auto-antigen in rare forms of familial congenital MGN (Table 1). Antibodies against neutral endopeptidase was first recognized in a newborn presenting with congenital nephrotic syndrome. Renal histology demonstrated MGN. The basis of the pathogenesis was the mother, carrying a genetic deficiency of neutral endopeptidase because of an homozygous deletion in *MME*, the corresponding gene. She became alloimmunized against neutral endopeptidase during a prior pregnancy, ended with miscarriage. Anti- neutral endopeptidase antibodies were then transferred to the fetus during the successive pregnancy and congenital MGN developed in the newborn while disappearing thereafter.

This elegant model could therefore demonstrate, for the first time, the pathogenic role of a podocyte antigen in human MGN. Similar mutations of *MME* were found in three further families that had in common at least one case of congenital MGN. Even if the presence and the involvement of antibodies against neutral endopeptidase was clearly demonstrated, the prevalence of this form of MGN is probably very low and these results cannot be translated directly in idiopathic MGN.

There is, in fact, now much debate about considering neutral endopeptidase an auto-antigen in non-familial MGN. In fact, circulating anti- neutral endopeptidase IgG4 can be detected in a minor part of patients with primary MGN but this antigen is not recognized by IgG_4 eluted from micro-dissected glomeruli (*Ghiggeri, personal observation*). Further studies are required to rule out the involvement of neutral endopeptidase in idiopathic MGN.

3.2 Technology advances for 'in vivo' studies

New technologies in the fields of tissue micro-dissection and protein characterization have recently played an essential role in discovering new auto-antigen in human MGN. They allowed for the first time the analysis of minute amounts of human tissue from a diagnostic renal biopsy. In fact, micro-dissection and proteomics are of fresh development but have been rapidly adapted to renal tissue studies (Murtas, et al., 2011).

The basic approach starts with the laser dissection of glomeruli from cryo-sections of renal tissue. This technique is highly specific and reproducible. It permits to obtain purified glomeruli from which antibodies can be eluted utilizing osmotic gradients and further characterizated.

Western blot analysis coupled with mass spectrometry is the second basic technique for characterizing auto-antibodies. In this case, podocyte proteins are first separated with mono-dimensional electrophoresis in both denaturing and non-denaturing conditions (a few proteins are not recognized after mild denaturing treatment) or with two-dimensional gel electrophoresis and they are then incubated with glomerular eluates. The binding of specific IgG_4 with podocyte antigens is detected with anti-IgG_4 antibodies and revealed with chemiluminescence. Finally, podocyte proteins recognized by IgG_4 are characterized by mass spectrometry.

Western-blot/mass spectrometry are also utilized for the characterization of circulating antibodies: serum replaces eluted antibodies.

3.3 Glomerular antigens in human MGN

In terms of general discussion it is rational to propose at least three basic characteristics that should be fulfilled by a protein when considered as an auto-antigen in idiopathic MGN. The first one is that the candidate auto-antigen is expressed by podocytes at least in pathological conditions and that it is recognized by IgG4 eluted from micro-dissected glomeruli. The second criterion is that the candidate antigen co-localizes with IgG_4 (and possibly with C5b-9) in glomerular sub-epithelial immune deposits. The final condition is that IgG_4 against the protein must be detected in MGN patients sera at least during the overt phase of the disease.

A question apart is specificity, that is a major issue of the consensus debate.

Therefore, characterizing an auto-antigen requires a multistep approach: first of all immunoglobulins are eluted from MGN glomeruli. Then their target is evaluated by western-blot against podocyte proteins. The evaluation of co-localization within the immune deposits, isotype analysis and titration of circulating antibodies are further steps of the same project. Following this scheme three podocyte proteins have been characterized as putative auto-antigens: phospholipase A2 receptor (PLA2r), Mn-superoxide dismutase (SOD2), aldose reductase (AR). Alpha enolase is a recent finding (Table 1 and Figure 1). Few others are still in progress.

PLA2r is a member of the mannose-receptor family that is normally expressed on the podocyte membrane in humans (East & Isacke, 2002; Lambeau & Lazdunski, 1999). It binds circulating phospholipase A2 but its physiological role is still uncertain. In MGN auto-antibodies recognize PLA2r only in its native configuration that is dependent on disulphide bonds and this is the reason why this protein requires stringent conditions of analysis rigorously in non-denaturing environment. It is reasonable that conformation of PLA2r plays a key role in auto-antibodies formation and binding. Studies (Beck, et al., 2009; Hofstra, et al., 2011) in limited groups of patients with idiopathic MGN revealed high circulating levels in a significant portion of patients and their absence in cases of secondary MGN suggesting a direct implication as causative factor.

SOD2 is a key anti-oxidant mitochondrial enzyme implicated in transformation of superoxide ions into hydrogen peroxide and diatomic oxygen (Son, et al.,2008). In the kidney, SOD2 is widely expressed in tubular epithelial cells, especially in the cortex, where it plays a central role in preserving the kidney during ischemia/reperfusion events but it has never been reported in normal glomeruli. In fact, SOD2 is neo-expressed in podocytes and in sub-epithelial immune deposits of patients with MGN. (Figure 1) (Prunotto, et al., 2010). This suggests that conditions associated with hyperexpression and membrane displacement may be implicated in the auto-immune process.

AR belongs to the family of aldo-keto reductases involved in catalysis of NADPH-dependent reduction of aliphatic and aromatic aldehydes and ketones. It is usually a cytoplasmic enzyme. It converts glucose into sorbitol and it is involved in regulation of tissue tonicity and osmolarity (Williamson, et al.,1993). As for SOD2, localization of AR within the normal kidney is limited to tubular epithelial cells of the medulla and it is absent in glomeruli. In MGN patients it become detectable in glomeruli and it co-localizes with deposed IgG_4 (Figure 1) (Barski, et al., 2005; Terubayashi, et al., 1989; Prunotto, et al. 2010).

The fourth antigen, **alpha enolase** (Bruschi, et al., 2011) is one of the most abundant proteins in cytosol where it participates in the glycolysis process as catalyst of the dehydration of 2-phosphoglycerate to phosphoenolpiruvate; it is particularly expressed in tubular kidney cells and in liver epithelia. A plasma membrane localization has also been described. Several autoimmune diseases are associated with circulating anti-alpha enolase antibodies; however a pathogenetic role has never been demonstrated in any pathological entity (Wistow, et al., 1988; Miles, et al., 1991; Aaronson, et al., 1995; Sabbatini, et al., 1997; Gitlits, et al., 2001). The presence of this kind of auto-antibodies in sera of MGN patients is not a new finding (Wakui, et al., 1999). However, alpha enolase neo-expression in MGN glomeruli and its co-localization with IgG_4 straighten the concept that it is another auto antigen implicated in MGN pathogenesis (Figure 1).

Glomerular immunoglobulin eluates interact with other podocyte membrane proteins (Figure 2). They need to be identified and they have to be tested with the approach described above. Probably, the list of MGN antigens will further increase in a few years.

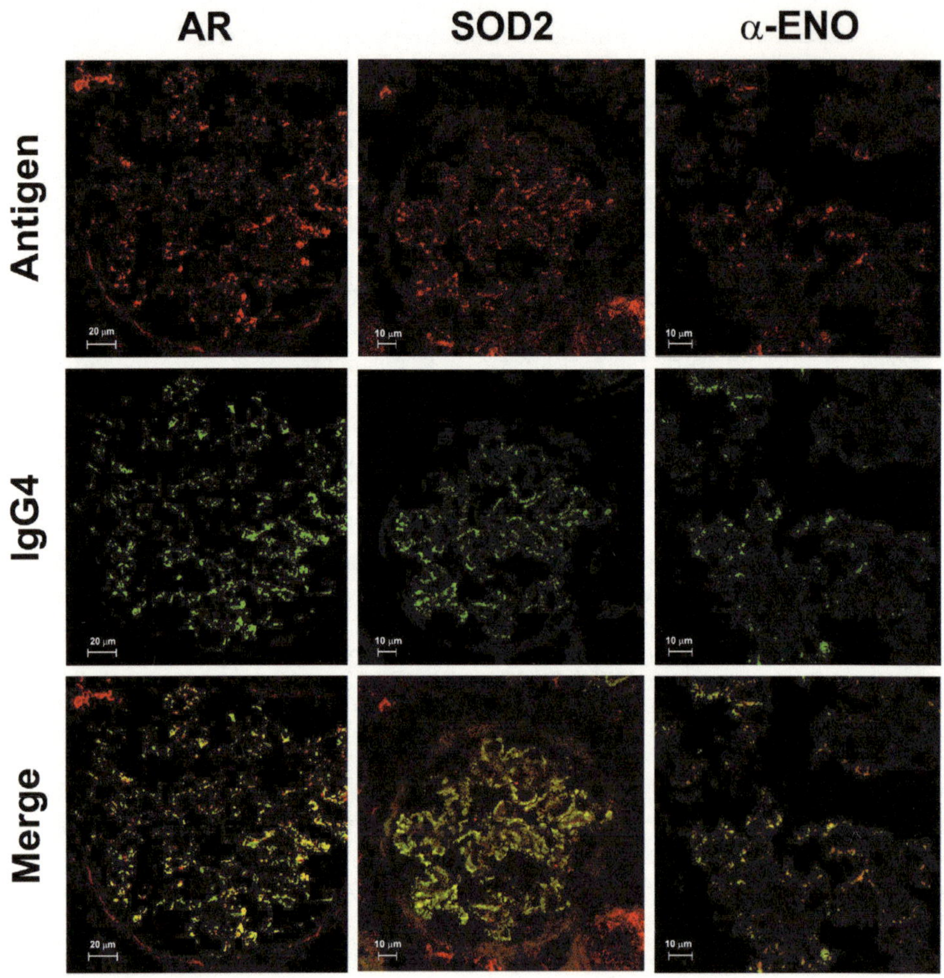

Fig. 1. Glomerular expression of aldose reductase, Mn-superoxide dismutase and alpha enolase in MGN patients. Immunofluorescence on renal cryo-sections analyzed with confocal microscopy. Merged images show co-localization between antigens and IgG_4.

3.4 Antibody isotypes and clinical correlations

IgG_4 typically represents the main body of immune deposits in both Heymann nephritis and human MGN. IgG_1 and IgG_2 are also present.

In sera IgG_4 against the described glomerular antigens are prevalent. However, also IgG_1 can be detected in case of auto-antibodies against alpha enolase. Circulating auto-antibodies are made up of the same he same IgG_4/IgG_1 isotypes indicating a good homology between the circulating and the renal counterparts (Figure 2). How the IgG isotype can influence pathogenesis of MGN is still matter of debate since a few issues are not clear. The first one is related to the described inability of IgG_4 to activate complement, that might suggests an independence between IgG_4 deposition and C5b-9 formation. Another concern is about IgG_1: their role in MGN need to be re-evaluated.

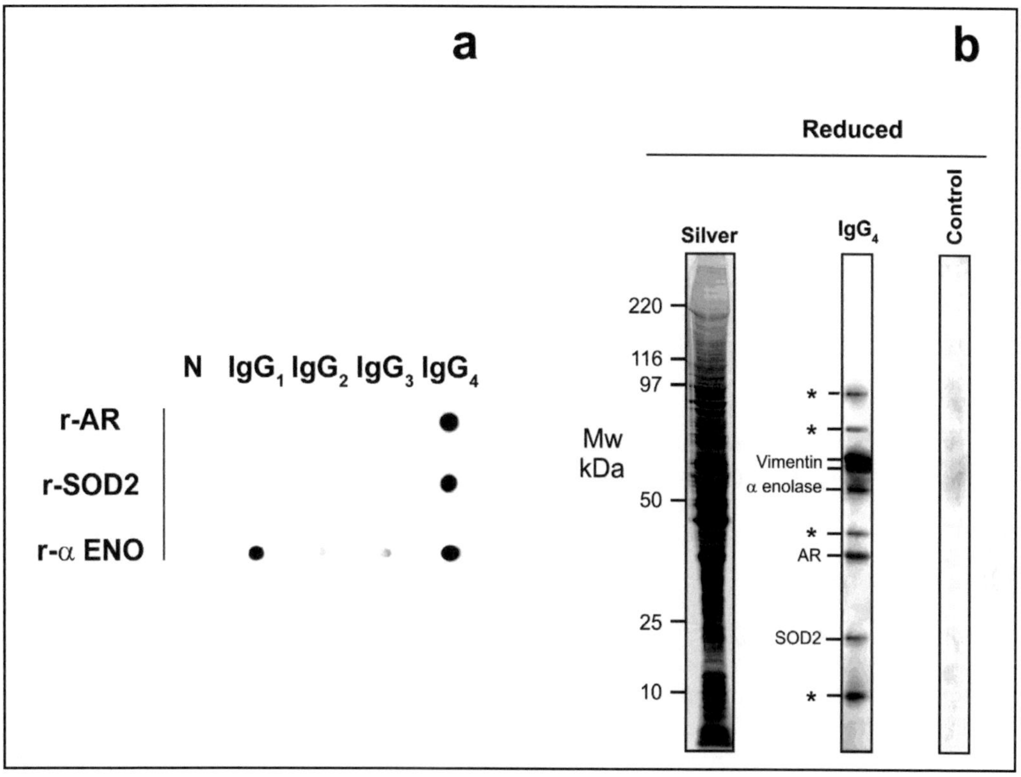

Fig. 2. (a) Circulating immunoglobulin isotypes referred to autoantibodies againsts AR, SOD2 and alpha enolase. In the former two cases the predominant isotype is IgG4, in the case of alpha enolase both IgG1 and IgG4 are detectable. (b) Western-blot with IgG_4 eluted from glomeruli of patients with MGN. A few podocyte proteins are recognized . Three of them have been characterized as aldose reductase (AR), Mn-superoxide dismutase (SOD2) and alpha enolase.

The determination of circulating levels of antibodies against auto-antigens and their clinical correlation is now in progress. Only small cohorts of patients have been evaluated. Moreover, in each population only one antigen have been tested (Beck, et al., 2009; Prunotto, et al., 2010; Debiec & Ronco, 2011; Hofstra, et al. 2011). A correlation of autoantibodies level with proteinuria has been proposed, suggesting that high circulating titers are in relationship with phases of immunological activity of the disease. A strong association with clinical outcome is still lacking. It is also an important issue to establish a correlation among antibodies against different antigens; such stuidies are on the way. Probably they will help in establishing a hierarchy between antigens, if it exists.
Another key aspect would be to find out a correlation between glomerular deposits and serum levels or clinical outome. Surrogate biomarkers are needed for guiding treatment and long-term follow-up in MGN patients.

3.5 Predisposing factors

Many immunological or infectious diseases, neoplasms and toxic or farmacological agents have been associated with MGN. In these situations MGN is considered "secondary" to the respective pathological entity, even if the presumptive antigen has never been isolated from the affected glomeruli. A classical pathogenetic theory affirms that the causative agent can initiate the pathological process in genetically susceptible individuals.

In primary MGN some association has been proved with HLA alleles: in particular HLA-B8, HLA-B18 and HLA-DR3. The latter has been described probably confering a threefold increased risk of the disease (Dyer, et al., 1992; Klouda, et al., 1979)

More recently a genomewide association study conducted in three white European population reported an evident association of MGN with single nucleotide polymorphism (SNP) in PLA2R gene and, more strongly, in HLA-DQ alpha chain 1 (HLA-DQA1). The authors do not report any association in AR and SOD2 genes. The MGN risk in relation with SNPs in PLA2R gene is proposed also in two other Asian studies (Stanescu, et al., 2011).

Even these data are not conclusive, they might suggest a "two hits" model also for the pathogenesis of MN. In fact, a variation in some component of the immune system (HLA-DQ variation) might confer an autoimmunity predisposition. Successively, an alteration, congenital or acquired, of the localization or of the structure of an antigen (PLA2R or others), can make the antigen itself became the target of the disregulated immune system.

4. Conclusions

Research on MGN pathogenesis restarted recently, after many years of frustrating findings. Technology evolution was the major incentive to new stuidies.

The finding of at least four auto-antigens implicated in the pathogenesis of MGN, needs an explanation in a complex pathogenetic theory. Nowadays, it seems reasonable that mechanisms related to the formation of auto-antibodies against membrane proteins, such as PLA2r, are different from auto-antibodies against antigens typically localized inside the cell, such as SOD2 (mitochondrial), and AR or alpha enolase (cytosolic). Antibody promiscuity can be in some way justified by mimicry in case of membrane proteins whereas, for molecules such as SOD2, AR or alpha enolase, mechanisms of de-localization should play a role.

Anyway, before a complete elucidation of MGN pathogenesis several studies have to be performed: more clinical data, new insights on cellular localization of antigens and , maybe, new animal models are needed.

There is a some kind of hierarchy between different targets of autoimmunity? The production of a first autoantibody stimulates podocyte expression of other auto-antigens and a new wave of immunization? There are types of autoantibody not correlated with clinical evolution that are only some kind of "epiphenomenon"? There are different clusters of MGN patients with different autoantibody profile?

Many questions raise when considering recent discoveries on MGN. They will be correctly answered only if scientific community proceeds with shared approach in discovering and testing candidate antigens. Exciting times are coming for the researches involved in studies on MGN and other renal auto-immune diseases.

5. Acknowledgements

This work was supported by the Italian Ministry of Health and by the Renal Child Foundation. Authors also acknowledge Fondazione Mara Wilma e Bianca Querci for financial support to the project "*Ruolo dello stress reticolare nella progressione del danno renale e*

tumorale", Fondazione La Nuova Speranza for supporting the project *'Progetto integrato per la definizione dei meccanismi implicati nella glomerulo sclerosi focale. Dalla predisposizione genetica alla regolazione della produzione di fattori cellulari e circolanti'* and Fondazione Compagnia di San Paolo for the project *'Nefropatia cronica del rene trapiantato'*
Data were critically discussed with Prof. Rosanna Gusmano before her death and this chapter is dedicated to her memory.

6. References

Aaronson, RM; Graven, KK; Tucci, M; McDonald, RJ & Farber, HW. (1995). Non-neuronal enolase is an endothelial hypoxic stress protein. *J Biol Chem*, Vol. 270, No. 46, (Nov 1995), pp. 27752-27757, ISSN 0021-9258

Allegri, L. (1997). Antigens in experimental models of membranous nephropathy: are they involved in human disease? *Nephrol Dial Transplant*, Vol. 12, No. 9, (Sep 1997), pp. 1801-1804, ISSN 0931-0509

Assmann, KJ; van Son, JP; Dijkman, HB & Koene, RA. (1992). A nephritogenic rat monoclonal antibody to mouse aminopeptidase A. Induction of massive albuminuria after a single intravenous injection. *J Exp Med*, Vol. 175, No. 3, (Mar 1992), pp. 623-635, ISSN 0022-1007

Barski, OA; Papusha, VZ; Ivanova, MM; Rudman, DM & Finegold, MJ. (2005). Developmental expression and function of aldehyde reductase in proximal tubules of the kidney. *Am J Physiol Renal Physiol*, Vol. 289, No. 1, (Jul 2005), pp. F200-207, ISSN 0363-6127

Beck, LH, Jr; Bonegio, RG; Lambeau, G; Beck, DM; Powell, DW; Cummins, TD; Klein, JB & Salant, DJ. (2009). M-type phospholipase A2 receptor as target antigen in idiopathic membranous nephropathy. *N Engl J Med*, Vol. 361, No. 1, (Jul 2009), pp. 11-21, ISSN 1533-4406

Bruschi, M; Candiano, G; Murtas, C; Prunotto, M; Santucci, L; Carnevali, ML; Scolari, F; Allegri, L & Ghiggeri, GM. (2009). Patients with primary membranous nephropathy lack auto-antibodies against LDL receptor, the homologue of megalin in human glomeruli. *NDT Plus*, (Jan 2009), 10.1093/ndtplus/sfp002

Bruschi, M; Carnevali, ML; Murtas, C; Candiano, G; Petretto, A; Prunotto, M; Gatti, R; Argentiero, L; Magistroni, R; Garibotto, G; Scolari, F; Ravani, P; Gesualdo, L; Allegri, L & Ghiggeri GM. (2011). Direct characterization of target podocyte antigens and auto-antibodies in human membranous glomerulonephritis: Alfa-enolase and borderline antigens. *J Proteomics*, (n.d.), 10.1016/j.jprot.2011.05.021

Couser, WG; Steinmuller, DR; Stilmant, MM; Salant, DJ & Lowenstein, LM. (1978). Experimental glomerulonephritis in the isolated perfused rat kidney. *J Clin Invest*, Vol. 62, No. 6, (Dec 1978), pp. 1275-1287, ISSN 0021-9738

Cybulsky, AV; Takano, T; Papillon, J & McTavish, AJ. (2000). Complement-induced phospholipase A2 activation in experimental membranous nephropathy. *Kidney Int*, Vol. 57, No. 3, (Mar 2000), pp. 1052-1062, ISSN 0085-2538

Debiec, H; Guigonis, V; Mougenot, B; Decobert, F; Haymann, JP; Bensman, A; Deschenes, G & Ronco, PM. (2002). Antenatal membranous glomerulonephritis due to anti-neutral endopeptidase antibodies. *N Engl J Med*, Vol. 346, No. 26, (Jun 2002), pp. 2053-2060, ISSN 0028-4793

Debiec, H; Nauta, J; Coulet, F; van der Burg, M; Guigonis, V; Schurmans, T; de Heer, E; Soubrier, F; Janssen, F & Ronco, P. (2004). Role of truncating mutations in MME gene in fetomaternal alloimmunisation and antenatal glomerulopathies. *Lancet*, Vol. 364, No. 9441, (Oct 2004), pp. 1252-1259, ISSN 0140-6736

Debiec, H & Ronco, P. (2011). PLA2R autoantibodies and PLA2R glomerular deposits in membranous nephropathy. *N Engl J Med*, Vol. 364, No. 7, (Feb 2011), pp. 689-690, ISSN 1533-4406

Dyer, PA; Short, CD; Clarke, EA & Mallick, NP. (1992). HLA antigen and gene polymorphisms and haplotypes established by family studies in membranous nephropathy. *Nephrol Dial Transplant*, Vol. 7 Suppl 1, pp. 42-47, ISSN 0931-0509

East, L & Isacke, CM. (2002). The mannose receptor family. *Biochim Biophys Acta*, Vol. 1572, No. 2-3, (Sep 2002), pp. 364-386, ISSN 0006-3002

Ghiggeri, GM; Bruschi, M; Candiano, G; Rastaldi, MP; Scolari, F; Passerini, P; Musante, L; Pertica, N; Caridi, G; Ferrario, F; Perfumo, F & Ponticelli, C. (2002). Depletion of clusterin in renal diseases causing nephrotic syndrome. *Kidney Int*, Vol. 62, No. 6, (Dec 2002), pp. 2184-2194, ISSN 0083-2538

Gitlits, VM; Toh, BH & Sentry, JW. (2001). Disease association, origin, and clinical relevance of autoantibodies to the glycolytic enzyme enolase. *J Investig Med*, Vol. 49, No. 2, (Mar 2001), pp. 138-45, ISSN 1081-5589

Heymann, W; Hackel, DB; Harwood, S; Wilson, SG & Hunter, JL. (1959). Production of nephrotic syndrome in rats by Freund's adjuvants and rat kidney suspensions. *Proc Soc Exp Biol Med*, Vol. 100, No. 4, (Apr 1959), pp. 660-664, ISSN 0037-9727

Heymann, W; Lund, HZ & Hackel, DB. (1952). The nephrotic syndrome in rats; with special reference to the progression of the glomerular lesion and to the use of nephrotoxic sera obtained from ducks. *J Lab Clin Med*, Vol. 39, No. 2, (Feb 1952), pp. 218-224, ISSN 0022-2143

Hofstra, JM; Beck, LH Jr; Beck, DM; Wetzels, JF & Salant, DJ. (2011). Anti-Phospholipase A2 Receptor Antibodies Correlate with Clinical Status in Idiopathic Membranous Nephropathy. *Clin J Am Soc Nephrol*, (n.d.), ISSN 1555-905X (Electronic)

Jones, DB. (1957). Nephrotic glomerulonephritis. *Am J Pathol*, Vol. 33, No. 2, (Mar-Apr 1957), pp. 313-329, ISSN 0002-9440

Kerjaschki, D. (2004). Pathomechanisms and molecular basis of membranous glomerulopathy. *Lancet*, Vol. 364, No. 9441, (Oct 2004), pp. 1194-1196, ISSN 0140-6736

Kerjaschki, D & Farquhar, MG. (1982). The pathogenic antigen of Heymann nephritis is a membrane glycoprotein of the renal proximal tubule brush border. *Proc Natl Acad Sci U S A*, Vol. 79, No. 18, (Sep 1982), pp. 5557-5561, ISSN 0027-8424

Kerjaschki, D; Horvat, R; Binder, S; Susani, M; Dekan, G; Ojha, PP; Hillemanns, P; Ulrich, W & Donini, U. (1987). Identification of a 400-kd protein in the brush borders of human kidney tubules that is similar to gp330, the nephritogenic antigen of rat Heymann nephritis. *Am J Pathol*, Vol. 129, No. 1, (Oct 1987), pp. 183-191, ISSN 0002-9440

Kerjaschki, D; Ullrich, R; Diem, K; Pietromonaco, S; Orlando, RA & Farquhar, MG. (1992). Identification of a pathogenic epitope involved in initiation of Heymann nephritis. *Proc Natl Acad Sci U S A*, Vol. 89, No. 23, (Dec 1992), pp. 11179-11183, ISSN 0027-8424

Klouda, PT; Manos, J; Acheson, EJ; Dyer, PA; Goldby, FS; Harris, R; Lawler, W; Mallick, NP & Williams, G. (1979). Strong association between idiopathic membranous nephropathy and HLA-DRW3. *Lancet*, Vol. 2, No. 8146, (Oct 1979), pp. 770-771, ISSN 0140-6736

Lambeau, G & Lazdunski, M. (1999). Receptors for a growing family of secreted phospholipases A2. *Trends Pharmacol Sci*, Vol. 20, No. 4, (Apr 1999), pp. 162-170, ISSN 0165-6147

Miles, LA: Dahlberg, CM; Plescia, J; Felez, J; Kato, K & Plow, EF. (1991). Role of cell-surface lysines in plasminogen binding to cells: identification of alpha-enolase as a candidate plasminogen receptor. *Biochemistry*, Vol. 30, No. 6, (Feb 1991), pp. 1682-1691, ISSN 0006-2960

Murtas, C; Bruschi, M; Carnevali, ML; Petretto, A; Corradini, E; Prunotto, M; Candiano, G; Degl'innocenti, ML; Ghiggeri, GM & Allegri, L. (2011). In vivo characterization of renal auto-antigens involved in human auto-immune diseases: The case of membranous glomerulonephritis. *Proteomics Clin Appl*, Vol. 5, No. 1-2, (Feb 2011), pp. 90-97, ISSN 1862-8354

Prunotto, M; Carnevali, ML; Candiano, G; Murtas, C; Bruschi, M; Corradini, E; Trivelli, A; Magnasco, A; Petretto, A; Santucci, L; Mattei, S; Gatti, R; Scolari, F; Kador, P; Allegri, L & Ghiggeri, GM. (2010). Autoimmunity in membranous nephropathy targets aldose reductase and SOD2. *J Am Soc Nephrol*, Vol. 21, No. 3, (Mar 2010), pp. 507-519, ISSN 1533-3450

Rastaldi, MP; Candiano, G; Musante, L; Bruschi, M; Armelloni, S; Rimoldi, L; Tardanico, R; Sanna-Cherchi, S; Ferrario, F; Montinaro, V; Haupt, R; Parodi, S; Carnevali, ML; Allegri, L; Camussi, G; Gesualdo, L; Scolari, F & Ghiggeri, GM. (2006). Glomerular clusterin is associated with PKC-alpha/beta regulation and good outcome of membranous glomerulonephritis in humans. *Kidney Int*, Vol. 70, No. 3, (Aug 2006), pp. 477-485, ISSN 0085-2538

Ronco, P; Allegri, L; Brianti, E; Chatelet, F; Van Leer, EH & Verroust, P. (1989). Antigenic targets in epimembranous glomerulonephritis. Experimental data and potential application in human pathology. *Appl Pathol*, Vol. 7, No. 2, pp. 85-98, ISSN 0252-1172

Sabbatini, A; Dolcher, MP; Marchini, B; Chimenti, D; Moscato, S; Pratesi, F; Bombardieri, S & Migliorini, P. (1997). Alpha-enolase is a renal-specific antigen associated with kidney involvement in mixed cryoglobulinemia. *Clin Exp Rheumatol*, Vol. 15, No. 6, (Nov-Dec 1997), pp. 655-658, ISSN 0392-856X

Saito, A; Pietromonaco, S; Loo, AK & Farquhar, MG. (1994). Complete cloning and sequencing of rat gp330/"megalin," a distinctive member of the low density lipoprotein receptor gene family. *Proc Natl Acad Sci U S A*, Vol. 91, No. 21, (Oct 1994), pp. 9725-9729, ISSN 0027-8424

Salant, DJ; Belok, S; Madaio, MP & Couser, WG. (1980a). A new role for complement in experimental membranous nephropathy in rats. *J Clin Invest*, Vol. 66, No. 6, (Dec 1980), pp. 1339-1350, ISSN 0021-9738

Salant, DJ; Darby, C & Couser, WG. (1980b). Experimental membranous glomerulonephritis in rats. Quantitative studies of glomerular immune deposit formation in isolated glomeruli and whole animals. *J Clin Invest*, Vol. 66, No. 1, (Jul 1980), pp. 71-81

Son, D; Kojima, I; Inagi, R; Matsumoto, M; Fujita, T & Nangaku, M. (2008). Chronic hypoxia aggravates renal injury via suppression of Cu/Zn-SOD: a proteomic analysis. *Am J Physiol Renal Physiol*, Vol. 294, No. 1, (Jan 2008), pp. F62-72, ISSN 0363-6127

Stanescu, HC; Arcos-Burgos, M; Medlar, A; Bockenhauer, D; Kottgen, A; Dragomirescu, L; Voinescu, C; Patel, N; Pearce, K; Hubank, M; Stephens, HA; Laundy, V; Padmanabhan, S; Zawadzka, A; Hofstra, JM; Coenen, MJ; den Heijer, M; Kiemeney, LA; Bacq-Daian, D; Stengel, B; Powis, SH; Brenchley, P; Feehally, J; Rees, AJ; Debiec, H; Wetzels, JF; Ronco, P; Mathieson, PW & Kleta, R. (2011). Risk HLA-DQA1 and PLA(2)R1 alleles in idiopathic membranous nephropathy. *N Engl J Med*, Vol. 364, No. 7, (Feb 2011), pp. 616-626, ISSN 1533-4406

Terubayashi, H; Sato, S; Nishimura, C; Kador, PF & Kinoshita, JH. (1989). Localization of aldose and aldehyde reductase in the kidney. *Kidney Int*, Vol. 36, No. 5, (Nov 1989), pp. 843-851, ISSN 0085-2538

Van Damme, BJ; Fleuren, GJ; Bakker, WW; Vernier, RL & Hoedemaeker, PJ. (1978). Experimental glomerulonephritis in the rat induced by antibodies directed against tubular antigens. V. Fixed glomerular antigens in the pathogenesis of heterologous immune complex glomerulonephritis. *Lab Invest*, Vol. 38, No. 4, (Apr 1978), pp. 502-510, ISSN 0023-6837

Williamson, JR; Chang, K; Frangos, M; Hasan, KS; Ido, Y; Kawamura, T; Nyengaard, JR; van den Enden, M; Kilo, C & Tilton, RG. (1993). Hyperglycemic pseudohypoxia and diabetic complications. *Diabetes*, Vol. 42, No. 6, (Jun 1993), pp. 801-813, ISSN 0012-1797

Wakui, H; Imai, H; Komatsuda, A & Miura, AB. (1999). Circulating antibodies against alpha-enolase in patients with primary membranous nephropathy (MN). *Clin Exp Immunol*, Vol. 118, No. 3, (Dec 1999), pp. 445-50, ISSN 0009-9104

Wistow, GJ; Lietman, T; Williams, LA; Stapel, SO; de Jong, WW; Horwitz, J & Piatigorsky, J. (1988). Tau-crystallin/alpha-enolase: one gene encodes both an enzyme and a lens structural protein. *J Cell Biol*, Vol. 107, No. 6 Pt 2, (Dec 1988), pp. 2729-2736, ISSN 0021-9525

3

Anti-Complement Autoantibodies in Membranoproliferative Glomerulonephritis and Dense Deposit Disease

Mihály Józsi
Junior Research Group Cellular Immunobiology,
Leibniz Institute for Natural Product Research and Infection Biology, Jena
Germany

1. Introduction

The complement system is an essential part of innate immunity by its role in protection against infections, but it is also involved in waste disposal and in modulating the adaptive immune response. Under physiological conditions complement activation is effectively regulated to restrain it to the required targets and extent, and to prevent collateral host tissue damage. An imbalance between complement activation and inhibition can lead to various diseases. Inappropriate regulation of complement activation, in particular that of the alternative pathway, is linked to kidney diseases. Mutations in complement components and regulatory molecules, and/or autoantibodies against complement proteins have been identified in patients with lupus nephritis, membranoproliferative glomerulonephritis (MPGN), dense deposit disease, C3 glomerulonephritis, CFHR5 nephropathy, and hemolytic uremic syndrome. This chapter summarizes the current knowledge on the role of complement dysregulation and of anti-complement autoantibodies in particular in dense deposit disease and MPGN.

2. Complement: Activation and regulation

The complement system plays a role in a variety of vital functions in the body, including the discrimination between self and nonself, the defense against invading pathogens, inflammation, disposal of cellular debris and apoptotic cells, immune complex clearance, developmental processes, and tissue regeneration. Complement is also involved in several pathophysiological processes, such as various renal disorders, age-related macular degeneration, rheumatoid arthritis, Alzheimer's disease, cancer, and other diseases (Ricklin et al., 2010). Complement is a complex network consisting of more than 40 molecules that are distributed in body fluids and/or appear on cell membranes. These include components that initiate and propagate the cascade, enzymatic components, soluble and cell membrane-bound regulators as well as cell surface receptors. The activated complement system exerts its functions through its components and their active fragments. These form enzymes to ensure the propagation of the cascade; deposit on activator surfaces such as microbes and dying host cells to mark them for phagocytosis (a process called opsonization); bind to complement receptors on several cell types and mediate adherence, phagocytosis or cell activation processes; the released anaphylatoxins C3a and C5a mediate inflammation; and the terminal components punch holes into target cell membranes and thus can cause cell lysis (Figure 1).

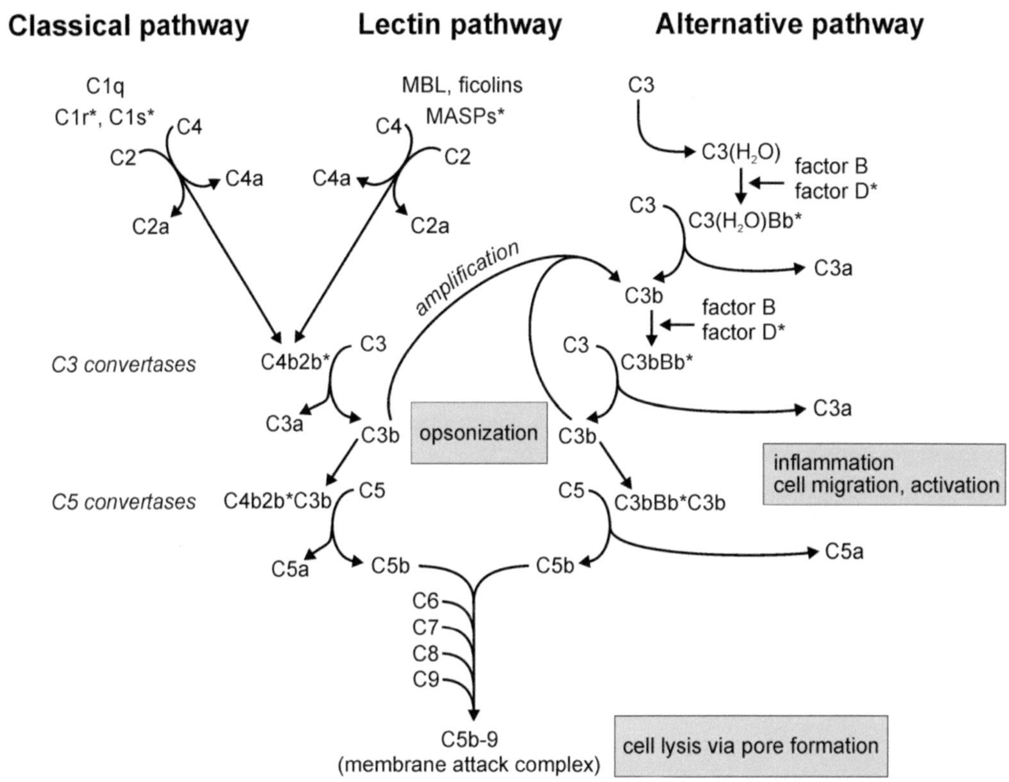

Fig. 1. Complement activation and its major functions. The three major pathways of complement activation are shown. Eventually, all three pathways lead to the formation of C3 convertases (C4b2b represents the classical/lectin pathway C3 convertase, and C3bBb the alternative pathway C3 convertase), which activate the central component C3. The C3b fragment can bind to the existing convertases and thus form the C5 convertases of the classical/lectin pathway (C4b2b3b) or the alternative pathway (C3bBbC3b). The latter are essential for the activation of the common terminal pathway, which leads to the generation of the lytic membrane attack complex. Note, that via the generation of active C3b fragments, which can interact with factors B and D, the classical/lectin pathways also lead to the activation of the alternative pathway ("amplification"). The C3b fragment is also a major opsonin, mediating phagocytosis via C3-fragment receptors on phagocytes. The generated C3a and C5a are potent anaphylatoxins that are involved in the activation of various cell types and mediate inflammatory processes. Asterisks denote enzymatic components. MBL, mannose-binding lectin; MASPs, MBL-associated serine proteases.

Complement can be activated via three major pathways (Figure 1). The classical pathway is activated by immune complexes or pentraxins, which bind the C1q molecule. The lectin pathway is activated by binding of mannose-binding lectin or ficolins to sugar patterns e.g. on microbes, but is also activated by pentraxins and by IgA. The alternative pathway can be activated by foreign surfaces such as microbes, by IgA, by properdin when it is bound to certain microbes or to apoptotic cells, and is also spontaneously activated by the hydrolysis of the internal thioester bond of C3 in plasma. All three pathways eventually lead to the formation of C3 convertases. These C3-converting enzymes cleave the central complement component C3 into C3a and C3b fragments. C3a is an anaphylatoxin and is involved in inflammation. The large C3b fragment can covalently bind to nearby molecules and surfaces via its thioester group, where it may further be degraded, and its fragments can bind to specific complement receptors on cells. C3b also binds factor B, and upon the action of factor D, the C3b-bound factor B is cleaved. The resulting C3bBb represents the alternative pathway C3 convertase that can generate further C3b. Because all three pathways lead to C3 activation, the formation of C3bBb allows an amplification of the cascade. The C3 convertases also allow the further propagation of the cascade by binding C3b, thus forming the C5 convertases and gaining the ability to cleave C5. This step is necessary for the generation of the C5a fragment, which has potent inflammatory activity, and the C5b fragment, which by interacting with the C6, C7, C8, and C9 components leads to the assembly of the so-called membrane attack complex that forms pores in target cell membranes and causes osmotic cell lysis.

Since each enzymatic step amplifies the activation of complement, this potentially leads to a systemic activation and total complement consumption which would be destructive to the host. The activated system may also be harmful because of its inflammatory and lytic effects in the host if not properly controlled. One of the means to avoid an overactivation of the complement cascade is that the human plasma contains several regulatory molecules that control the various activation steps in order to limit the activation to target surfaces and to the necessary extent (Zipfel and Skerka, 2009). Similarly, cells and tissues carry surface complement regulators in various combinations that help them protect themselves from complement attack. Deficiencies in complement components and disturbances in the proper function and regulation of the complement cascade cause severe diseases (Walport, 2001a, 2001b; Markiewski and Lambris, 2007).

2.1 The alternative pathway C3 convertase and its regulation

When the thioester bond is hydrolyzed in C3, the resulting C3(H_2O) molecule (also called "C3b-like C3") gains the ability to interact with factor B (Pangburn et al., 1981). The bound factor B is cleaved by factor D. The resulting initial alternative pathway convertase C3(H_2O)Bb can cleave plasma C3 into C3a and C3b. C3b in turn can form the C3bBb convertase upon interacting with factors B and D. This enzyme cleaves additional C3 molecules and thus amplifies the cascade. The convertase is not a stable enzyme and decays spontaneously. The plasma protein properdin stabilizes the convertase, thus positively regulates the alternative pathway. On the other hand, the plasma regulator factor H, and the membrane proteins decay accelerating factor and complement receptor type 1 destabilize the convertase. In addition, the plasma serine protease factor I can cleave C3b in the presence of one of its cofactors (factor H, membrane cofactor protein, complement receptor type 1), and the inactivated C3b (iC3b) can no longer form a convertase (Figure 2).

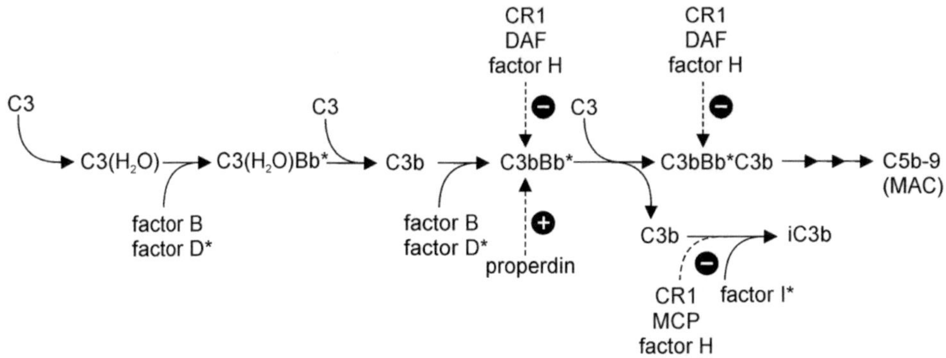

Fig. 2. Activation and regulation of the alternative pathway and the C3 convertase. The spontaneous activation of the alternative pathway is due to a low rate of hydrolysis of the thioester bond in C3. The resulting C3(H_2O) can bind factor B, and after the action of factor D, the C3(H_2O)Bb forms an initial C3 convertase enzyme. This cleaves C3 into C3a and C3b. C3b upon its interaction with factor B generates the C3bBb convertase that further amplifies the alternative pathway. Properdin stabilizes the C3 convertase, whereas CR1, DAF and factor H destabilize the convertase. In addition, C3b is inactivated by factor I in the presence of CR1, MCP or factor H. Asterisks denote enzymes. CR1, complement receptor type 1; DAF, decay accelerating factor; iC3b, inactivated C3b; MAC, membrane attack complex; MCP, membrane cofactor protein.

2.2 Complement and kidney diseases

The importance of a finely tuned balance between the protective and damaging effects of the complement system has clearly been demonstrated in recent years (Ricklin et al., 2010). Complement is implicated in various forms and aspects of renal pathology (Berger and Daha, 2007; Trouw et al., 2003). Deficiencies, mutations and polymorphisms in complement components and regulators, as well as anti-complement autoantibodies have been linked to renal diseases such as lupus nephritis, hemolytic uremic syndrome, MPGN, dense deposit disease, and C3 glomerulonephritis.

Alternative pathway dysregulation in particular is associated with renal disorders (Meri, 2007; Zipfel et al., 2006). Recent data on the genetics and pathophysiology led to a better understanding of underlying pathomechanisms and the role of complement especially in atypical hemolytic uremic syndrome and dense deposit disease, and also to the identification of new disease entities, such as the CFHR5 glomerulopathy (Gale et al., 2010; Pickering and Cook, 2011). Identified mutations affect the activity of complement proteins that are either part of the C3 convertase (C3 and factor B) or that are regulators (factor H, factor I, membrane cofactor protein, CFHR5) of complement activation.

In addition, complement dysregulation caused by anti-complement autoantibodies is involved in the pathophysiology of a number of diseases, several of them affecting the kidney, such as MPGN, dense deposit disease, C3 glomerulonephritis, and atypical hemolytic uremic syndrome (Trouw et al., 2001; Servais et al., 2007; Skerka et al., 2009). Autoantibodies against the complement regulator factor H are detected in some patients with atypical hemolytic uremic syndrome and patients with dense deposit disease, and autoantibodies against the C3 convertase (C3 nephritic factor [C3NeF] or anti-factor B) in patients with MPGN, dense deposit disease and C3 glomerulonephritis.

3. The role of complement in membranoproliferative glomerulonephritis and dense deposit disease

Complement deposition in the presence or absence of immunoglobulins is observed in the glomeruli of patients with MPGN and dense deposit disease. Fluorescence microscopic analyses show staining for C3 fragments in the glomeruli together with immunoglobulins in MPGN I and in MPGN III, or usually in the absence of immunoglobulins in dense deposit disease (Benz and Amann, 2009). MPGN I is characterized with subendothelial glomerular basement membrane deposits, whereas MPGN III is associated with both subendothelial and subepithelial electron-dense glomerular basement membrane deposits. The characteristic of dense deposit disease is electron-dense deposits within the glomerular basement membrane. Dense deposit disease was formerly termed MPGN II; however, an MPGN pattern is not seen in many cases. Dense deposit disease is associated with defective complement alternative pathway regulation, and hypocomplementemia is often observed in the patients (Smith et al., 2007). The glomerular deposits contain components of the alternative and the terminal activation pathways (Sethi et al., 2009). Genetic and acquired factors (i.e., autoantibodies) have been described in MPGN, in C3 glomerulonephritis with or without MPGN, and in dense deposit disease (Licht and Frémeaux-Bacchi, 2009; Pickering and Cook, 2008; Servais et al., 2007, 2011). Recent research provided fresh insights into mechanisms of pathologic complement activation in these diseases. First, some aspects of genetic complement defects related to glomerular disease will be summarized, followed by an overview of autoantibodies associated with MPGN and dense deposit disease.

3.1 Insights from human complement mutations

Deficiency of the major alternative pathway regulator factor H has been associated with MPGN I, dense deposit disease, and C3 glomerulonephritis (Dragon-Durey et al., 2004; Pickering and Cook, 2008; Servais et al., 2011). Several reports described patients with mutations in cysteine residues that are essential for disulfide bridge formation and thus the proper folding and stabilization of the SCR domains. This leads to defective protein folding and a retainment of factor H intracellularly (Ault et al., 1997; Servais et al., 2011). A case was also reported where the Cys431Tyr amino acid exchange caused factor H aggregation and a likely reduced protein half-life (Montes et al., 2008). In these cases, the resulting quantitative factor H deficiency leads to a lack of proper complement regulation in body fluids. In addition, a functional factor H deficiency due to a deletion of one amino acid in SCR4 of factor H causing a defect in the regulatory activity was described (Licht et al., 2006). All these factor H abnormalities lead to a defective C3 regulation in both plasma and at cell surfaces. Sequence variations in the genes coding for factor H and the CFHR5 protein have also been linked to dense deposit disease (Abrera-Abeleda et al., 2006), although it is not clear if and how these allele variants are related to the pathophysiology of the disease.

Recently, a C3 mutation in dense deposit disease was described that results in the deletion of two amino acids in the molecule ($C3_{923delDG}$). This mutant C3 protein generates a convertase that is resistant to decay by factor H, and is also resistant to cleavage by factor I when factor H is the cofactor (Martínez-Barricarte et al., 2010). Dysfunctional C3 was also associated with MPGN III (Marder et al., 1983).

These data indicate that the tipping of the tightly regulated balance between complement activation and inhibition can lead to glomerular disease.

3.2 Insights from animal models

Factor H deficiency was described in pigs that died of kidney failure due to membranoproliferative glomerulonephritis (Høgåsen et al., 1995). The factor H deficiency was caused by a mutation that led to the retention of this protein intracellularly (Hegasy et al., 2002).

The essential role of a failed C3 regulation in plasma in the development of glomerulonephritis was demonstrated in genetically engineered factor H-deficient mice (Pickering et al., 2002). These factor H-deficient mice spontaneously developed membranoproliferative glomerulonephritis and 23% of them died by 8 months. If the gene coding for factor B was also knocked out, no deposits at the glomerular basement membrane and no MPGN were observed, indicating the essential role of the alternative pathway (Pickering et al., 2002). Also, mice with combined factor H and factor I deficiency, despite uncontrolled alternative pathway activation, did not develop dense deposit disease because of the lack of C3b degradation in the absence of factor I. Reconstitution with exogenous factor I, however, caused C3 fragment deposition, which was derived from plasma, along the glomerular basement membrane (Rose et al., 2008). These data provide evidence that the development of dense deposit disease critically depends on activated C3 fragments generated in plasma. Additional studies showed that mice deficient in both factor H and C5, i.e., lacking activation of the terminal complement pathway, still develop membranoproliferative glomerulonephritis, although with less glomerular inflammation and cellular infiltration (Pickering et al., 2006). Thus, an impaired regulation of C3 is enough to develop the disease.

4. Anti-complement autoantibodies in membranoproliferative glomerulonephritis and dense deposit disease

Autoantibodies against complement proteins have been associated with various forms of MPGN and with dense deposit disease. Whereas C3NeF is commonly detected in patients with MPGN, so far there are only one and two cases reported for anti-factor B and anti-factor H autoantibodies, respectively. These antibodies affect complement regulation and are implicated in the pathophysiology of renal disease, even though a direct pathogenic role for the autoantibodies was rarely demonstrated.

4.1 C3 nephritic factor

C3NeF is an IgG or IgM autoantibody against the alternative pathway C3 convertase enzyme (Spitzer et al., 1969), and is the most common autoantibody detected in patients with MPGN. It can be detected in up to 50% of patients with MPGN I and MPGN III, and up to 80% in dense deposit disease (Appel et al., 2005; Schwertz et al., 2001). C3NeF was also found in C3 glomerulonephritis with or without MPGN (Servais et al., 2007). However, C3NeF was reported in patients with partial lipodystrophy (Mathieson et al., 1993; Sissons et al., 1976), and even in healthy individuals (Spitzer et al., 1990, 1992). Therefore, and because of the lack of a clear correlation between the presence and amounts of C3NeF, C3 levels, and renal pathology, a nephritogenic role of C3NeF is unclear. This may partly be related to the heterogeneity of C3NeF and the problematic of C3NeF detection assays, as discussed below. It is possible that C3NeF appears secondarily due to otherwise present complement activation products and thus a prolonged exposure of neoantigenic sites.

C3NeF binds to a neoepitope appearing on the newly formed alternative pathway C3 convertase, and stabilizes the convertase against intrinsic (natural) and extrinsic (e.g., factor H-mediated) decay, thus significantly increasing the half-life of the convertase (Daha et al., 1976; Daha and van Es, 1981). This leads to an enhanced C3 activation in the plasma of the patients (Figure 3A and 3B). Hypocomplementemia is indeed often observed (Ruley et al., 1973; Smith et al., 2007), and glomerular deposits of patients with C3NeF contain C3 fragments, and may also contain C5 (West et al., 2001).

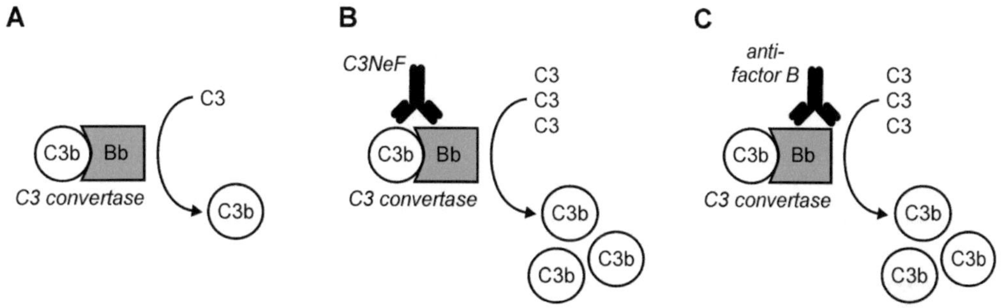

Fig. 3. The effect of autoantibodies on the alternative pathway C3 convertase. (A) The C3bBb convertase cleaves C3 and thus generates C3b fragments, which participate in opsonization and in the propagation of the cascade by forming additional convertases. The enzyme has a short half-life, which is influenced by positive (properdin) and negative (e.g., factor H) regulators. (B) C3NeF binds to a neoepitope on C3bBb and stabilizes this enzyme against intrinsic and extrinsic decay, thus the convertase can cleave more C3. (C) The anti-factor B autoantibody binds to the Bb portion of the convertase, and stabilizes it against both natural and factor H-mediated decay.

The term C3NeF describes a heterogeneous group of autoantibodies (Davis et al., 1977; Daha et al., 1978), which can be different in their functional effects. It was reported that C3NeFs that were not associated with hypocomplementemia did not stabilize the C3 convertase against extrinsic decay, while still acting against natural convertase decay (Ohi et al., 1992). C3NeF may also be properdin-dependent (Clardy et al., 1989; Tanuma et al., 1990), and such a C3NeF:P slowly activates C3 and the terminal pathway (Clardy et al., 1989). By contrast, some C3NeFs appear to inhibit the generation of C5 convertases and therefore do not cause terminal pathway activation (Mollnes et al., 1986). Thus, C3NeFs can be directed against different epitopes and have distinct effects on complement activation.

C3NeF may change over time, disappear and reappear; moreover, reports supporting both a relationship and also indicating a lack of correlation between C3NeF, C3 plasma levels and clinical course are published (Appel et al., 2005). C3NeF may also occur together with C4 nephritic factor and/or anti-C1q (Tanuma et al., 1989; Ohi and Yasugi, 1994; Strife et al., 1990), and may present together with heterozygous mutations of factor H or factor I (Leroy et al., 2011). It is still not clear if C3NeF is directly nephritogenic or it rather appears due to a prolonged or increased presence of the C3 convertase enzyme and complement activation fragments in plasma. Nevertheless, once present, C3NeF by stabilizing the convertase further contributes to an abnormally increased complement activation. As the animal models demonstrated, the generated C3 fragments are involved in glomerular injury, without the requirement of terminal pathway activation, although the latter (also increased by most C3NeFs) exacerbates glomerular inflammation and damage.

C3NeF determination is not very reliable, partly because of the heterogeneous nature of C3NeFs and because commonly used methods are indirect measurements based on hemolysis (López-Trascasa et al., 1987; Rother et al., 1982; West, 2008). Immunoglobulins are most often not directly measured and functional assays for C3NeF based on lysis of sheep erythrocytes may not necessarily detect antibodies. On the other hand, it is possible to measure C3NeF by ELISA (Seino et al., 1987). The lack of a readily available and simple assay that makes C3NeF measurements truly comparable between laboratories makes interpretation of literature data and the assessment of the pathogenic relevance of these autoantibodies difficult. C3NeF diagnostics should be improved, and the autoantibodies functionally characterized using modern methods (e.g., surface plasmon resonance), in order to unravel the role of C3NeF in renal pathology.

4.2 Anti-factor B autoantibody

Recently, we have identified an anti-factor B autoantibody in dense deposit disease. This autoantibody also targets the alternative pathway C3 convertase but has some features that distinguishes it from C3NeF (Strobel et al., 2010a). The patient showed signs of systemic complement activation and enhanced amounts of the alternative pathway activation product Bb were present in the patient's plasma. Whereas the traditional assay to detect C3NeF (Rother, 1982) failed to identify a convertase-specific antibody, an anti-factor B IgG was readily detectable by ELISA. The anti-factor B antibody bound to the alternative pathway C3 convertase and, by stabilizing it, enhanced the turnover of C3 (Figure 3C). The anti-factor B autoantibody stabilized the convertase against both spontaneous and factor H-mediated decay. However, the anti-factor B antibody inhibited the activation of the terminal pathway, likely by interfering with the formation of the C5 convertase. Differences from C3NeF include binding of the autoantibody to native factor B in plasma, as well as to the Bb fragment incorporated into the C3 convertase, and interference with C5 convertase activity, even though the latter may also be characteristic to some types of C3NeF (Mollnes et al., 1986). Future studies need to determine the frequency of anti-factor B antibodies in dense deposit disease and evaluate its diagnostic and prognostic relevance.

4.3 C4 nephritic factor

Similar to the C3 convertase of the alternative pathway, the classical pathway C3 convertase (C4b2b) can also be a target for autoantibodies. These IgG autoantibodies termed C4 nephritic factor (C4NeF) were first described in patients with post-infectious glomerulonephritis (Halbwachs et al., 1980) and in patients with SLE (Daha and van Es, 1980). C4NeF stabilizes the C4b2b convertase and thus causes an enhanced classical pathway mediated complement activation, leading to C3 consumption. The binding of this antibody renders the convertase resistant against both the intrinsic and the extrinsic decay, mediated by C4b-binding protein, and the C4b portion of the convertase is protected from the proteolytic inactivation by factor I (Gigli et al., 1981). In a case report of a patient with chronic glomerulonephritis the C4NeF was analyzed for binding to the convertase and shown to recognize a neoepitope on the convertase but not C4b (Fujita et al., 1987). C4NeF and C3NeF can also be present together in patients (Ohi and Yasugi, 1994; Tanuma et al., 1989). To date, only few studies have addressed the presence and role of C4NeF in glomerulonephritis, and patients with MPGN or dense deposit disease are not routinely tested for this kind of autoantibody. This is partly due to the difficulties with the detection method, applying hemolytic assays or ELISA (Seino et al., 1990).

4.4 Anti-factor H autoantibody

An anti-factor H autoantibody was described in a patient with hypocomplementemic MPGN and characterized in detail. The antibody was isolated as a monoclonal lambda light chain dimer from the patient's serum and urine. It was shown to bind to factor H and cause alternative pathway activation in the fluid phase (Meri et al., 1992). The binding site of the antibody was localized to SCR3 of factor H, i.e., within the part responsible for complement regulatory activity (Figure 4), and the autoantibody inhibited the interaction of factor H with C3b. In functional assays, this "miniautoantibody" led to defective complement control by functionally blocking factor H and thus leading to uncontrolled alternative pathway activation and enhanced C3 conversion (Jokiranta et al., 1999). Thus, the anti-factor H autoantibody led to an acquired functional factor H deficiency in the patient. Because the antibody affects the regulatory activity of factor H, factor H activity is impaired in both the fluid phase and on surfaces. Although not tested, the antibody likely also inhibits the function of factor H-like protein 1, which shares the N-terminal seven domains with factor H. Since this original description there is only one additional report of an anti-factor H antibody in C3 glomerulonephritis, but the antibody was not further characterized (Sethi et al., 2011). Apparently, anti-factor H antibodies are relatively rare in glomerulonephritis, especially in comparison with the occurrence of C3NeF.

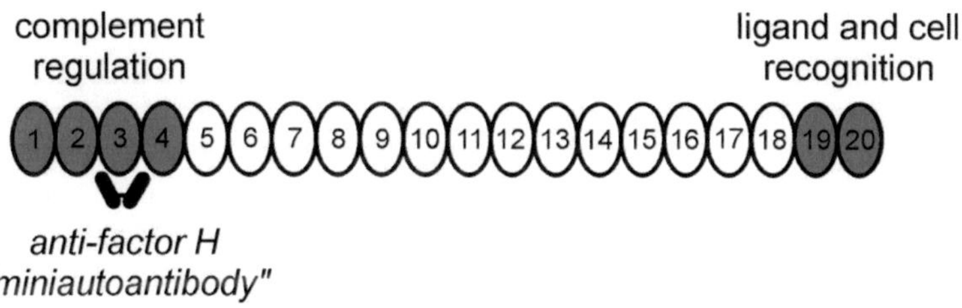

Fig. 4. Anti-factor H autoantibody inhibits the complement regulatory activity of factor H in MPGN. Factor H consists of 20 domains termed short consensus repeats (SCRs). The N-terminal four SCRs mediate the cofactor and convertase decay accelerating activities of factor H, whereas the C-terminal domains (SCRs 19 and 20) are responsible for targeting the molecule to host surfaces. The anti-factor H lambda light chain dimer causes alternative pathway activation in plasma due to its inhibitory effect on factor H function (Jokiranta et al., 1999; Meri et al., 1992).

By contrast, approximately 10% of the patients with atypical hemolytic uremic syndrome have circulating anti-factor H antibodies, most of which bind to the C-terminal recognition domains (i.e., SCRs 19-20) of factor H, thus impairing the ability of factor H to protect self surfaces, whereas the activity in plasma is usually not compromized (Dragon-Durey et al., 2005; Józsi et al., 2007; Moore et al., 2010; Strobel et al., 2010b). Further studies are needed to systematically screen patients with dense deposit disease and MPGN for anti-factor H autoantibodies, and to characterize such antibodies in detail.

4.5 Anti-C1q autoantibody

Anti-C1q antibodies against a neoepitope on the collagen-like region of C1q have also been identified in patients with MPGN I, MPGN III and dense deposit disease (Strife et al., 1989, 1990), and such antibodies can occur together with C3NeF. Interestingly, in most cases of MPGN I the anti-C1q autoantibodies were IgG3, which is considered an antibody subclass that efficiently activates the classical pathway. The patient with dense deposit disease and anti-factor B antibody also had detectable anti-C1q that activated the classical pathway as demonstrated by antigen microarray analysis (Strobel et al., 2010a). The relevance of such anti-C1q antibodies for the pathophysiology of MPGN and dense deposit disease is unclear.

5. Conclusion

Our current understanding of the role of anti-complement autoantibodies in MPGN and dense deposit disease is insufficient. Even though C3NeF is known for long, its relationship with disease manifestation is still unclear. The heterogeneic nature of MPGN/dense deposit disease-associated autoantibodies makes diagnostics and interpretation of results difficult. More detailed studies into the functional effects of these autoantibodies are necessary to be able to assess their role and relevance. There is much need for improvement of autoantibody diagnostics and functional analyses. Novel assays, such as antigen arrays to detect the presence of autoantibodies in parallel with their complement activating capacity, could be invaluable tools in characterizing autoantibodies in patients' samples (Papp et al., 2008).

Recent genetic, functional and structural studies provided fresh mechanistic insights into the regulation of the alternative complement pathway and into the formation and regulation of the alternative pathway C3 convertase (Fakhouri et al., 2010a; Forneris et al, 2010; Martínez-Barricarte et al., 2010; Torreira et al., 2009). New autoantibodies and the concurrence of acquired and genetic defects in MPGN and dense deposit disease have been described (Leroy et al., 2011; Strobel et al., 2010a). Patients should be analyzed for the presence of such autoantibodies and complement mutations to determine their diagnostic and clinical significance. Additional autoantibodies and genetic changes affecting the complement system are likely to join the list of those associated with MPGN and/or dense deposit disease.

There is no general therapy for MPGN and dense deposit disease. Treatment should be tailored to individual patients based on diagnosis and the identified complement defect(s). Better and more comprehensive diagnostics, and an increased understanding of the underlying pathomechanism could in the future improve the treatment of the patients. Patients with complement abnormalities may benefit from novel therapeutic complement inhibitors such as anti-C5 antibody or recombinant complement regulatory proteins (Wagner and Frank, 2010). Additional options include immunosuppressive therapies to patients with autoantibodies, plasma exchange, and factor H replacement in the case of inherited or acquired factor H deficiency (Fakhouri et al., 2010b; Noris and Remuzzi, 2008; Smith et al., 2007). Improved diagnostic tools are also useful to assess the efficacy of treatments and to monitor autoantibody levels during therapy.

There has been significant advancement in our understanding of the role of complement and in particular that of the alternative pathway in kidney diseases in recent years. There is hope that the improved diagnostic and therapeutic tools can be applied to translate this knowledge into personalized treatment for the benefit of the patients.

6. Acknowledgment

I thank laboratory members, especially Stefanie Strobel, collaboration partners and in particular the patients, their relatives and clinicians for contributing to the work on anti-complement autoantibodies. The German Science Fund (Deutsche Forschungsgemeinschaft) is gratefully acknowledged for supporting the research on autoantibodies in kidney diseases (JO 844/1-1). I also thank Barbara Uzonyi for helpful suggestions.

7. References

Abrera-Abeleda, M.A., Nishimura, C., Smith, J.L., Sethi, S., McRae, J.L., Murphy, B.F., Silvestri, G., Skerka, C., Józsi, M., Zipfel, P.F., Hageman, G.S. & Smith, R.J. (2006) Variations in the complement regulatory genes factor H (CFH) and factor H related 5 (CFHR5) are associated with membranoproliferative glomerulonephritis type II (dense deposit disease). *J. Med. Genet.*, 43:582-589.

Appel, G.B., Cook, H.T., Hageman, G., Jennette, J.C., Kashgarian, M., Kirschfink, M., Lambris, J.D., Lanning, L., Lutz, H.U., Meri, S., Rose, N.R., Salant, D.J., Sethi, S., Smith, R.J., Smoyer, W., Tully, H.F., Tully, S.P., Walker, P., Welsh, M., Würzner, R. & Zipfel, P.F. (2005) Membranoproliferative glomerulonephritis type II (dense deposit disease): an update. *J. Am. Soc. Nephrol.*, 16:1392-1403.

Ault, B.H., Schmidt, B.Z., Fowler, N.L., Kashtan, C.E., Ahmed, A.E., Vogt, B.A. & Colten, H.R. (1997) Human factor H deficiency. Mutations in framework cysteine residues and block in H protein secretion and intracellular catabolism. *J. Biol. Chem.*, 272:25168-25175.

Benz, K. & Amann, K. (2009) Pathological aspects of membranoproliferative glomerulonephritis (MPGN) and haemolytic uraemic syndrome (HUS) / thrombocytic thrombopenic purpura (TTP). *Thromb. Haemost.*, 101:265-270.

Berger, S.P. & Daha, M.R. (2007) Complement in glomerular injury. *Semin. Immunopathol.*, 29:375-384.

Clardy, C.W., Forristal, J., Strife, C.F. & West, C.D. (1989) A properdin dependent nephritic factor slowly activating C3, C5, and C9 in membranoproliferative glomerulonephritis, types I and III. *Clin. Immunol. Immunopathol.*, 50:333-347.

Daha, M.R., Fearon, D.T. & Austen, K.F. (1976) C3 nephritic factor (C3NeF): stabilization of fluid phase and cell-bound alternative pathway convertase. *J. Immunol.*, 116:1-7.

Daha, M.R., Austen, K.F. & Fearon, D.T. (1978) Heterogeneity, polypeptide chain composition and antigenic reactivity of C3 nephritic factor. *J. Immunol.*, 120:1389-1394.

Daha, M.R. & van Es, L.A. (1980) Relative resistance of the F-42-stabilized classical pathway C3 convertase to inactivation by C4-binding protein. *J. Immunol.*, 125:2051-2054.

Daha, M.R. & van Es, L.A. (1981) Stabilization of homologous and heterologous cell-bound amplification convertases, C3bBb, by C3 nephritic factor. *Immunology*, 43:33-38.

Davis, A.E., Ziegler, J.B., Gelfand, E.W., Rosen, F.S. & Alper, C.A. (1977) Heterogeneity of nephritic factor and its identification as an immunoglobulin. *Proc. Natl. Acad. Sci. U S A*, 74:3980-3983.

Dragon-Durey, M.A., Frémeaux-Bacchi, V., Loirat, C., Blouin, J., Niaudet, P., Deschenes, G., Coppo, P., Herman Fridman, W. & Weiss, L. (2004) Heterozygous and homozygous factor H deficiencies associated with hemolytic uremic syndrome or membranoproliferative glomerulonephritis: report and genetic analysis of 16 cases. *J. Am. Soc. Nephrol.*, 15:787-795.

Dragon-Durey, M.A., Loirat, C., Cloarec, S., Macher, M.A., Blouin, J., Nivet, H., Weiss, L., Fridman, W.H. & Frémeaux-Bacchi, V. (2005) Anti-Factor H autoantibodies associated with atypical hemolytic uremic syndrome. *J. Am. Soc. Nephrol.*, 16:555-563.

Fakhouri, F., Frémeaux-Bacchi, V., Noël, L.H., Cook, H.T. & Pickering, M.C. (2010a) C3 glomerulopathy: a new classification. *Nat. Rev. Nephrol.*, 6:494-499.

Fakhouri, F., de Jorge, E.G., Brune, F., Azam, P., Cook, H.T. & Pickering, M.C. (2010b) Treatment with human complement factor H rapidly reverses renal complement deposition in factor H-deficient mice. *Kidney Int.*, 78:279-286.

Forneris, F., Ricklin, D., Wu, J., Tzekou, A., Wallace, R.S., Lambris, J.D. & Gros, P. (2010) Structures of C3b in complex with factors B and D give insight into complement convertase formation. *Science*, 330:1816-1820.

Fujita, T., Sumita, T., Yoshida, S., Ito, S. & Tamura, N. (1987) C4 nephritic factor in a patient with chronic glomerulonephritis. *J. Clin. Lab. Immunol.*, 22:65-70.

Gale, D.P., de Jorge, E.G., Cook, H.T., Martinez-Barricarte, R., Hadjisavvas, A., McLean, A.G., Pusey, C.D., Pierides, A., Kyriacou, K., Athanasiou, Y., Voskarides, K., Deltas, C., Palmer, A., Frémeaux-Bacchi, V., de Cordoba, S.R., Maxwell, P.H. & Pickering, M.C. (2010) Identification of a mutation in complement factor H-related protein 5 in patients of Cypriot origin with glomerulonephritis. *Lancet*, 376:794-801.

Gigli, I., Sorvillo, J., Mecarelli-Halbwachs, L. & Leibowitch, J. (1981) Mechanism of action of the C4 nephritic factor. Deregulation of the classical pathway of C3 convertase. *J. Exp. Med.*, 154:1-12.

Halbwachs, L., Leveillé, M., Lesavre, P., Wattel, S. & Leibowitch, J. (1980) Nephritic factor of the classical pathway of complement: immunoglobulin G autoantibody directed against the classical pathway C3 convetase enzyme. *J. Clin. Invest.*, 65:1249-1256.

Hegasy, G.A., Manuelian, T., Høgåsen, K., Jansen, J.H. & Zipfel, P.F. (2002) The molecular basis for hereditary porcine membranoproliferative glomerulonephritis type II: point mutations in the factor H coding sequence block protein secretion. *Am. J. Pathol.*, 161:2027-2034.

Høgåsen, K., Jansen, J.H., Mollnes, T.E., Hovdenes, J. & Harboe, M. (1995) Hereditary porcine membranoproliferative glomerulonephritis type II is caused by factor H deficiency. *J. Clin. Invest.*, 95:1054-1061.

Jokiranta, T.S., Solomon, A., Pangburn, M.K., Zipfel, P.F. & Meri, S. (1999) Nephritogenic lambda light chain dimer: a unique human miniautoantibody against complement factor H. *J. Immunol.*, 163:4590-4596.

Józsi, M., Strobel, S., Dahse, H.M., Liu, W.S., Hoyer, P.F., Oppermann, M., Skerka, C. & Zipfel, P.F. (2007) Anti-factor H autoantibodies block C-terminal recognition function of factor H in hemolytic uremic syndrome. *Blood*, 110:1516-1518.

Leroy, V., Fremeaux-Bacchi, V., Peuchmaur, M., Baudouin, V., Deschênes, G., Macher, M.A. & Loirat, C. (2011) Membranoproliferative glomerulonephritis with C3NeF and genetic complement dysregulation. *Pediatr. Nephrol.*, 26:419-424.

Licht, C., Heinen, S., Józsi, M., Löschmann, I., Saunders, R.E., Perkins, S.J., Waldherr, R., Skerka, C., Kirschfink, M., Hoppe, B. & Zipfel, P.F. (2006) Deletion of Lys224 in regulatory domain 4 of Factor H reveals a novel pathomechanism for dense deposit disease (MPGN II). *Kidney Int.*, 70:42-50.

Licht, C. & Fremeaux-Bacchi, V. (2009) Hereditary and acquired complement dysregulation in membranoproliferative glomerulonephritis. *Thromb. Haemost.*, 101:271-278.

López-Trascasa, M., Marín, M.A. & Fontán, G. (1987) C3 nephritic factor determination. A comparison between two methods. *J. Immunol. Methods*, 98:77-82.

Marder, H.K., Coleman, T.H., Forristal, J., Beischel, L. & West, C.D. (1983) An inherited defect in the C3 convertase, C3b,Bb, associated with glomerulonephritis. *Kidney Int.*, 23:749-758.

Markiewski, M.M. & Lambris, J.D. (2007) The role of complement in inflammatory diseases: from behind the scenes into the spotlight. *Am. J. Pathol.*, 171:715-727.

Martínez-Barricarte, R., Heurich, M., Valdes-Cañedo, F., Vazquez-Martul, E., Torreira, E., Montes, T., Tortajada, A., Pinto, S., Lopez-Trascasa, M., Morgan, B.P., Llorca, O., Harris, C.L. & Rodríguez de Córdoba, S. (2010) Human C3 mutation reveals a mechanism of dense deposit disease pathogenesis and provides insights into complement activation and regulation. *J. Clin. Invest.*, 120:3702-3712.

Mathieson, P.W., Würzner, R., Oliveria, D.B., Lachmann, P.J. & Peters, D.K. (1993) Complement-mediated adipocyte lysis by nephritic factor sera. *J. Exp. Med.*, 177:1827-1831.

Meri, S., Koistinen, V., Miettinen, A., Törnroth, T. & Seppälä, I.J. (1992) Activation of the alternative pathway of complement by monoclonal lambda light chains in membranoproliferative glomerulonephritis. *J. Exp. Med.*, 175:939-950.

Meri, S. (2007) Loss of self-control in the complement system and innate autoreactivity. *Ann. N. Y. Acad. Sci.*, 1109:93-105.

Mollnes, T.E., Ng, Y.C., Peters, D.K., Lea, T., Tschopp, J. & Harboe, M. (1986) Effect of nephritic factor on C3 and on the terminal pathway of complement in vivo and in vitro. *Clin. Exp. Immunol.*, 65:73-79.

Montes, T., Goicoechea de Jorge, E., Ramos, R., Gomà, M., Pujol, O., Sánchez-Corral, P. & Rodríguez de Córdoba S. (2008) Genetic deficiency of complement factor H in a patient with age-related macular degeneration and membranoproliferative glomerulonephritis. *Mol. Immunol.*, 45:2897-2904.

Moore, I., Strain, L., Pappworth, I., Kavanagh, D., Barlow, P.N., Herbert, A.P., Schmidt, C.Q., Staniforth, S.J., Holmes, L.V., Ward, R., Morgan, L., Goodship, T.H. & Marchbank, K.J. (2010) Association of factor H autoantibodies with deletions of CFHR1, CFHR3, CFHR4, and with mutations in CFH, CFI, CD46, and C3 in patients with atypical hemolytic uremic syndrome. *Blood*, 115:379-387.

Noris, M. & Remuzzi, G. (2008) Translational mini-review series on complement factor H: therapies of renal diseases associated with complement factor H abnormalities: atypical haemolytic uraemic syndrome and membranoproliferative glomerulonephritis. *Clin. Exp. Immunol.*, 151:199-209.

Ohi, H., Watanabe, S., Fujita, T. & Yasugi, T. (1992) Significance of C3 nephritic factor (C3NeF) in non-hypocomplementaemic serum with membranoproliferative glomerulonephritis (MPGN). *Clin. Exp. Immunol.*, 89:479-484.

Ohi, H. & Yasugi, T. (1994) Occurrence of C3 nephritic factor and C4 nephritic factor in membranoproliferative glomerulonephritis (MPGN). *Clin. Exp. Immunol.*, 95:316-321.

Pangburn, M.K., Schreiber, R.D. & Müller-Eberhard, H.J. (1981) Formation of the initial C3 convertase of the alternative complement pathway. Acquisition of C3b-like activities by spontaneous hydrolysis of the putative thioester in native C3. *J. Exp. Med.*, 154:856-867.

Papp, K., Végh, P., Miklós, K., Németh, J., Rásky, K., Péterfy, F., Erdei, A. & Prechl, J. (2008) Detection of complement activation on antigen microarrays generates functional antibody profiles and helps characterization of disease-associated changes of the antibody repertoire. *J. Immunol.*, 181:8162-8169.

Pickering, M.C., Cook, H.T., Warren, J., Bygrave, A.E., Moss, J., Walport, M.J. & Botto, M. (2002) Uncontrolled C3 activation causes membranoproliferative glomerulonephritis in mice deficient in complement factor H. *Nat. Genet.*, 31:424-428.

Pickering, M.C., Warren, J., Rose, K.L., Carlucci, F., Wang, Y., Walport, M.J., Cook, H.T. & Botto, M. (2006) Prevention of C5 activation ameliorates spontaneous and experimental glomerulonephritis in factor H-deficient mice. *Proc. Natl. Acad. Sci. U S A*, 103:9649-9654.

Pickering, M.C. & Cook, H.T. (2008) Translational mini-review series on complement factor H: renal diseases associated with complement factor H: novel insights from humans and animals. *Clin. Exp. Immunol.*, 151:210-230.

Pickering, M. & Cook, H.T. (2011) Complement and glomerular disease: new insights. *Curr. Opin. Nephrol. Hypertens.*, 20:271-277.

Ricklin, D., Hajishengallis, G., Yang, K. & Lambris, J.D. (2010) Complement: a key system for immune surveillance and homeostasis. *Nat. Immunol.*, 11:785-797.

Rose, K.L., Paixao-Cavalcante, D., Fish, J., Manderson, A.P., Malik, T.H., Bygrave, A.E., Lin, T., Sacks, S.H., Walport, M.J., Cook, H.T., Botto, M. & Pickering, M.C. (2008) Factor I is required for the development of membranoproliferative glomerulonephritis in factor H-deficient mice. *J. Clin. Invest.*, 118:608-618.

Rother, U. (1982) A new screening test for C3 nephritis factor based on a stable cell bound convertase on sheep erythrocytes. *J. Immunol. Methods*, 51:101-107.

Ruley, E.J., Forristal, J., Davis, N.C., Andres, C. & West, C.D. (1973) Hypocomplementemia of membranoproliferative nephritis. Dependence of the nephritic factor reaction on properdin factor B. *J. Clin. Invest.*, 52:896-904.

Schwertz, R., Rother, U., Anders, D., Gretz, N., Schärer, K. & Kirschfink, M. (2001) Complement analysis in children with idiopathic membranoproliferative glomerulonephritis: a long-term follow-up. *Pediatr. Allergy Immunol.*, 12:166-172.

Seino, J., Fukuda, K., Kinoshita, Y., Sudo, K., Horigome, I., Sato, H., Saito, T., Furuyama, T. & Yoshinaga, K. (1987) Quantitation of C3 nephritic factor of alternative complement pathway by an enzyme-linked immunosorbent assay. *J. Immunol. Methods*, 105:119-125.

Seino, J., Kinoshita, Y., Sudo, K., Horigome, I., Sato, H., Narita, M., Noshiro, H., Kudo, K., Fukuda, K., Saito, T. & Yoshinaga K. (1990) Quantitation of C4 nephritic factor by an enzyme-linked immunosorbent assay. *J. Immunol. Methods*, 128:101-108.

Servais, A., Frémeaux-Bacchi, V., Lequintrec, M., Salomon, R., Blouin, J., Knebelmann, B., Grünfeld, J.P., Lesavre, P., Noël, L.H. & Fakhouri, F. (2007) Primary glomerulonephritis with isolated C3 deposits: a new entity which shares common genetic risk factors with haemolytic uraemic syndrome. *J. Med. Genet.*, 44:193-199.

Servais, A., Noël, L.H., Dragon-Durey, M.A., Gübler, M.C., Rémy, P., Buob, D., Cordonnier, C., Makdassi, R., Jaber, W., Boulanger, E., Lesavre, P. & Frémeaux-Bacchi, V. (2011) Heterogeneous pattern of renal disease associated with homozygous Factor H deficiency. *Hum. Pathol.*, 2011 Mar 9. [Epub ahead of print] doi:10.1016/j.humpath.2010.11.023

Sethi, S., Gamez, J.D., Vrana, J.A., Theis, J.D., Bergen, H.R. 3rd, Zipfel, P.F., Dogan, A. & Smith, R.J. (2009) Glomeruli of Dense Deposit Disease contain components of the alternative and terminal complement pathway. *Kidney Int.*, 75:952-960.

Sethi, S., Fervenza, F.C., Zhang, Y., Nasr, S.H., Leung, N., Vrana, J., Cramer, C., Nester, C.M. & Smith, R.J. (2011) Proliferative Glomerulonephritis Secondary to Dysfunction of the Alternative Pathway of Complement. *Clin. J. Am. Soc. Nephrol.*, 6:1009-1017.

Sissons, J.G., West, R.J., Fallows, J., Williams, D.G., Boucher, B.J., Amos, N. & Peters, D.K. (1976) The complement abnormalities of lipodystrophy. *N. Engl. J. Med.*, 294:461-465.

Skerka, C., Licht, C., Mengel, M., Uzonyi, B., Strobel, S., Zipfel, P.F. & Józsi, M. (2009) Autoimmune forms of thrombotic microangiopathy and membranoproliferative glomerulonephritis: Indications for a disease spectrum and common pathogenic principles. *Mol. Immunol.*, 46:2801-2807.

Smith, R.J., Alexander, J., Barlow, P.N., Botto, M., Cassavant, T.L., Cook, H.T., Rodríguez de Córdoba, S., Hageman, G.S., Jokiranta, T.S., Kimberling, W.J., Lambris, J.D., Lanning, L.D., Levidiotis, V., Licht, C., Lutz, H.U., Meri, S., Pickering, M.C., Quigg, R.J., Rops, A.L., Salant, D.J., Sethi, S., Thurman, J.M., Tully, H.F., Tully, S.P., van der Vlag, J., Walker, P.D., Würzner, R. & Zipfel, P.F.; Dense Deposit Disease Focus Group. (2007) New approaches to the treatment of dense deposit disease. *J. Am. Soc. Nephrol.*, 18:2447-2456.

Spitzer, R.E., Vallota, E.H., Forristal, J., Sudora, E., Stitzel, A., Davis, N.C. & West, C.D. (1969) Serum C'3 lytic system in patients with glomerulonephritis. *Science*, 164:436-437.

Spitzer, R.E., Stitzel, A.E. & Tsokos, G.C. (1990) Evidence that production of autoantibody to the alternative pathway C3 convertase is a normal physiologic event. *J. Pediatr.*, 116:S103-108.

Spitzer, R.E., Stitzel, A.E. & Tsokos, G. (1992) On the origin of C3 nephritic factor (antibody to the alternative pathway C3 convertase): evidence for the Adam and Eve concept of autoantibody production. *Clin. Immunol. Immunopathol.*, 64:177-183.

Strife, C.F., Leahy, A.E. & West, C.D. (1989) Antibody to a cryptic, solid phase C1Q antigen in membranoproliferative nephritis. *Kidney Int.*, 35:836-842.

Strife, C.F., Prada, A.L., Clardy, C.W., Jackson, E. & Forristal, J. (1990) Autoantibody to complement neoantigens in membranoproliferative glomerulonephritis. *J. Pediatr.*, 116:S98-102.

Strobel, S., Zimmering, M., Papp, K., Prechl, J. & Józsi, M. (2010a) Anti-factor B autoantibody in dense deposit disease. *Mol. Immunol.*, 47:1476-1483.

Strobel, S., Hoyer, P.F., Mache, C.J., Sulyok, E., Liu, W.S., Richter, H., Oppermann, M., Zipfel, P.F. & Józsi, M. (2010b) Functional analyses indicate a pathogenic role of factor H autoantibodies in atypical haemolytic uraemic syndrome. *Nephrol. Dial. Transplant.*, 25:136-144.

Tanuma, Y., Ohi, H., Watanabe, S., Seki, M. & Hatano, M. (1989) C3 nephritic factor and C4 nephritic factor in the serum of two patients with hypocomplementaemic membranoproliferative glomerulonephritis. *Clin. Exp. Immunol.*, 76:82-85.

Tanuma, Y., Ohi, H. & Hatano, M. (1990) Two types of C3 nephritic factor: properdin-dependent C3NeF and properdin-independent C3NeF. *Clin. Immunol. Immunopathol.*, 56:226-238.

Torreira, E., Tortajada, A., Montes, T., Rodríguez de Córdoba, S. & Llorca O. (2009) 3D structure of the C3bB complex provides insights into the activation and regulation of the complement alternative pathway convertase. *Proc. Natl. Acad. Sci. U S A*, 106:882-887

Trouw, L.A., Roos, A. & Daha, M.R. (2001) Autoantibodies to complement components. *Mol. Immunol.*, 38:199-206.

Trouw, L.A., Seelen, M.A. & Daha, M.R. (2003) Complement and renal disease. *Mol. Immunol.*, 40:125-134.

Wagner, E. & Frank, M.M. (2010) Therapeutic potential of complement modulation. *Nat. Rev. Drug Discov.*, 9:43-56.

Walport, M.J. (2001a) Complement. First of two parts. *N. Engl. J. Med.*, 344:1058-1066.

Walport, M.J. (2001b) Complement. Second of two parts. *N. Engl. J. Med.*, 344:1140-1144.

West, C.D., Witte, D.P. & McAdams, A.J. (2001) Composition of nephritic factor-generated glomerular deposits in membranoproliferative glomerulonephritis type 2. *Am. J. Kidney Dis.*, 37:1120-1130.

West, C.D. (2008) A hemolytic method for the measurement of nephritic factor. *J. Immunol. Methods*, 335:1-7.

Zipfel, P.F., Heinen, S., Józsi, M. & Skerka, C. (2006) Complement and diseases: defective alternative pathway control results in kidney and eye diseases. *Mol. Immunol.*, 43:97-106.

Zipfel, P.F. & Skerka, C. (2009) Complement regulators and inhibitory proteins. *Nat. Rev. Immunol.*, 9:729-740.

Part 2

Animal Models of Glomerulonephritis

4

The Experimental Model of the Autoimmune Glomerulonephritis Induced by the Chronic Graft versus Host Reaction

O.T. Kudaeva et al.*
Institute of Clinical Immunology,
Siberian Branch of Russian Academy of Medical Sciences
Russian Federation

1. Introduction

Graft-versus-host reaction (GVHR) is a cellular immune reaction developed by transplanting mature T-lymphocytes to tissue incompatible recipients. As it has been stated by R.E. Billingham in a Harvey Lecture, there are three requirements for the development of GVHR: the graft must contain immunologically competent cells; the recipient must be incapable of rejecting the transplanted cells; the recipient must express tissue antigens that are not present in the donor (Billingham, 1966, as cited in Sun et al., 2007). There are several situations in which it's possible: the introduction of incompatible lymphocytes to newborn or adult immunocompromised recipients or the transfer parental lymphocytes to F1 hybrids. A recipient with a normal immune system will usually reject cells from a foreign donor.

At the present time there are described and characterized two forms of graft-versus-host reaction: acute and chronic. The mechanisms of acute and chronic GVHR are distinguished by participating of $CD8^{+}$T-cells. If the $CD8^{+}$T-cells are involved in the development of immune processes, a primary stimulating phase of reaction (activation of the donor cell by recipient alloantigens) is followed by a cytotoxic phase including a generation of effector cells - cytotoxic T lymphocytes (CTL), directed against recipient alloantigens, and the reaction ends with destruction of host tissues. In general, it can be called a normal physiological immune reaction "graft versus host" - accomplished immune response of mature donor cells against allogeneic recipient. From this viewpoint chronic GVHR is an incomplete ("defective") GVHR: the reaction does not lead to formation of $CD8^{+}$T-effector cells and to a development of a cytotoxic phase, as it should be, but «freezes» at a primary stimulating stage and ends with lymphoproliferation. Such type of the reaction may be caused by different situations: removal or inactivation of some inoculum T cells subpopulations, the suppression of the reaction by pharmacological agents at early stages, or the lack of donor T cells stimulation through the absence of MHC class I incompatibility.

---

* O.P. Kolesnikova, E.V. Goiman, V.O. Tkachev, N.N. Volsky, O.M. Perminova, E.D. Gavrilova and V.A. Kozlov.
Institute of Clinical Immunology, Siberian Branch of Russian Academy of Medical Sciences, Russian Federation.

Acute GVHR leads to severe cytotoxic reaction of transplanted cells against host tissues. It's characterized by thymic involution, pronounced hypoplasia of the lympho-hemopoietic tissue, including aplastic anemia, immunodeficiency, hypogammaglobulinemia, and sepsis. Acute GVHR often ends with the death of the recipient. Chronic GVHR is characterized by a long incubation period and relatively low mortality. It's manifested by lymphoid hyperplasia, hypergammaglobulinemia, autoantibody formation. Chronic GVHR is more diverse in the immune mechanisms and accordingly in the clinical manifestations: it may be observed the development of immunodeficiency, the formation of different variants of autoimmune pathologies, lymphoproliferative processes, skin lesions, disorders of intestines (enteritis, colitis) and other internal organs (Gleichmann et al., 1984; Via & Shearer, 1988; Mori et al., 1998; Chu & Gress, 2008).

It has been shown that GVHR may be useful model for study various human disorders. In mouse models of GVHR a reaction may be directed to MHC class I, MHC class II, or both or to isolated multiple minor histocompatibility antigens (miHA) alone. In each case the reaction is dependent on either $CD8^+$T cells, $CD4^+$T cells, or both, depending on the strain combination of donor and recipient. When donor and recipient are distinguished by MHC I and II classes acute GVHR occurs, whereas in the case of only MHC class II differences chronic GVHR is formed. Initially acute GVHR was considered Th1-dependent and chronic GVHR - Th2-dependent form of reaction (Krenger & Ferrara, 1996; Okamoto et al., 2000; Shustov et al., 2000; Kataoka et al., 2001). Now it has become evident that this is an oversimplification and a situation is much more complicated. Currently it has been shown involvement either Th1- and Th2-subpopulation in the development of acute and chronic GVHR, and thus there are many unresolved issues concerning of GVHR mechanisms and participating of different cytokines and cell subpopulations, particularly with regard to the chronic form of the reaction (Koreth & Antin, 2008; Reddy & Ferrara, 2009).

2. Experimental model of glomerulonephritis induced by chronic GVHR

Graft-versus-host reaction leads to the development of immunopathological states (graft-versus-host disease - GVHD), in some cases similar to human disease which are caused by immune abnormalities. Primarily it refers to autoimmune diseases. The transfer parental lymphocytes to F1 hybrids is particularly appealing for use as models of human diseases. In this case it does not require to expose recipients previously to irradiation or cytotoxic drugs suppressing its ability to graft reject.

In semiallogeneic system C57Bl/6→(C57Bl/6xDBA/2)F1 donor and recipient are differ in the MHC class I and II and an acute form of reaction develops in accordance with a general rule. However if cells of the second parental line DBA/2 use for transplantation (the semiallogeneic system DBA/2→(C57Bl/6xDBA/2)F1) chronic GVHD develops despite differences between donor and recipient by MHC classes I and II and miHAs (Gleichmann et al., 1984; Reddy et al., 2008; Kim et al., 2010). The inability of DBA/2 mice lymphocytes to induce acute GVHD may be explained by different production of inflammatory cytokines such as IFNγ , TNFα, IL-6, which play an important role in the activation of CTL, in mice with $H2^b$ and $H2^d$ haplotype (De Maeyer-Guignard et al., 1986; Raj et al., 1992). Moreover, it has been shown that the population of $CD8^+$lymphocytes in DBA/2 mice is quantitatively and qualitatively defective. $CD8^+$T-cells of DBA/2 mice generate a weak response to BDF1 alloantigen in vitro and the frequency of CTL precursors in DBA/2 mice is many times less than one in C57Bl/6 mice (Via et al., 1987; Tschetter et al., 2000). Thus induction of GVHR in transfer system DBA/2→(C57Bl/6xDBA/2)F1 does not lead to an acute form as it should be due genetic donor-recipient differences but causes a chronic GVHD dependent on $CD4^+$ donor cells (Gleichmann et al., 1984; Reddy et al., 2008). There are a polyclonal activation of B cells, an increase of a total IgG level, a formation of multiple autoantibodies including antibodies to DNA. Autoantibodies found in this GVHR are of the IgG class whereas antibodies binding to a variety of self antigens and found in the peripheral blood of normal individuals are of the IgM class (Rolink et al., 1987). Chronic GVHD results in a development of autoimmune disorder similar human systemic lupus erythematosis (SLE) and in a formation of lupus-like immune complex glomerulonephritis (Via & Shearer, 1988).

2.1 Two variants of GVHD induced in transfer system DBA/2→(C57Bl/6xDBA/2)F1

Studying this model we have discovered that although the typical chronic GVHR develops in all recipients reaction can proceed in two different directions despite the genetic homogeneity of recipients - (C57Bl/6xDBA/2)F1 mice. The development of chronic GVHR is sustained by increased spleen cell number and polyclonal B-cell activation in the absence of thymus destruction (Kozlov et al., 2002). The absence of destruction of lymphoid tissue, in particular, atrophy of the thymus is a sharp-cut distinctive feature of chronic GVHD from its acute form. Chronic GVHD is not accompanied by marked disruptions of thymus tissue, infiltration of the thymus by donor T-cells, pronounced structural changes, signs of local inflammation and disorders of cell proliferation (Krenger et al., 2000).

2.1.1 Development of chronic GVHR

The formation of glomerulonephritis is going on for 6 - 12 weeks (Fig. 1). The autoimmune glomerulonephritis develops in 50-60% recipients (a *lupus* group), whereas marked disorders of kidney are absent in the rest ones (a *nonlupus* group) (Fig. 2).

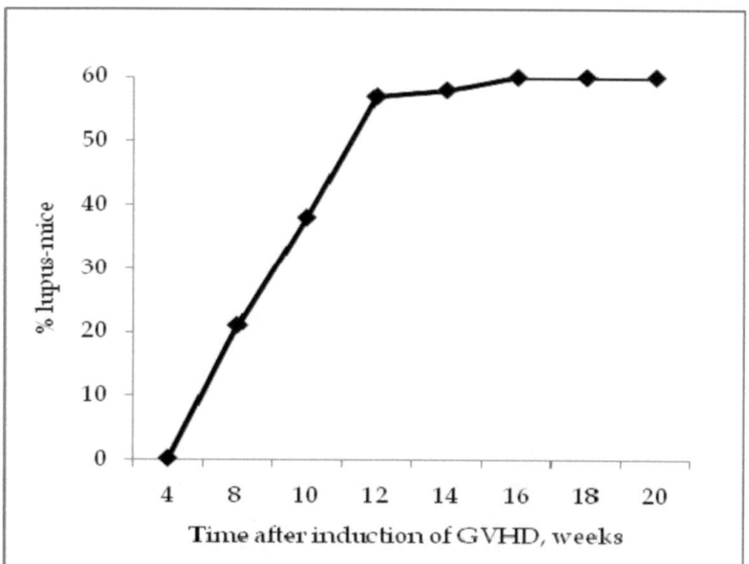

Fig. 1. Frequency of lupus-like nephritis in the course of chronic GVHD development

The availability of the autoimmune glomerulonephritis has been tested by the urine protein level that has been strictly correlated with the appearance of immune complex deposits in kidney and morphological manifestations of kidney disorders as it has been verified previously (Kolesnikova et al., 1991).
The development of the reaction is accompanied by the increase of total IgG level and the appearance of autoantibodies to own tissues components (dsDNA, erythrocytes) in the peripheral blood (Fig. 3) (Kudaeva et al., 2005a).

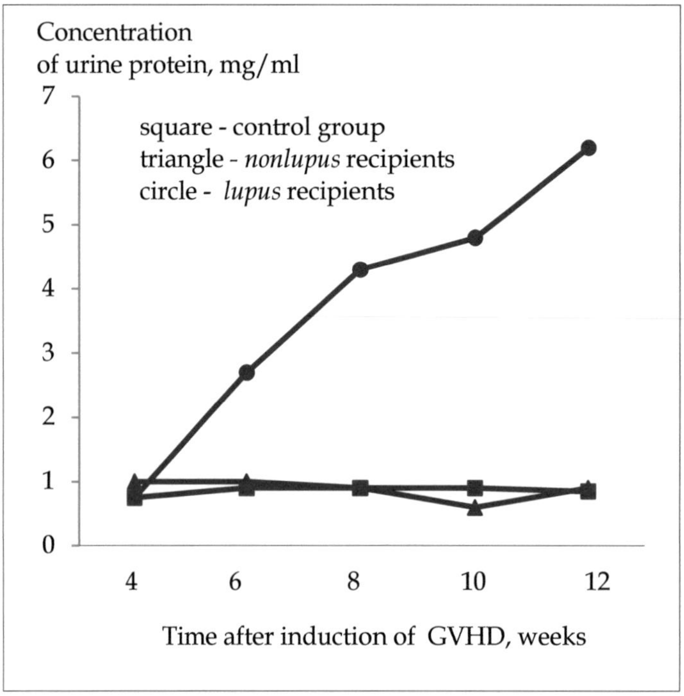

Fig. 2. Formation of glomerulonephritis in the course of chronic GVHD development

2.1.2 Kidney morphology

The severity of the pathological process in the kidneys is evaluated by a 4-marks scale depending on the number of glomeruli involved in the pathological process and the extent of their damage (Yoshioka et al., 1989; Muracami et al., 1995).
Morphological study has shown that animals without proteinuria (a *nonlupus* group) have slight pathomorphological changes in the form of proliferative mesangium in some glomeruli, expressed in increasing in the number of mesangial cells and in the size of the glomerular capillaries. A weak proliferation of mesangial cells combines with dust-like deposits of IgG in the glomeruli and small proteinosis of tubular epithelium. It is observed small periglomerular lymphoid infiltrates. The kidney structure is saved. Tubules dystrophy is absent. Morphological characteristics of renal pathology correspond to 1 in *nonlupus* recipients.
In the group of animals with proteinuria (a *lupus* group) it is observed gross changes in renal tissue. Changes in the glomeruli become diffuse and are expressed in increasing the number of mesangial cells with mesangial matrix deposition, diffuse wall thickening of

capillary loops until the hyalinosis lesions. Glomeruli become "gripping" look. Periglomerular lymphoid infiltrates meet constantly. Proteinosis of convoluted tubule epithelium is expressed sharply. In some cases there is the phenomenon of glomerular sclerosis. Deposits of IgG in the glomeruli have linear and granular character. Morphological characteristics of renal pathology correspond to 3.5 in *lupus* recipients. At 6-7 months of illness proteinuria attains a high level and coarse sclerotic changes dominate in kidney tissue: multiple sclerosis and hyalinosis of many glomeruli, proliferation of renal capsule epithelium with the formation of "crescent", expressed tubular atrophy with cystic enlargement of the lumen, lymphoid infiltration of the interstitium. It is found granular IgG deposits in sclerosal glomeruli; content of cystic tubules are positive stained for IgG also. Thus the induction of chronic GVHD in genetically identical recipients leads to the development of autoimmune glomerulonephritis in the part of the recipients.

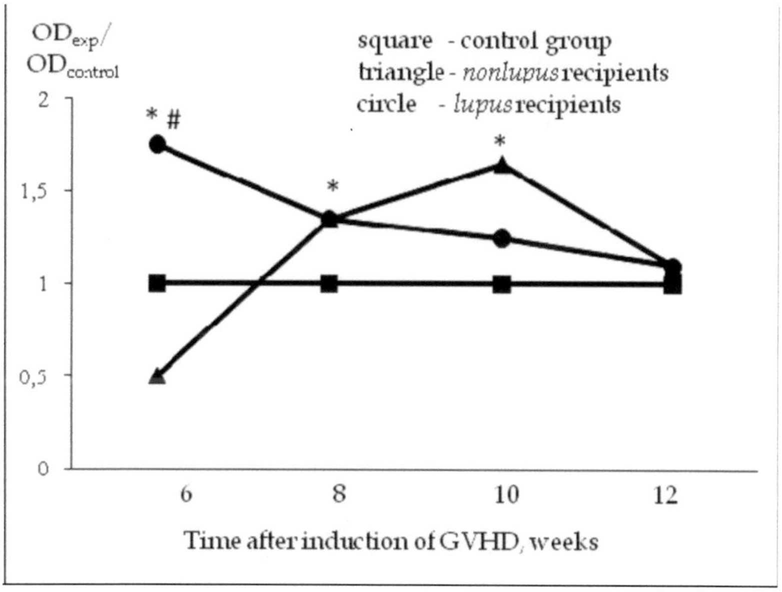

* - $p < 0.05$ compared between control and experimental group; # - $p < 0.05$ between experimental groups

Fig. 3. The level of antibodies to dsDNA in recipients in the course of chronic GVHD development

2.1.3 The Th1/Th2 balance

The further study has revealed that different Th1/Th2 ratio is the main distinction between *nonlupus* and *lupus* recipients. Existence of two Th-subpopulations producing different cytokine sets and exerting opposing influence upon basic links of immune response has been described among murine $CD4^{+}$T-cells in 1986 and then among human T-lymphocytes (Mosmann et al., 1986; Del Prete et al., 1991). It has led to conception of immune polarization: Th1/Th2 balance is the basic parameter of regulation of immune processes (Mosmann & Sad, 1996; Allen & Maizels, 1997; O'Gor et al., 2003). The Th-cell fate decision depends on specific Th1 or Th2 factors of transcription that is determined by a set of external epigenetic factors (Glimcher & Murphy, 2000; Wilson & Makarb, 2002; Agnello et al., 2003). Choosing of each Th-cell differential way is subjected to influence of abundant factors connecting immune reactions with the current condition of a whole organism. The GVHD is among the processes in which Th1/Th2 balance plays the pivotal role.

Application of this paradigm for studying the regulation of immunity in both normal physiological conditions and immune pathological states has proved fruitful, and today is widely used in the study of processes such as bacterial and viral infections, allergic diseases, immune responses during carcinogenesis, autoimmune disorders, immune conflicts in pregnancy (Fresno et al., 1997; Kunzendorf et al., 1998; Chaouat et al., 2003; Wilczynski, 2005). Not all the currently known experimental facts and clinical observations perfectly fit into this concept. There are many new data on the participation of other T-cell subpopulations in the regulation of immune processes (Th17, Treg, ThF, Th9) (Mosmann et al., 2009). However the application of this paradigm remains useful to solve contemporary problems of the immune regulation.

The following points indicate that Th1- or Th2-subpopulation is predominant in *nonlupus*- or *lupus*-mice respectively (Vlasov et al., 2002; Kozlov et al., 2002; Kudaeva et al., 2005b). It is known that in mice Th1-dependent immune response is characterized by increased IgG2a subclass level, whereas activation of Th2-cells is accompanied by an increase of IgG1 one (Snapper & Paul, 1987; Morris et al., 1994). Ratio of Th1- and Th2-dependent IgG subclasses in peripheral blood of mice with GVHD shows a pronounced shift toward IgG2a (Th1-dependent subclass) in *nonlupus* mice and toward IgG1 (Th2-dependent subclass) in the *lupus* mice. Differences emerge at the early stages of reaction (1 month) and amplify over time (6 months) (Fig. 4).

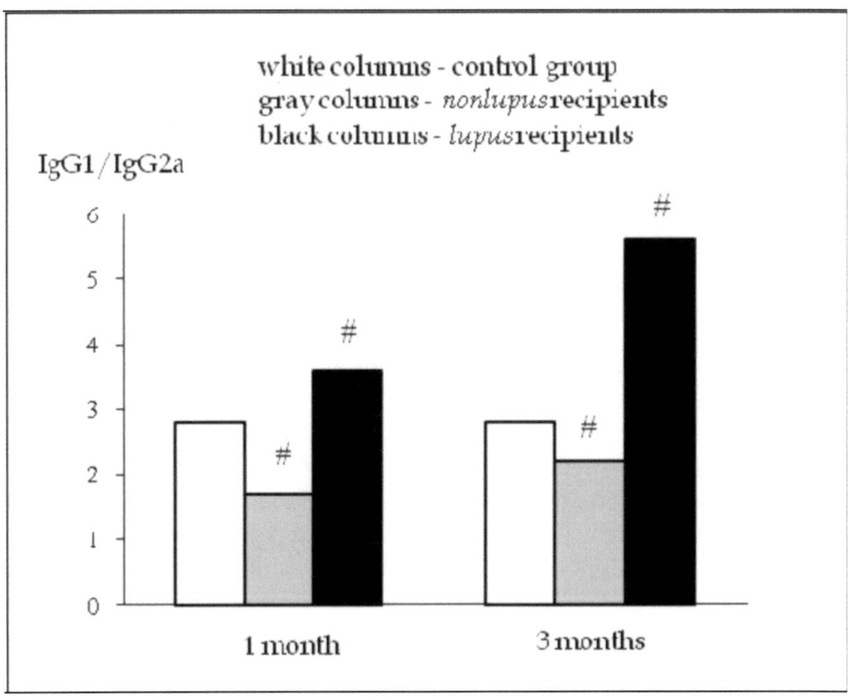

- $p < 0.05$ compared between *nonlupus* and *lupus*

Fig. 4. IgG1/IgG2a ratio in the serum of mice with chronic GVHD

There are many observations about the intimate direct correlation between the concentration of IgE and the level of the key Th2-cell cytokine IL-4 (Doutrelepont et al., 1991; Umland et al., 1992; Ushiyama et al., 1995). Determination of the IgE concentration in peripheral blood of recipients has shown a high IgE level during the development of chronic GVHD and the formation of glomerulonephritis. IgE content sharply increases at the initial stages of reaction, then reduces but remains significantly higher than one of intact animals. IgE levels in *lupus* mice is considerably superior to one in *nonlupus* recipients at all stages of reaction (Tabl. 1) (Goiman et al., 2009).

	Control	*Nonlupus*	*Lupus*
10 days	6.95 (2.2 - 10.6)	20.0* (8.4 - 30.2)	24.9* (8.2 - 41.9)
24 days		132.5* (54.2 - 348.6)	232.1* (63.0 - 396.2)
3 months		24.3* # (15.0 - 36.6)	69.2* # (22.5 - 166.4)

* - $p < 0.05$ compared between control and experimental group; # - $p < 0.05$ between experimental groups

Table 1. The IgE content in peripheral blood of recipients in the course of GVHD development (M, (min-max), μg/ml)

2.2 Characteristics of recipients with glomerulonephritis

2.2.1 The homeostatic proliferation

Homeostatic proliferation is a compensatory repair of quantitative deficit of lymphocytes by triggering their proliferation at the periphery. Homeostatic proliferation decreases the variety of antigen recognizing receptors and leads to the appearance of an appreciable amount of autoreactive effector cells (Baccala & Theofilopoulos, 2005; Marleau & Sarvetnick, 2005). Now homeostatic proliferation is regarded as a possible mechanism of the development of autoimmune disease (Khoruts & Fraser, 2005; Surth & Sprent, 2008).

Acute GVHR is associated with a drop of lymphocyte count. Chronic GVHR is called immunostimulatory, because lymphoproliferative reaction is indicative of it (Via & Shearer, 1988). However measure of lymphocyte counts in the recipient peripheral blood over the course of reaction has revealed its drastic decrease at the early stage of chronic GVHR in this model. This decrease persists throughout the first two weeks and then is replaced by lymphocytosis followed by normalization of lymphocyte count in the peripheral blood against the background of developing splenomegaly (Tkachev et al., 2006). Hence it has been studied the possible involvement of homeostatic proliferation in the development of autoimmune disease - glomerulonephritis in this model (Goiman et al., 2010).

An obligatory condition for homeostatic proliferation of naive and memory $CD4^+$ T-cell is high concentration of IL-7 (Schluns et al., 2000; Boyman et al., 2008). It has been shown the significantly increased level of endogenous splenic IL-7 mRNA in irradiated recipients with acute GVHR (Gendelman et al., 2004). The content of IL-7 in the peripheral blood of recipients with chronic GVHR sharply increases during the early period (25.5 pg/ml) and remains high within 3 months after induction of GVHD in *lupus* recipients (6.5 pg/ml) in comparison with control animals (lower the verge of method) and *nonlupus* recipients (lower the verge of method) (Goiman et al., 2010).

The key characteristic of homeostatic proliferation is taking T memory cell phenotype ($CD4^+CD45RB^{low}$ and $CD8^+CD45RB^{low}$) by naïve T cells ($CD4^+CD45RB^{high}$ and $CD8^+CD45RB^{high}$). Despite the increase in both $CD4^+$ subpopulations (naïve and memory) its proportion is shifted towards memory cells in *lupus* recipients. The T-cell donor chimerism is just 2% in chronic GVHR in this model (Via & Shearer, 1988). Hence, the $CD4^+CD45RB^{low}$ and $CD8^+CD45RB^{low}$ cells in the spleens of *lupus* mice are mainly recipient cells.
It can be assumed that lymphopenia at the early stages of chronic GVHR causes homeostatic proliferation of T lymphocytes in *lupus* recipients, which participates in the development of autoimmune pathology in this model.

2.2.2 The immune response of recipients

GVHR is accompanied by immunosuppression. The mechanism of immunodeficiency has been well studied in case of acute reaction: it's a destruction of the recipient's immune system by donor immune cells. The mechanism of immunosuppression in the chronic form of GVHR remains unclear (Kimura & Gleichmann, 1987; Haridas & Kamat, 1997; Kataoka et al, 2001; Chu & Gress, 2008).
In spite of the occurrence of two different variants of chronic GVHR in this model the suppression of primary immune response to T-dependent antigen is observed in all recipients (Fig. 5) (Kozlov et al., 2002; Kudaeva et al., 2010b). The decrease of the primary response is significantly heavier in *nonlupus* recipients.

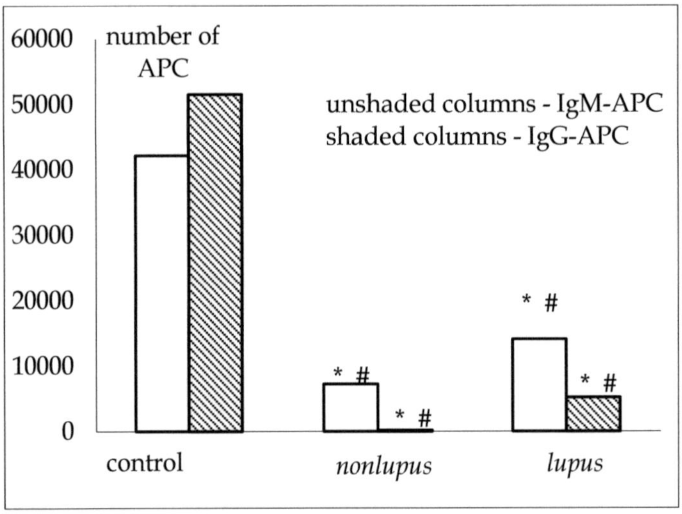

* - $p < 0.05$ compared between control and experimental group; # - $p < 0.05$ between experimental groups

Fig. 5. The level of primary humoral immune response in recipients with chronic GVHD

An enhancement of the suppressive activity of regulatory T cells, a disruption of the antigen-presenting cells, an increase of specific Th-cells apoptosis are considered as a possible reasons. Experiments in vitro indicate the possible inability of B lymphocytes in chronic GVHR to respond to T-dependent antigen. The latter can be explained by the abundance of activating factors leading to the ultimate differentiation of the few antigen specific B-cell and thus excluding its proliferation (Kimura & Gleichmann, 1987).

The inhibition of humoral immune response may be due to hyperactivation of the B-lymphocytes. Indeed, the development of chronic GVHD is accompanied by a marked polyclonal activation of B-lymphocytes, which is known to impede an adequate response to new stimulus (Reina-San-Martin et al., 2000; Spera et al., 2006; Montes et al., 2007; Marques et al., 2008).

At the same time a decrease of the secondary immune response is less marked especially in the *lupus* recipients (Fig. 6). Perhaps, it indicates that a formation of immune memory is more rigidly processes, resistant to the action of various factors. Explanation of this discordance between the level of primary and secondary response under chronic GVHD requires further investigation.

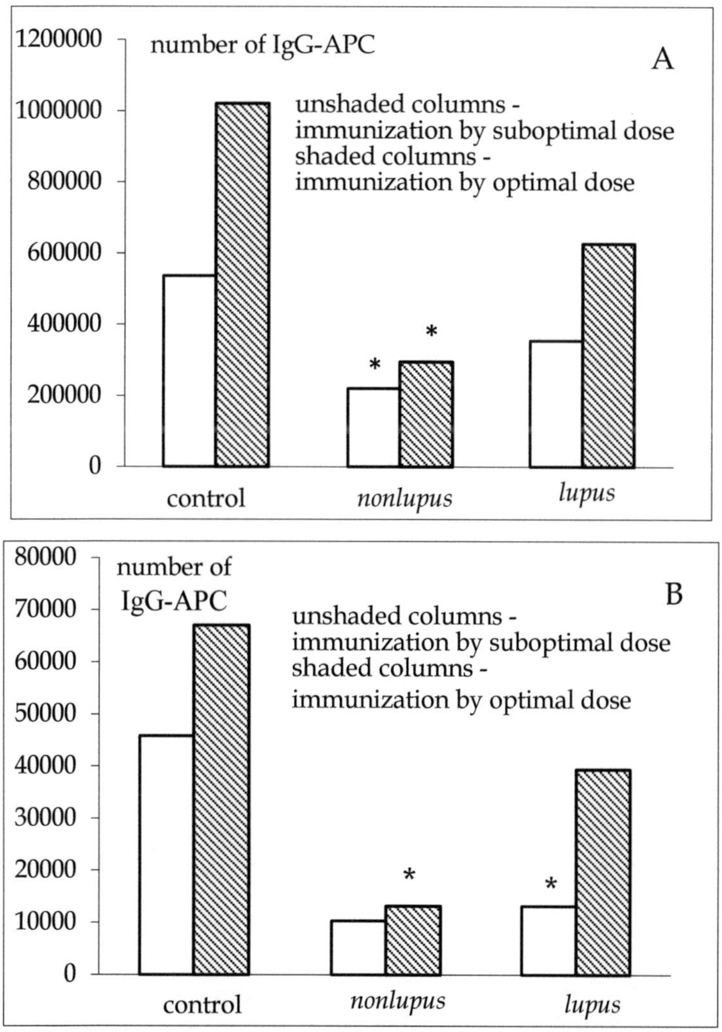

* - $p < 0.05$ compared between control and experimental group

Fig. 6. The level of the secondary humoral immune response in recipients with chronic GVHD (A – spleen; B – bone marrow)

The suppression of humoral immune response to T-dependent antigen is observed in all recipients (*nonlupus* and *lupus*) and by this means is not specific feature of autoimmune disorder in this model.

2.2.3 Anemia

Hematological abnormalities are common in systemic lupus erythematosus and may be manifested in anemia of different pathogenesis. In SLE many factors are produced which disturb the hematological balance both on the peripheral level and in the bone marrow. It is assumed that the autoantibodies produced in SLE are the main cause of autoimmune hemolytic anemia. However it should be considered that quantitative changes in the number of erythrocytes observed in this disease are also caused by chronic inflammatory condition, which impairs the endocrine function of the kidneys in erythropoietin production as the element of autoimmune disease.

Parameters	control	*lupus*
Hemoglobin, g/l	199.5 ± 3.5	137.3 ± 6.9 **
Hematocrit, per cent	49.2 ± 0.4	39.7 ± 1.4 **
Reticulocytes, pro mille	10.0 ± 1.3	26.2 ± 4.7 **

M±m, * - $p < 0.05$ and ** - $p < 0.01$ compared between control and experimental group

Table 2. Hematological parameters of *lupus* mice

It has been shown that acute GVHD (C57BL/6→(C57BL/6xDBA/2)F1) reduces the peripheral blood cell counts, the number of bone marrow cells, and colony forming unit-granulocyte macrophage (CFU-GM), whereas the host hematopoiesis in chronic GVHD (DBA/2→(C57BL/6xDBA/2)F1) is not affected within 2 weeks after the transfer of parental splenocytes (Mori et al., 1998). However study of the host hematopoiesis at late stages of GVHD has revealed the set of immune- and hemopoiesis disorders (Kozlov et al., 1995).
The results presented in Table 2 show that *lupus* mice have a significant decrease of hemoglobin and hematocrit levels in comparison with intact animals. Marked reticulocytosis corresponds to the expression of anemic syndrome and gives evidence of a quite regenerative ability of the *lupus* bone marrow. To clarify the nature of anemia assessment of early and late erythropoietic progenitors has been studied. Data on the number of erythroid precursors in the myelogram and the number of erythroid burst forming units (BFU-E) and colony forming unit-granulocyte macrophage in bone marrow are shown in Table 3.

Parameters	control	*lupus*
Nucleated erythroid precursors, per cent	28.3 ± 1.2	37.6 ± 2.9 *
BFU-E per 10^5 bone marrow cells	7.8 ± 0.9	21.3 ± 1.8 **
CFU- GM per $5x10^4$ bone marrow cells	8.7 ± 0.7 (10)	4.7 ± 0.5*

M ± m, * - $p < 0.05$ and ** - $p < 0.01$ compared between control and *lupus*

Table 3. Assessment of erythropoiesis at the level of early and late hematopoietic precursors in *lupus* mice

Changes in bone marrow smears of SLE patients with autoimmune hemolytic anemia and ones of *lupus* recipients are similar. The relative and absolute number of BFU-E in the bone marrow increases in *lupus* recipients compared with intact animals.

The decrease of hemoglobin and hematocrit in *lupus* recipients is accompanied by reticulocytosis and hypertrophy of erythropoiesis in the bone marrow, thus it becomes apparent that anemia develops as a result of increased destruction of erythrocytes.

Increasing the number of BFU-E and nucleated erythroid precursors suggests hypertrophy of erythron in *lupus* mice. Similar changes of erythron are observed in mice NZB, whose autoimmune hemolytic anemia is accompanied by increased numbers of early erythroid precursors in the bone marrow and spleen (Orlovskaja & Kozlov, 2001).

Autoimmune hemolytic anemia is diagnosed in the presence of variable intensity of anemia (usually macrocytic), reticulocytosis, and a positive direct and/or indirect antiglobulin test after ruling out other types of hemolytic anemia.

Coombs test (direct antiglobulin test) is used to verify the occurrence of erythrocyte-bound antibodies which mediate red cell destruction in anemic mice. Autoantibodies to erythrocytes have been determined by this test at weekly intervals, starting at week 1 and lasting until week 12 after the initiation of the GVHR. Coombs-positive erythrocytes begin to appear at early stages of reaction. It has been established that the frequency of Coombs-positive results within 1-2 months after induction of GVHD achieves 60%. In mice with positive results of Coombs-test hematocrit is reduced by 26%, hemoglobin by 33%. Immune complex glomerulonephritis develops in 52% of mice with positive Coombs test at the early stages of GVHR. However a positive direct antiglobulin test alone is not sufficient to diagnose of autoimmune hemolytic anemia and may be positive in many patients without anemia or negative in some patients with one.

It has been studied the possibility of correction of impaired erythropoiesis by hypoxia (Table 4). Hypoxia has had favorable effect on anemia, significantly increasing hematocrit and hemoglobin levels and reducing the increased number of reticulocytes (Kolesnikova et al., 2001).

Parameters	control		*lupus*	
	intact	hypoxia	without hypoxia	hypoxia
Hemoglobin, g/l	197.5 ± 3.5	224.5 ± 7.8	137.3 ± 6.9**	186.0 ± 4.6##
Hematocrit, per cent	49.2 ± 0.4	50.0 ± 1.3	34.2 ± 0.9 **	39.5 ± 0.9 #
Reticulocytes, per mille	10.0 ± 1.3	-	26.2 ± 4.7 **	12.3 ± 1.1##

(M ± m, ** - $p < 0.01$ compared between control and *lupus*, # - $p < 0.05$ and ## - $p < 0.01$ compared between *lupus* without hypoxia and *lupus* with hypoxia

Table 4. The influence of hypoxia on hemoglobin and hematocrit levels, reticulocyte number in *lupus* mice

It is known that hypoxia stimulates the production of erythropoietin by kidney. It is used for treatment anemia with a decrease of erythropoiesis (Eckardt et al., 1989). There are no available data on the use of chronic hypoxia for treatment of moderate hemolytic anemia with increase of bone marrow erythropoiesis combined with immunopathology. In this model it has been shown some positive effect of chronic hypoxia on GVHR induced immunopathology: hypoxia increases humoral immune response, abolishes anemia and corrects of early and late committed hemopoietic precursors number (Kolesnikova et al., 2001). Apparently initial increase of erythropoietin synthesis leads to the growth of hemoglobin level in blood. When a level of hemoglobin in blood is restored, the hyperplasia of bone marrow hemopoietic cells stops.

2.2.4 Macrophages

Macrophages play a pivotal role in development of immune response and inflammatory reactions, acting as effectors and regulatory cells. Their participation in renal development, damage and repair has been well described (Williams et al., 2010). In pathogenesis of immune-mediated kidney injury different types of macrophages take part. There are resident renal macrophages (mesangial cells), macrophages differentiated from blood monocytes migrating in site of inflammation, and macrophages located in other organs (e.g. spleen and lymph nodes macrophages).

Resident renal macrophages are supposed to play protective role in mechanism of glomerular damage induced by immune complexes via scavenging and preventing immune complexes depositions in glomeruli. This "physiologic" clearance of immune complexes is nonphlogistic and does not lead to increased production of inflammatory mediators (Duffield, 2003; Serhan & Savill, 2005; Bergtold et al., 2006; Castano et al., 2009). But if these mechanism is overwhelmed it results in deposit formation on glomerular basal membrane causing leukocytes activation, liberation of cytotoxic and chemoattracting products, local kidney injury and recruitment of further leukocytes (Gomez-Guerrero et al., 2004, 2005; Berger & Daha, 2010). These processes contribute a progressive loss of renal functions.

Severity of clinical manifestation of kidney diseases closely correlates with intensity of macrophages infiltration (Van Goor et al., 1994; Duffield, 2010). Transfer of semiallogeneic lymphoid cells from DBA/2 mice to (C57Bl/6xDBA/2)F1 hybrids leads to rapid accumulation of CD11a-positive leukocytes in renal glomeruli which is maximal within 4 weeks after GVHD induction and is synchronized with the time of proteinuria onset (Kootstra et al., 1998). Moreover in the murine model of proliferative glomerulonephritis caused by deposition of immune complexes at the glomerular basal membrane it has been shown that macrophages ablation ameliorates severity of injury (Guo et al., 2009).

Role of macrophages in kidney injury and repair can also depend on the mechanism of their activation. It is suggested that macrophages can polarize and differentiate into different subpopulations of activated cells according to a type of stimuli. In common, polarized macrophages can be divided into 2 basic groups: classical activated macrophages (they are named M1 cells, reminiscent of T-lymphocyte subsets) differentiate by Th1-associated cytokine IFNγ and microbe component such as LPS and alternatively activated macrophages (M2) including subpopulations of M2a (activated by Th2-dependent cytokines IL-4 and IL-13), M2b (activated via FcR) and M2c (requiring IL-10, TGFβ or glucocorticoids). These subpopulations of activated and polarized macrophages have different phenotypes and spectrum of secreting chemokines/cytokines (Martinez et al., 2008, 2009; Gordon & Martinez, 2010) and play different roles in mechanism of immunologic inflammation of the kidney (Williams et al., 2010). It is commonly accepted that M1 cells producing large amount of nitric oxide and reactive oxygen species by NO synthase and NADPH oxidase, respectively, mediate renal tissue damage while M2 cells producing significant amounts of proline and polyamines stimulate cells proliferation and sclerotic processes.

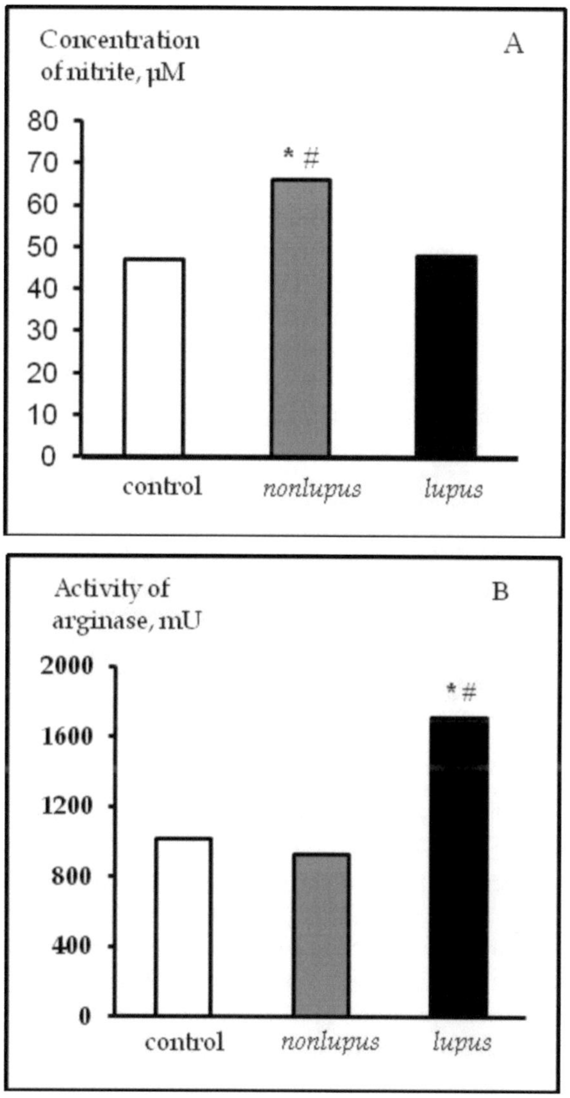

* - $p < 0.05$ compared between control and experimental group; # - $p < 0.05$ between experimental groups

Fig. 7. Activity of NO synthase (A) and arginase (B) in recipients

It is established that M1 and M2 cells are significantly differ from each other by the ways of arginine metabolism, which is a substrate of both NO synthase and arginase. M1 macrophages are characterized by high production of NO in combination with low activity of arginase, while for M2 it is typical an inverse relationship, since the balance in this subpopulation of macrophages shifts toward the reaction catalyzed by arginase (Munder et al., 1998). Thus determining the ratio of NO synthase and arginase activities in the culture of macrophages can evaluate the M1 and M2 subpopulations balance and its changes under influence of various agents.

Study of arginine metabolism in peritoneal macrophages of recipients has been shown that macrophages isolated from *lupus* mice expose high arginase activity and macrophages isolated from *nonlupus* mice without clinical symptoms of kidney disease produce large amount of nitric oxide upon LPS/IFNγ stimulation (Fig. 7).
According their metabolic properties it has been supposed that Th1-dependent variant of chronic GVHD is associated with classical macrophages activation with NO synthase prevalence, while Th2-dependent variant of chronic GVHD is characterized by alternative macrophages activation with arginase domination. Since it has been researched on peritoneal macrophages not directly involved into renal inflammation, these differences of arginine metabolism have systemic nature and may characterize metabolic changes in whole immune system. Preferential activation of M1 or M2 cells may be one of the key points of chronic GVHD-induced immunopathological processes. In Th2-associated type of chronic GVHD there are immune complexes forming deposits in renal glomeruli and causing their inflammatory damage. In this case high arginase activity of M2 macrophages can promote via enhanced polyamine synthesis the proliferation of polyclonally activated B cells and the increase of autoantibody production. Moreover, the local increase of arginase activity in renal macrophages (mesangial cells) contributes proliferative forms of glomerulonephritis and amplifies collagen synthesis causing glomerular sclerosis. It have been also shown that lowering of local NO production in glomeruli exacerbates renal injury induced by different ways and enforces proteinuria via glomerular hemodynamics disturbances (Cattell, 2002; Waddington, 2002). Controversially, high activity of macrophagal NO synthase decreases proliferation of T- and B-lymphocytes and amplifies activated cells apoptosis preventing autoimmunity expansion (Kim et al., 1999; Hoffman et al., 2002; Koide et al., 2003).

2.2.5 Cytokines

The key cytokines for Th1 and Th2 subpopulations are IFNγ and IL-4, relatively. Unfortunately, its concentrations have fallen outside of the bottom value of used test system. The concentration of IL-10, IL-15, IL-17A has been on the verge of method sensitivity or lower also. Data on IL-7 is presented in chapter 2.2.1. Determination of cytokines content in peripheral blood has reveals the increase of IL-6 and TNFα levels in *lupus* recipients (Table 5). It has been shown that serum Il-6 and IL-10 levels increase and are closely associated with disease activity in SLE (Chun et al., 2007). Today it's known the Janus-faced role of IL-6 as pro- and antiinflammatory cytokine. IL-6 participates in the acute phase response, B cell maturation and macrophage differentiation. Furthermore it has been shown that IL-6 can promote Th1/Th2 ratio towards Th2 inducing IL-4-dependent differentiation of Th2 and simultaneously inhibiting Th1 polarization through IL-4-independent mechanism (Diehl & Rincon, 2002). Thus, the high level of IL-6 coincides with the increase of $CD19^+$ B lymphocytes in spleen of *lupus* recipients and does not contradict to shifting their Th1/Th2 balance towards Th2 (Fig. 8). TNFα is also multifunctional cytokine and is involved in the different immune processes. Except proinflammatory effects it is likewise an important factor of physiologic processes of B cells growth and activation. It has been shown that its level is increased in the blood and in the inflamed kidneys of systemic lupus erythematosus patients (Aringer & Smolen, 2003) although its role in human SLE is controversial (Aringer & Smolen, 2008; Zhu et al., 2010). The high level of TNFα likely accounts for processes of inflammation in kidney; a possible cause of its increase is discussed in chapter 2.2.6.

	IL-2	IL-6	TNFα
control	2.3 (2.0 - 2.6)	4.4 (1.6 - 9.5)	7.9 (6.0 - 10.2)
nonlupus	2.6 (2.0 - 2.9)	2.3 (0 - 4.8)	9,03 (0 - 15.7)
lupus	2.9 (2.3 - 3.6)	8.9# (0 - 17.4)	19.1*# (7.1 - 40.6)

(M, min - max; pg/ml; * - $p < 0.05$ between control and experimental group; # - $p < 0.05$ between experimental groups

Table 5. The cytokines concentration in serum of recipients

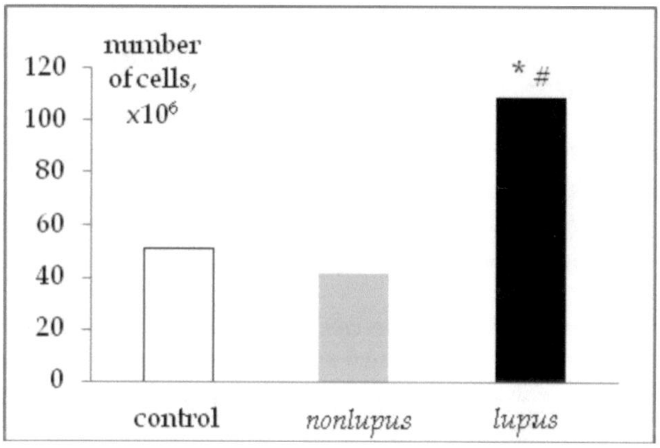

* - $p < 0.05$ between control and experimental group; # - $p < 0.05$ between experimental groups

Fig. 8. The content of $CD19^{+}$ cells in the spleen of recipients with chronic GVHD

2.2.6 Change of cholesterol metabolism in recipients with glomerulonephritis

The development of lupus-like nephritis in described experimental model of chronic GVHD is associated with severe hyperlipidemia (Xiao et al., 2007; Perminova et al., 2009). According to our experimental data (Fig. 9) increase of serum cholesterol level in mice with autoimmune glomerulonephritis is most pronounced in the period corresponding to the formation of kidney damage and the appearance of proteinuria (about within 3 months after induction of chronic GVHD), however, and after 5 months, and even after 12 months concentration of cholesterol in the blood of these animals remains significantly elevated. It has been also found that in these mice the triglyceride level in serum is significantly increased (from 1.72 mM in intact control to 5.25 mM in *lupus* recipients; $p < 0.01$). At the same time *nonlupus* mice have normal cholesterol and triglyceride levels. Our results of the study blood cholesterol levels in the dynamics of chronic GVHD indicate that hypercholesterolemia and formation of autoimmune glomerulonephritis occur simultaneously (Fig. 10). In the initial stages of induction of GVHD individual animals with opposite variants of the immunopathological process do not significantly differ from each other, and only after 8-12 weeks serum cholesterol level begins to increase in mice with a lupus-like nephritis. Thus, the formation of kidney damage and lipid metabolism disturbance in described experimental model are parallel to each other and appear in the same time.

The coincidence between kidney diseases and changes in lipid metabolism has been known for a long time. As stated in one of modern articles: "Historically, Virchow first suggested the association between lipids and renal disease in 1858 when he described successive stages of fatty metamorphosis and fatty detritus in the renal epithelium in Bright's disease" (Jiang et al., 2005). Now the combination of different forms of nephritis and nephrotic syndrome with hypercholesterolemia is well known in the clinic and is described in various forms of experimental nephritis in animals. It has been found experimentally that kidney disease combines not only with changes serum lipid levels, but also with a variety of disorders of lipid metabolism in tissues. In clinical and experimental works it has been evidenced that nephrotic syndrome is accompanied by significant changes in activity of some enzymes involved in cholesterol metabolism (such as HMG-CoA reductase, acyl-CoA:cholesterol acyltransferase, lecithin-cholesterol acyltransferase and other), by decreased expression of LDL receptors on membranes of hepatocytes, by decline of apolipoprotein E, and by impaired reverse cell cholesterol transport (Subbaiah & Rodby, 1994; Deighan et al., 2000; Vaziri & Liang, 2002; Shearer et al., 2005; Vaziri et al., 2011). Undoubtedly, these data are very important for deep understanding of the pathogenesis of hypercholesterolemia in nephrotic syndrome, but they do not clarify the question what are mechanisms linking kidney disease and changes in lipid metabolism. Initial assumption that the level of serum lipoproteins increases compensatory in answer to decline of serum albumin concentration, today is rejected as not supported by clinical and experimental data. It has been found that it is not correlation between serum lipid profiles and serum albumin levels while the severity of lipid abnormalities correlates with the degree of proteinuria and hence with extent of kidney damage (Vaziri & Liang, 2002; Hu et al., 2009). Thus, the question of the primary cause of the hypercholesterolemia development in renal disease remains not completely resolved.

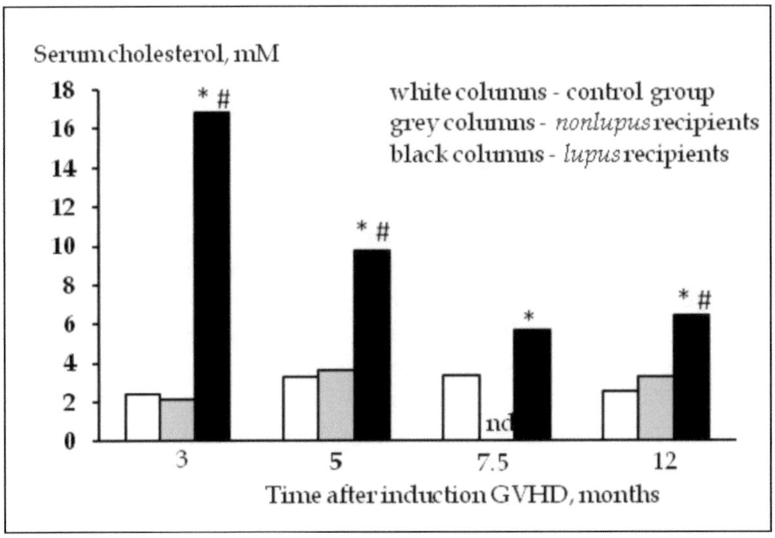

* - $p < 0.05$ between control and experimental group; # - $p < 0.05$ between experimental groups; nd - data are not available

Fig. 9. Serum cholesterol concentrations in mice with *lupus*-like nephritis and in *nonlupus* mice

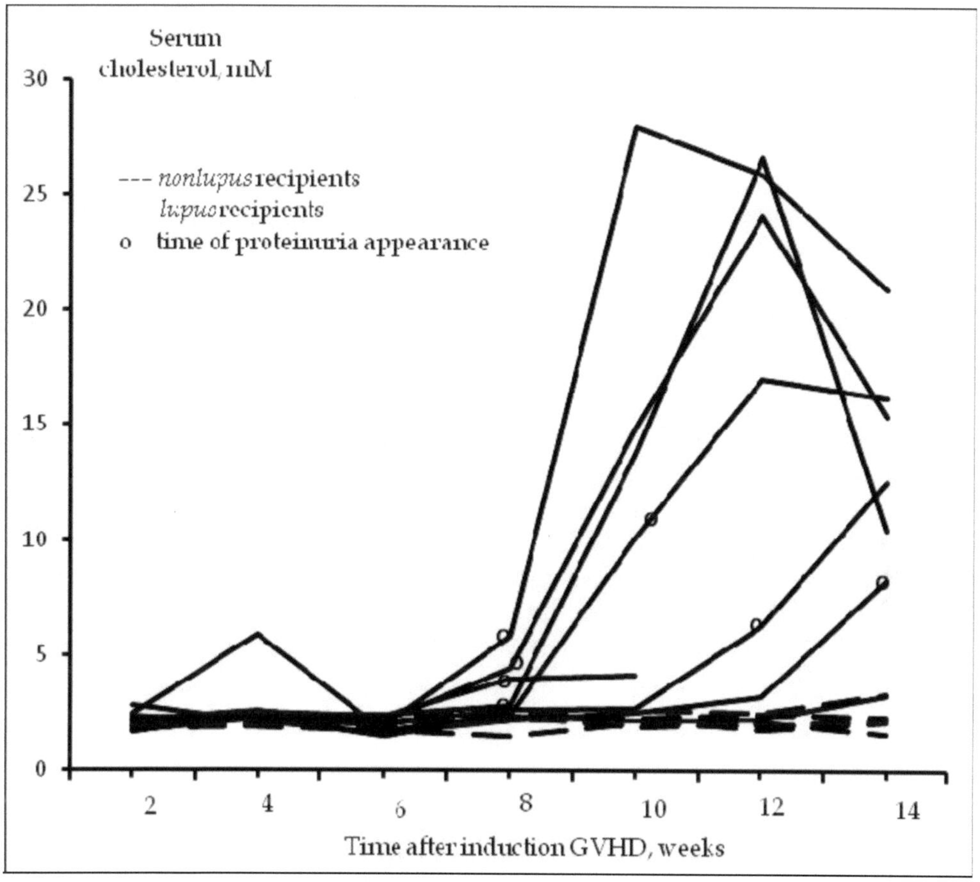

Fig. 10. Development of hypercholesterolemia in individual animals in the dynamics of chronic GVHD

It is generally accepted that the main pathogenetic point of such diseases is a massive production of specific autoantibodies and the formation of immune complexes which deposite in kidney tissues and serve as trigger for the chronic inflammatory process. In our experiments we also have found a gradual increase in the number of antibodies to DNA at the early stages of nephritis development (see 2.1.1). As it would be expected greater number of antibodies to DNA has been detected in those animals in which lupus-like nephritis develops. Based on this fact and on the currently available literary data, we assume that an accumulation of immune complexes in tissues may be act as a connecting link between kidney damage and hypercholesterolemia and that cell production of oxysterols is a key element of this association.

In vitro experiments demonstrate (Reiss et al., 2001) that adding of immune complexes to macrophages and endothelial cells inhibits the activity of mitochondrial sterol 27-hydroxylase – a key enzyme of cholesterol metabolism present in most tissues of the body and converting cholesterol to 27-hydroxycholesterol which is endogenous ligand for nuclear liver X receptors (LXRs) (Fu et al., 2001). *In vivo* this effect of immune complexes must be resulted in the decrease of 27-hydroxycholesterol concentrations in the body and therefore in the decline of the activation degree of LXRs. Since the LXR activation is associated with the inhibition of cholesterol synthesis *de novo* and with the increase of the rate of its degradation to bile acids (Björkhem & Diczfalusy, 2002; Wang et al., 2008), reduced LXR activity would be reflected by accumulation of cholesterol in the tissues and by hypercholesterolemia. Schematic representation of these relationships is shown in Figure 11.

As of now, this assumption presents a pure speculative construction, but there are experimental evidences counting in favour of this hypothesis. In particular, it has long been known that many of the autoimmune diseases accompanied by increased formation of immune complexes are associated with pronounced hypercholesterolemia. A classical examples of such illnesses are autoimmune injuries of kidneys and systemic lupus erythematosus (McMahon & Hahn, 2007). According to literary data, the close relation between accumulation of immune complexes in tissues and hypercholesterolemia is the characteristic feature of the murine lupus-like syndromes developing spontaneously in (NZB x NZW)F1 mice, in MRL/lpr, BXSB and other relevant mouse strains (Ogura et al., 1989; Itoh et al., 1994; Gu et al., 1999; Kono et al., 2000; Lawman et al., 2004). Similar association has come to light also in experimental investigations of a various immune complex renal injuries induced in animals by the administration of $HgCl_2$, cationic bovine serum albumin and antibodies to renal proteins (Couser et al., 1978; Bagenstose et al., 1999; Shi et al., 2005; Wu et al., 2008).

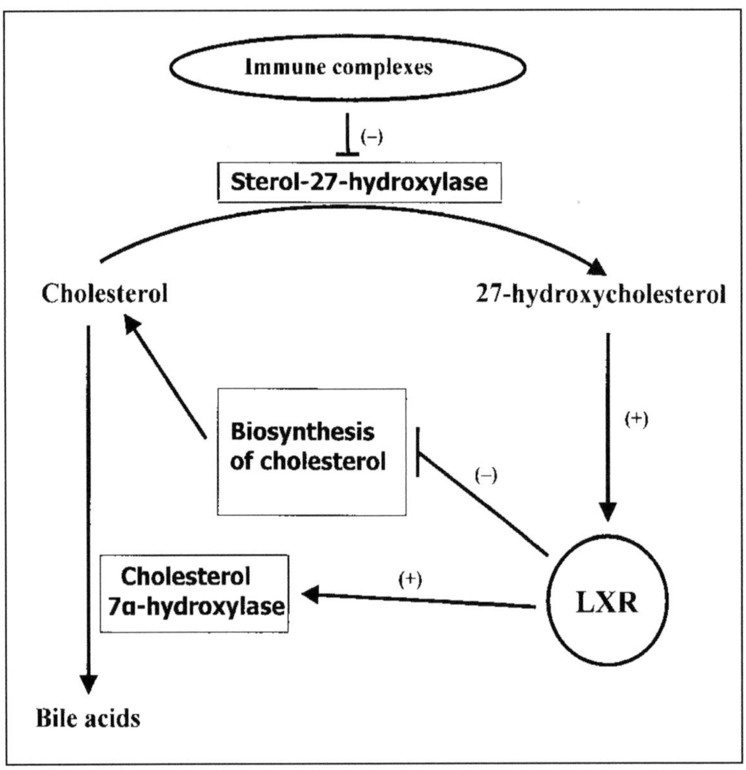

Fig. 11. A schematic representation of possible impact of immune complexes on the biosynthesis and catabolism of cholesterol

Described in this paper (see Table 5) increase of TNFα in the serum of *lupus* mice emerging simultaneously with the appearance of proteinuria and hypercholesterolemia, also can be attributed to decreased production of 27-hydroxycholesterol since oxysterols (via LXR) inhibit an expression and synthesis of proinflammatory cytokines (Dushkin et al., 1998; Hong et al., 2011). These currently available indirect evidences are in good agreement with the foregoing hypothesis, however its proof requires further experimental investigations.

2.2.7 Sex differences of autoimmune glomerulonephritis formation in the experimental model

As it's known there is a pronounced sexual dimorphism in the incidence of many human autoimmune pathologies, particularly systemic lupus erythematosus (Whitacre, 2001). It has been shown that the induction of chronic GVHD in the semiallogeneic system DBA/2→(C57Bl/10xDBA/2)F1 causes the formation of autoimmune pathology only in female recipients for up to 6 weeks (Van Griensven et al., 1997).

Parameter	Females		Males	
	control	*lupus*	control	*lupus*
renal cortex				
Tubules	90.2 (88-91)	66.3*#(50-81)	90.8 (89-93)	88.1# (79-96)
Glomeruli	3.4 (3-5)	1.5* (1-3)	3.9 (3-5)	2.0* (1-4)
Blood vessels	5.9 (5-7)	2.1*# (1-3)	5.3 (3-7)	3.4*# (2-5)
Leukocyte infiltration	0.2 (0-2)	13.2*# (5-19)	0	0#
Cylinders	0	7.4* (2-15)	0	3.6* (0-9)
Cysts and cavities with liquid	0	9.5* (3-21)	0	2.9* (0-7)
renal medulla				
Tubules and ducts	95.8 (95-96)	94.9 (93-97)	97.5 (97-99)	97.3 (95-99)
Blood vessels	4.0 (3-5)	1.3*# (1-2)	2.5 (1-4)	2.2# (1-4)
Cylinders	0	3.8*# (3-5)	0	0.5*# (0-1)

(M, (min-max); * - $p < 0.05$ between control and experimental group; # - $p < 0.05$ between experimental groups

Table 6. The relative area of the structures on the cut renal cortex and renal medulla (% of section area)

In case of DBA/2→(C57BL/6xDBA/2)F1 model it has been observed that induction of GVHD using female donor and host mice causes more severe glomerulonephritis than one using male donor and host. This is not due to differences in splenic homing, alloreactive precursor frequency, initial proliferation rates, or apoptotic rates but rather to sustained high proliferative activity at early stage of GVHR. Crossover studies (female donor and

male host; male donor and female host) has revealed that this effect is depended on the host sex (Lang et al., 2003). In our experiments chronic GVHD induced by transfer of female donor cells leads to the development of glomerulonephritis in recipients of both sexes by the end of 3 months. Kidney pathological picture in male recipients is characterized by less pronounced glomerular and tubular lesions, the absence of leukocyte infiltration and vessel walls damage compared with females littermates (Table 6) (Kudaeva et al., 2009). Determination of the testosterone level in the peripheral blood of female *lupus* mice has shown an increase of its concentration (6.1 nM compared with 4.8 nM in intact females of the same age, $p < 0.05$). It may be explained by the compensatory response to kidney damage, taking into account renotropic effect of testosterone. However testosterone level in female *nonlupus* recipients is also increased (7.7 nM, $p < 0.05$).
Currently great attention is paid to sex hormones as regulators of immune responses. Higher incidence of autoimmune pathologies in women, its changing during pregnancy, sex differences of immune response, the influence of sex hormones on Th1/Th2 balance identify the role of sex hormones, mainly estrogen, progesterone and testosterone, as mediators of sexual dimorphism in the immune system (Erlandsson et al., 2003; Soldan et al., 2003; Cutolo et al., 2004; Matejuk et al., 2004). Less pronounced renal damage in males and increase of testosterone level in female recipients suggest testosterone as a factor of regulation, suppressed autoimmune processes during chronic GVHD.

2.3 Modulation by Th1/Th2 balance shifting

Currently, there is evidence of the possibility of Th1/Th2 balance changing through a variety of factors under the immunopathological situations, in particular, under the development of allergic diseases (Kato et al., 1999; Raz & Spiegelberg, 1999; Tipping & Kitching, 2005). Since a formation of autoimmune glomerulonephritis induced by chronic GVHR is a Th2-dependent process whereas a development of chronic GVHR without a kidney damage is a Th1-dependent one it has been studied the possibility to change the direction of reaction by agents shifting Th1/Th2 ratio towards Th1 or Th2. Drugs have been administered during the induction of the reaction (the first and second week of GVHR). Results have assessed by the change in the proportion of *lupus* recipients at the end of the experiment (within 3 months after the transfer semiallogeneic cells).

2.3.1 Shifting Th1/Th2 ratio towards Th1

DNA with immunostimulating properties (pUC19 plasmid DNA) and hormone dehydroepiandrosterone (in its transport form - dehydroepiandrosterone sulfate) are used as agents stimulating Th1 subpopulation.
It has been shown that injection of bacterial DNA containing nonmethylated CpG-plots stimulates production of Th1 cells activating cytokines: TNFα, IL-1, IL-12, IFNγ (Klinman et al., 1996; Carson & Raz, 1997; Krieg, 1999). pUC19 plasmid DNA is injected intravenously twice in dose 5 mg/kg. Calf thymus DNA in the same dose and scheme is used as a control.
Dehydroepiandrosterone sulfate is taken as Th1 activator (Stam et al., 1993; Rook et al., 1994; Sudo et al., 2001). Dehydroepiandrosterone sulfate restores production of Th1-dependent cytokines by old female mice (Araghi-Niknam et al., 1997). Dehydroepiandrosterone sulfate (Aldrich) has been injected subcutaneously 4 times in dose 37.5 mg/kg.
Results are shown in Figure 12. Both pUC19 plasmid DNA and dehydroepiandrosterone sulfate decrease the proportion of *lupus* recipients directing the reaction to Th1-dependent *nonlupus* variant (Vlasov et al., 2002; Tkachev et al., 2009).

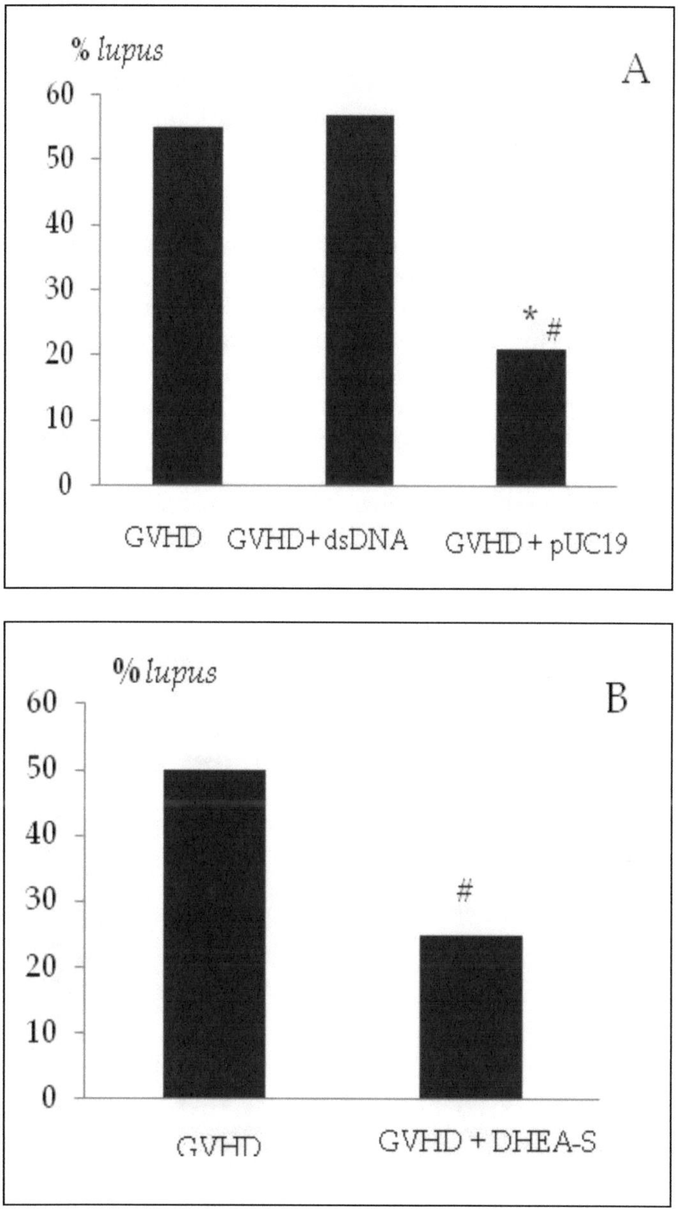

* - $p < 0.05$ compared to GVHD; # - $p < 0.05$ compared to GVHD+dsDNA)

Fig. 12. Frequency of *lupus* mice among the recipients upon the effect of pUC19 plasmid DNA (A) and DHEA-S (B)

2.3.2 Shifting Th1/Th2 ratio towards Th2

It has been studied the possibility of modifying the course of reaction towards Th2-dependent processes also (Kudaeva et al., 2005b). Compounds with different mechanisms of action shifting the Th1/Th2 ratio towards Th2 cells have been used as immunomodulators: muramyl dipeptide, bisphenol A, and pentoxifylline. Muramyl dipeptide, a bacterial cell wall derivative characterized by adjuvant effect, causes polyclonal activation of B-cells, and potentiates the stimulatory effect of IL-4 on activated B-lymphocytes (Souvannavong et al., 1990). Muramyl dipeptide (ICN) has been injected intraperitoneally in a dose of 1.0 mg/kg twice ten days apart. Bisphenol A widely used in the industrial manufacture of plastics binds to estrogen receptors despite structural differences from the hormone. It decreases production of IFNγ and synthesis of IgG2a (Sawai et al., 2003). Bisphenol A (ICN) has been given intraperitoneally in a daily dose of 2.5 μg/kg for 2 weeks. Pentoxifylline (a drug improving microcirculation and blood rheology) inhibits production of proinflammatory cytokines including IFNγ and suppresses the development of Th1-dependent experimental allergic encephalomyelitis in mice (Okuda & Sakoda, 1996). Pentoxifylline (Aventis Pharma Ltd.) has been given per os in a daily dose of 50 mg/kg for 1 week.

All these drugs cause an increased protein concentration in the urine of *lupus* recipients (Fig. 13) that strictly correlates with the severity of kidney damage (Kolesnikova et al., 1991). Moreover these drugs increase the incidence of lupus-like glomerulonephritis among recipients (Kudaeva et al., 2005b). Hence they deteriorate a course of a disease.

So, in this experimental model the change of the Th1/Th2 balance by introduction of immunomodulating drugs causes the amelioration or the progression of kidney damage.

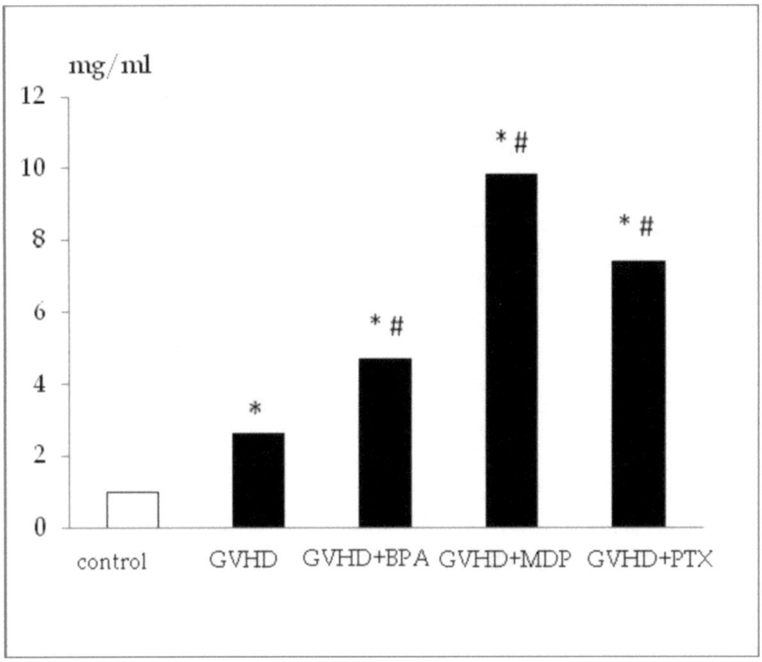

* - $p < 0.05$ compared with control; # - $p < 0.05$ compared with GVHD; BPA - bisphenol A; MDP – muramyl dipeptide; PTX - pentoxifylline

Fig. 13. Protein concentration in urine of recipients

2.4 Correction of glomerulonephritis

In addition to studying the pathogenesis of autoimmune glomerulonephritis, it has been also investigated the possibility of correcting fully developed disease in this experimental model (Kudaeva et al., 2010a).

Lupus recipients have been lethally irradiated and then injected of bone marrow cells from intact syngeneic donors into a vein. Monitoring of follow-up processes have been included regular determination of the protein concentration in the urine. It has been found that such treatment of *lupus* recipients leads to a gradual decrease in the protein concentration in urine, the level of which is not differ from control values at the end of the experiment (Fig. 14). This result can be regarded as evidence of the positive effect of the therapy.

2.4.1 Immune parameters

At the end of the experiment it has been studied kidney morphology and measured body, thymus and spleen weight, cell number and the levels of total IgG and IgG-antibodies to DNA in peripheral blood.

Mice with chronic GVHD are characterized by severe splenomegaly and polyclonal activation of B cells, leading to high levels of IgG in peripheral blood and the appearance of antibodies to components of its own tissues (Via & Shearer, 1988; Morris et al., 1990). After treatment spleen cells number and the concentration of IgG in peripheral blood of *lupus* recipients are not differ from the appropriate values of control (intact animals lethally irradiated and then injected of bone marrow cells from syngeneic donors). Correction of clinical manifestations of glomerulonephritis has been also accompanied by the disappearance of IgG antibodies to DNA from peripheral blood (Fig. 15).

It has not been significant difference in thymus weight between *lupus* mice before the treatment and control intact animals of the same sex and age. After the treatment its value in *lupus* recipients has diminished but has been not differ from irradiated and restored control. It may be due to slowing thymus recovery in mice of such age.

2.4.2 Kidney morphology

The results of morphological study of kidneys are presented in Tables 7-9. Formation of glomerulonephritis in *lupus* mice has been accompanied by development of inflammatory reaction with leukocyte infiltration, microcirculation change (an impairment of the permeability, a blockade of the venous capillaries) and lymphostasis in the renal parenchyma. All the pathological changes of the kidneys in *lupus* recipients indicate the active acute glomerulonephritis lasting for a long time (a different cell composition of leukocyte infiltrates, a large number of cylinders in the tubules and destructive changes in the glomeruli). After lethal irradiation and injection of syngeneic bone marrow cells it has been observed a fall in edema, in a severity of inflammation, in a leukocyte infiltration. In addition, a sharp decrease in the number of plasma cells in the leukocyte infiltrates, a large number of those present in *lupus* mice has been observed after therapy. At the end of the experiment number of plasma cells has been not differ from intact control values. Individual recipients have had various intensity of these changes. It has been no reverse development of pathological changes of glomeruli except of the reduction of leukocyte infiltration and edema. Restoration of structures of impaired glomeruli has been no observed. The latter is in agreement with the observation that regeneration of mammals kidney structure is demonstrated for renal tubular epithelium only (Hishikawa & Fujita, 2006; Poulsom et al., 2006; Bi et al., 2007). Another results have been obtained in a model of autosomally recessive Alport syndrome. Mice that lack the 3 chain of collagen IV fail to synthesize normal glomerular basement membrane and develop progressive glomerular damage leading to renal failure; bone marrow transplantation can rectify this podocyte defect but the mechanisms underlying repopulation of glomerular podocytes by bone marrow-derived cells are not yet clear (Prodromidi et al., 2006).

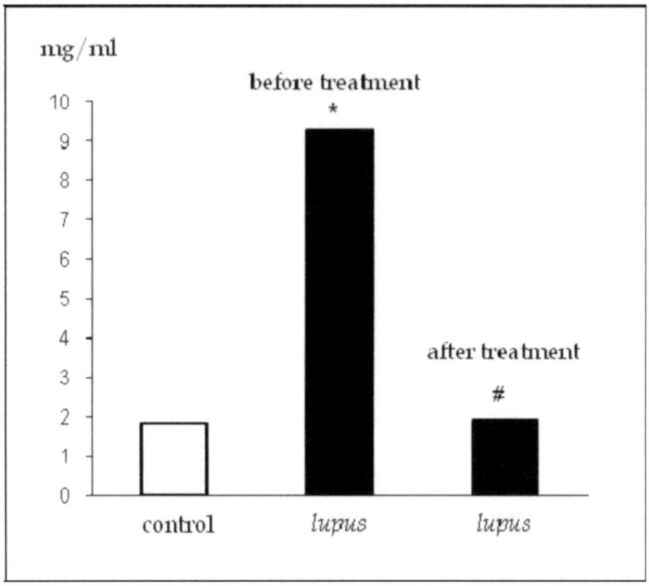

* - $p < 0.05$ between control and experimental group, # - $p < 0.05$ between experimental groups

Fig. 14. Protein content in urine of recipients

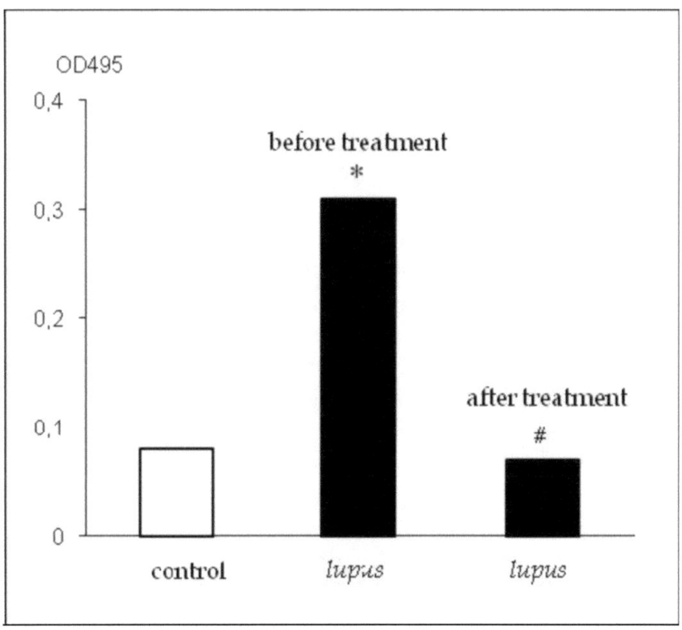

* - $p < 0.05$ between control and experimental group; # - $p < 0.05$ between experimental groups

Fig. 15. The level of antibodies to dsDNA in peripheral blood of *lupus* recipients

Parameter	groups of animals *			
	1	2	3	4
Tubules	$90.2^{3,4**}$ (88-92)	88.9^{4} (82-94)	$66.3^{1,4}$ (50-81)	$78.5^{1,2,3}$ (61-89)
Glomeruli	$3.4^{3,4}$ (3-5)	3.7^{4} (3-5)	1.5^{1} (1-3)	$1.4^{1,2}$ (0-3)
Blood vessels	$5.9^{2,3,4}$ (5-7)	$3.7^{1,4}$ (3-5)	$2.1^{1,4}$ (1-3)	$4.9^{1,2,3}$ (3-7)
Connective tissue	0	0	0	0
Leukocyte infiltration	$0.2^{2,3,4}$ (0-2)	$1.9^{1,4}$ (0-5)	13.2^{1} (5-21)	$9.8^{1,2}$ (6-14)
Cylinders	$0^{3,4}$	0^{4}	$7.4^{1,4}$ (3-15)	$1.1^{1,2,3}$ (0-3)
Cysts and cavities with liquid	$0^{2,3,4}$	1.8^{1} (0-5)	$9.5^{1,4}$ (3-21)	$3.6^{1,3}$ (0-18)
Hemorrhage	0.3 (0-10)	0	0	0.7 (0-5)

M, (min-max); * the groups of animals: 1 – control, intact mouse; 2 – the control, irradiation and transfer of bone marrow cells; 3 – the mouse with chronic GVHD, *lupus*; 4 – the mouse with chronic GVHD, *lupus*, irradiation and transfer of bone marrow cells; * ^{1,2,3,4}– the groups that have significant differences among themselves

Table 7. The relative area of the structures on the cut renal cortex (% of section area)

Parameter	groups of animals*			
	1	2	3	4
Tubules and ducts	$95.8^{2,4**}$ (95-97)	96.6^{1} (96-97)	94.9^{4} (93-97)	$97.1^{1,3}$ (96-98)
Blood vessels	$4.0^{2,3,4}$ (3-4)	$3.4^{1,4}$ (3-4)	$1.3^{1,4}$ (1-2)	$2.7^{1,2,3}$ (2-4)
Connective tissue	0	0	0	0
Leukocyte infiltration	0	0	0	0
Cylinders	0^{3}	0	$3.8^{1,4}$ (2-5)	0.2^{3} (0-1)
Cysts and cavities with liquid	0	0	0	0
Hemorrhage	0	0	0	0

M, (min-max); * the groups of animals as in table 7; * ^{1,2,3,4}– the groups that have significant differences among themselves

Table 8. The relative area of the structures on the cut renal medulla (% of section area)

		groups of animals *			
		1	2	3	4
Number (N) of renal infiltrates (%)		10	60	100	100
Area cut infiltration	A_A****	$0.2^{3,4}$** (0-2)	1.9^{4} (0-5)	13.2^{1} (6-18)	$9.8^{1,2}$ (6-14)
	A*****	$7500^{2,3,4}$	13500^{1} (6875-26250)	$37625^{1,4}$ (26875-51875)	$19375^{1,3}$ (6250-42500)
Numerical density leukocytes (N_A***)		19.0	28.0 (16-37)	28.2 (19-40)	30.4 (21-37)
Neutrophils	%	0	0.8^{4} (0-20)	2.3 (1-3)	2.1^{2} (0-5)
	N_A	0	0.239^{4} (0-0.68)	0.66 (0.24-1.14)	0.611^{2} (0-1.11)
Monocytes	%	3	4.4 (2-7)	4.1 (3-5)	3.1 (1-4)
	N_A	0.57	1.18 (0.57-1.92)	1.17 (0.57-1.9)	0.931 (0.63-1.36)
Macrophages	%	48.0	22.4 (9-41)	24.8 (15-35)	23.7 (9-42)
	N_A	9.12	5.65 (2.43-7.68)	7.03 (3.15-13.3)	7.39 (2.1-14.28)
Fibroblasts and fibrocytes	%	18	8 (0-34)	1.2^{4} (0-3)	9.6^{3} (0-34)
	N_A	3.42	2.51 (0-10.2)	0.306^{4} (0-0.96)	3.24^{3} (0-12.58)
Plasma cells	%	0	10 (0-42)	17.7^{4} (8-33)	2.1^{3} (0-6)
	N_A	0	2.63 (0-8.96)	5.35^{4} (1.9-13.2)	0.66^{3} (0-1.92)

M, (min-max); * the groups of animals as in table 7; ** ^{1,2,3,4}– the groups that have significant differences among themselves;

***N_A - numerical density of cells per 10^3 μm^2;

****A_A - relative area of infiltration at the cut renal cortex (% of section area);

***** A - area of leukocyte infiltration (μm^2).

Table 9. Characteristics of leukocyte infiltration in renal cortex

The data allow to conclude that induced by chronic GVHD immune complex glomerulonephritis of autoimmune genesis is maintained in the recipients by prolonged activity of immune cells. This inference is supported by data that the alloreactive donor T cells maintaining hyperplasia of host B lymphocytes with production of lupus-like antibodies persist in GVHD F1 mice for a long time after the induction of chronic GVHR (Rozendaal et al., 1990). Lethal irradiation interrupts the autoimmune process confirmed by disappearance of antibodies to DNA in peripheral blood and plasma cells in the kidney leukocyte infiltrates and consequently reduces the severity of kidney damage and leads to disappearance of clinical manifestations of glomerulonephritis - proteinuria.

3. Conclusion

Epigenetic mechanisms are long-term but reversible changes of gene activity not connected with DNA nucleotide sequence. Now it isn't doubted that epigenetic mechanisms play the important role in determination of individual immune reactions. A purposeful integration of immune reactions with adaptive processes of whole organism is achieved by epigenetic regulation (Vercelli, 2004; Reiner, 2005; Wilson et al., 2005). Consequently, the character of immune reactions and their final effects are not defined by the animal genotype and parameters of antigenic action on an organism only but are determined by its «epigenetic component» taking during ontogenesis also. In such a manner individual living conditions form the current stable state of immune system modifying immune characteristics of individual predetermined by genotype. Accompanied by genetic heterogeneity of natural populations these variations of immune parameters, based on epigenetic mechanisms, provide the observed diversity of individual responses to antigenic stimuli and form the perceptivity to infections and different diseases in developing of which functional activity of immune cells plays an appreciable role.

Th1 and Th2 activation has been shown to be affected in antagonist manner by numerous regulatory factors including hormones, mediators, and other biologically active substances (Rook et al., 1994; Piccini et al., 1995; Elenkov et al., 2000; Elenkov, 2004). The dissimilar level of biologically active molecules in recipient's organism may cause predominantly stimulation of Th1- or Th2-cells and as a consequence directs the GVHD development for Th1- or Th2-dependent ways and initiates predominantly the development of *nonlupus* or *lupus* variants respectively.

Experimental animals are a genetic homogenous group; transplanted cells have been identical for all recipients; the animal keeping conditions and transplanting procedure have been constant and the same for all mice in our work. Nonetheless there are two different variants of GVHD in our experiments. It is undoubtedly that even when experimental animals have identical genotype, there is always the dispersion of results that is usually considered as methodic imperfection. It is quite possible that such dispersion is rather an adequate reflection of the really existing situation: in spite of initial genetic identity animals are taking some stable distinctive properties in response to environmental influences by epigenetic mechanisms during ontogenesis (Jaenisch & Bird, 2003; Anway et al., 2005; Horsthemke & Ludwig, 2005; Reiner, 2005; Wong et al., 2005).

Thus, in spite of the genetic, sexual and age uniformity of recipients, the same living conditions and the standard transfer procedure, the trend of the chronic GVH disease can proceed in the classical Th2- or early not described Th1-dependent pathways in the DBA/2→(C57Bl/6xDBA/2)F1 system that eventually causes the development of two variants of immunopathology, only one of them results in the autoimmune disorder - lupus-like immune complex glomerulonephritis. This model of the immunopathology permits the study of lupus-like nephritis pathogenesis. Furthermore it allows to use of GVHD in the DBA/2→(C57Bl/6xDBA/2)F1 system for devise practicable drugs and regimens of treatment during all stages of disease.

4. References

Agnello D., Lankford C., Bream J., Morinobu A., Gadina M., O'Shea J., & Frucht D. (2003). Cytokines and transcription factors that regulate T helper cell differentiation: new players and new insight. *J. Clin. Immunol.*, Vol. 23, No. 3, pp. 147-161

Allen J. & Maizels R. (1997). Th1-Th2: reliable paradigm or dangerous dogma. *Immunol. Today*, Vol. 18, No. 8, pp. 387-392

Anway M., Cupp A., Uzumcu M., & Skinner M. (2005). Epigenetic transgenerational actions of endocrine disruptors and male fertility. *Science*, Vol. 308, No. 5727, pp. 1466-1469

Araghi-Niknam M., Liang B., Zhang Z., Ardestani S., & Watson R. (1997). Modulation of immune dysfunction during murine leukaemia retrovirus infection of old mice by dehydroepiandrosterone sulphate (DHEAS). *Immunology*, Vol. 90, No. 3, pp. 344-349

Aringer M. & Smolen J.S. (2003). SLE-complex cytokine effects in a complex autoimmune disease: tumor necrosis factor in systemic lupus erythematosus. *Artritis Res. Ther.*, Vol. 5, No. 4, pp. 172-177

Aringer M. & Smolen J.S. (2008). The role of tumor necrosis factor-alpha in systemic lupus erythematosus. *Arthritis Res Ther.*, Vol. 10, No. 1 : 202

Baccala R. & Theofilopoulos A.N. (2005). The new paradigm of T-cell homeostatic proliferation-induced autoimmunity. *Trends Immunol.*, Vol. 26, No. 1, pp. 5-8

Bagenstose L.M., Salgame P., & Monestier M. (1999). Cytokine regulation of a rodent model of mercuric chloride-induced autoimmunity. *Environ. Health Perspect.*, Vol. 107, Suppl. 5, pp. 807-810

Berger S.P. & Daha M.R. (2010). Pattern recognition and renal defence in crescentic glomerulonephritis. *Nephrol. Dial. Transplant.*, Vol. 25, No. 9, pp. 2876-2878

Bergtold A., Gavhane A., D'Agati V., Madaio M., & Clynes R. (2006). FcR-bearing myeloid cells are responsible for triggering murine lupus nephritis. *J. Immunol.*, Vol. 177, No. 10, pp. 7287-7295

Bi B., Schmitt R., Israilova M., Nishio H., & Cantley L.G. (2007). Stromal cells protect against acute tubular injury via an endocrine effect. *J. Am. Soc. Nephrol.*, Vol. 18, No. 9, pp. 2486-2496

Björkhem I. & Diczfalusy U. (2002). Oxysterols: friends, foes, or just fellow passengers? *Arterioscler. Thromb. Vasc. Biol.*, Vol. 22, No. 5, pp. 734-742

Boyman O., Ramsey C., Kim D.M., Sprent J., & Surh C.D. (2008). IL-7/anti-IL-7 mAb complexes restore T cell development and induce homeostatic T cell expansion without lymphopenia. *J.Immunol.*, Vol. 180, No. 11, 7265-7275

Carson D. & Raz E. (1997). Oligonucleotide adjuvants for T helper (Th1)-specific vaccination. *J. Exp. Med.*, Vol. 186, No. 10, pp. 1621-1622

Castano A.P., Lin S.L., Surowy T., Nowlin B.T., Turlapati S.A., Patel T., Singh A., Li S., Lupher M.L.Jr., & Duffield J.S. (2009). Serum amyloid P inhibits fibrosis through Fc-

R-dependent monocyte-macrophage regulation in vivo. *Science Transl. Med.*, Vol. 1, No. 5, 5ra13

Cattell V. (2002). Nitric oxide and glomerulonephritis. *Kidney Int.*, Vol. 61, No. 3, pp. 816–821

Chaouat G., Ledee-Bataille N., Dubanchet S., Zourbas S., Sandra O., & Martal J. (2004). Reproductive immunology 2003: reassessing the Th1/Th2 paradigm? *Immunol. Let.*, Vol. 92, No. 3, pp. 207-214

Chu Y.-W. & Gress R.E. (2008). Murine models of chronic graft-versus-host disease: insights and unresolved issues. *Biol. Blood Marrow Transplant.*, Vol. 14, No. 4, pp. 365-378

Chun H.Y., Chung J.W., Kim H.A., Yun J.M., Jeon J.Y., Ye Y.M., Kim S.H., Park H.S., & Suh C.H. (2007). Cytokine IL-6 and IL-10 as biomarkers in systemic lupus erythematosus. *J. Clin. Immunol.*, Vol. 27, No. 5, pp. 461-466

Couser W.G., Jernianovich N.B., Belok S., Stilmant M.M., & Hoyer J.R. (1978). Effect of aminonucleoside nephrosis on immune complex localization in autologous immune complex nephropathy in rats. *J. Clin. Invest.*, Vol. 61, No. 3, pp. 561-572

Cutolo M., Sulli A., Capellino S., Villaggio B., Montagna P., Seriolo B., & Straub R. (2004). Sex hormones influence on the immune system: basic and clinical aspects in autoimmunity. *Lupus*, Vol. 13, No. 9, pp. 635-638

Deighan C.J., Caslake M.J., McConnell M., Boulton-Jones J.M., & Packard C.J. (2000). Patients with nephrotic-range proteinuria have apolipoprotein C and E deficient $VLDL_1$. *Kidney Int.*, Vol. 58, No. 3, pp. 1238-1246

Del Prete G., De Carli M., Ricci M., & Romagnani S. (1991). Helper activity for immunoglobulin synthesis of T helper type 1 (Th1) and Th2 human T cell clones: the help of Th1 clones is limited by their cytolytic capacity. *J. Exp. Med.*, Vol. 174, No. 4, pp. 809-813

De Maeyer-Guignard J., Dandoy F., Bailey D., & De Maeyer E. (1986). Interferon structural genes do not participate in quantitative regulation of interferon production by If loci as shown in C57Bl/6 mice that are congenic with Balb/c mice at the interferon-alpha gene cluster. *J. Virol.*, Vol. 58, No. 3, pp. 743-747

Diehl S. & Rincon M. The two faces of IL-6 on Th1/Th2 differentiation. (2002). *Mol. Immunol.*, Vol. 39, No. 9, pp. 531-536

Doutrelepont J.M., Moser M., Leo O., Abramowicz D., Vanderhaegen M.L., Urbain J., & Goldman M. (1991). Hyper IgE in stimulatory graft-*versus*-host disease: role of interleukin-4. *Clin. Exp. Immunol.*, Vol. 83, No. 1, pp. 133-136

Duffield J.S. (2003). The inflammatory macrophage: a story of Jekyll and Hyde. *Clin. Sci. (London)*, Vol. 104, No. 1, pp. 27-38

Duffield J.S. (2010). Macrophages and immunologic inflammation of the kidney. *Semin. Nephrol.*, Vol. 30, No. 3, pp. 234-254

Dushkin M., Schwartz Y., Volsky N., Musatov M., Vereschagin E., Ragino J., Perminova O., & Kozlov V. (1998). Effects of oxysterols upon macrophage and lymphocyte functions in vitro. *Prostaglandins Other Lipid Mediat.*, Vol. 55, No. 4, pp. 219-236

Eckardt K., Kurtz A., & Bauer C. (1989). Regulation of erythropoietin production is related to proximal tubular function. *Amer. J. Physiol.*, Vol. 256, No. 5, pp. 942-947

Elenkov I., Wilder R., Chrousos G., & Vizi E. (2000). The sympathetic nerve - an integrative interface between two supersystems: the brain and the immune system. *Pharmacol. Rev.*, Vol. 52, No. 4, pp. 595-638

Elenkov I. (2004). Glucocorticoids and Th1/Th2 balance. *Ann. N.Y. Acad. Sci.*, Vol. 1024, pp. 138-146

Erlandsson M., Jonsson C., Islander U., Ohlsson C., & Carlsten H. (2003). Oestrogen receptor specificity in oestradiol-mediated effects on B lymphopoiesis and immunoglobulin production in male mice. *Immunology*, Vol. 108, No. 3, pp. 346-351

Espinouse D. & Souteyrand P. (1982). Manifestation hematologigues. *Cah. Med.*, Vol. 8, No. 10, pp. 581-583

Fresno M., Kopf M., & Rivas L. (1997). Cytokimes and infectious diseases. *Immunol. Today*, Vol. 18, No. 2, pp. 56-58.

Horsthemke B.& Ludwig M. (2005). Assisted reproduction: the epigenetic perspective. *Human Reprod. Update*, Vol. 11, No. 5, pp. 473-482

Fu X., Menke J.G., Chen Y., Zhou G., MacNaul K.L., Wright S.D., Sparrow C.P., & Lund E.G. (2001). 27-hydroxycholesterol is an endogenous ligand for liver X receptor in cholesterol-loaded cells. *J. Biol. Chem.*, Vol. 276, No. 42, pp. 38378-38387

Gendelman M., Hecht T., Logan B., Vodanovic-Jankovic S., Komorowski R., & Drobyski W.R. (2004). Host conditioning is a primary determinant in modulating the effect of IL-7 on murine graft-versus-host disease. *J. Immunol.*, Vol. 172, No. 5, pp. 3328-3336

Gleichmann E., Pals S.T., Rolink A.G., Radaszkiewicz T., & Gleichmann H. (1984). Graft-versus-host reactions: clues to the etiopathology of a spectrum of immunological diseases. *Immunol. Today*, Vol 5, pp. 324-332

Glimcher L. & Murphy K. (2000). Lineage commitment in the immune system: the T helper lymphocyte grows up. *Gene Development*, Vol. 14, No. 14, pp. 1693-1711

Goiman E.V., Gavrilova E.D., Kudaeva O.T., & Kolesnikova O.P. (2009). Level of the IgE in the dynamics of development of different variants of chronic graft-versus-host. *Vestnik Uralskoi meditsinskoi akademicheskoi nauki*, No. 2/1, pp. 27-28

Goiman E.V., Kudaeva O.T., Ilina N.A., Borisov V.I., Kozhevnikov V.C., Kolesnikova O.P., & Kozlov V.A. (2010). Processes of homeostatic proliferation in the pathogenesis of autoimmune glomerulonephritis induced by chronic graft-versus-host disease. *Bull. Exp. Biol. Med.*, Vol. 149, No. 1, pp. 54-56

Gomez-Guerrero C., Lopez-Franco O., Sanjuan G., Hernandez-Vargas P., Suzuki Y., Ortiz-Munoz G., Blanco J., & Egido J. (2004). Suppressors of cytokine signaling regulate Fc receptor signaling and cell activation during immune renal injury. *J. Immunol.*, Vol. 172, No. 11, pp. 6969-6977

Gomez-Guerrero C., Hernandez-Vargas P., Lopez-Franco O., Ortiz-Munoz G., & Egido J. (2005). Mesangial cells and glomerular inflammation: from the pathogenesis to novel therapeutic approaches. *Curr. Drug Targets Inflamm. Allergy*, Vol. 4, No. 3, pp. 341-351

Gordon S. & Martinez F.O. (2010). Alternative activation of macrophages: mechanism and functions. *Immunity*, Vol. 32, No. 5, pp. 593-604

Gu L., Johnson M.W., & Lusis A.J. (1999). Quantitative trait locus analysis of plasma lipoprotein levels in an autoimmune mouse model: interactions between lipoprotein metabolism, autoimmune disease, and atherogenesis. *Arterioscler. Thromb. Vasc. Biol.*, Vol. 19, No. 2, 442-453

Guo S., Mühlfeld A.S., Wietecha T.A., Peutz-Kootstra C.J., Kowalewska J., Yi K., Spencer M., Pichaiwong W., Nimmerjahn F., Hudkins K.L., & Alpers C.E. (2009). Deletion of activating Fcgamma receptors does not confer protection in murine cryoglobulinemia-associated membranoproliferative glomerulonephritis. *Am. J. Pathol.*, Vol. 175, No. 1, pp. 107-118

Haridas V. & Kamat R.S. (1997). Antigen-presenting cells (APC) of mice with chronic graft-versus-host disease (GVHD) cause excessive activation-induced death of T helper cells. *Clin. Exp. Immunol*, Vol. 110, No. 3, pp. 454-463.

Hishikawa K. & Fujita T. (2006). Stem cells and kidney disease. *Hypertens Res.*, Vol. 29, No. 10, pp. 745-749

Hoffman R.A., Mahidhara R.S., Wolf-Johnston A.S., Lu L., Thomson A.W., & Simmons R.L. (2002). Differential modulation of CD4 and CD8 T-cell proliferation by induction of nitric oxide synthesis in antigen presenting cells. *Transplantation*, Vol. 74, No. 6, pp. 836-845

Hong C., Walczak R., Dhamko H., Bradley M.N., Marathe C., Boyadjian R., Salazar J.V., & Tontonoz P. (2011). Constitutive activation of LXR in macrophages regulates metabolic and inflammatory gene expression: identification of ARL7 as a direct target. *J. Lipid Res.*, Vol. 52, No. 3, pp. 531-539

Hu P., Lu L., Hu B., & Du P.F. (2009). Characteristics of lipid metabolism under different urinary protein excretion in children with primary nephrotic syndrome. *Scand. J. Clin. Lab. Invest.*, Vol. 69, No. 6, pp. 680-686

Itoh J., Takahashi S., Ono M., Yamamoto T., Nose M., & Kyogoku M. (1994). Nephritogenic antibodies in MRL/lpr lupus mice: molecular characteristics in pathological and genetic aspects. *Tohoku J. Exp. Med.*, Vol. 173, No. 1, pp. 65-74

Jaenisch R. & Bird A. (2003). Epigenetic regulation of gene expression: how the genome integrates intrinsic and environmental signals. *Nature Gen.*, Vol. 33, Suppl., pp. 245-254

Jiang T., Wang Z., Proctor G., Moskowitz S., Liebman S.E., Rogers T., Lucia M.S., Li J., & Levi M. (2005). Diet-induced obesity in C57BL/6J mice causes increased renal lipid accumulation and glomerulosclerosis via a sterol regulatory element-binding protein-1c-dependent pathway. *J. Biol. Chem.*, Vol. 280, No. 37, pp. 32317-32325

Kataoka Y., Iwasaki T., & Kuroiwa T. (2001). The role of donor T cells for target organ injuries in acute and chronic graft-versus-host disease. *Immunology*, Vol. 103, No. 3, pp. 310-318

Kato Y., Manabe T., Tanaka Y., & Mochizuki H. (1999). Effect of an orally active Th1/Th2 balance modulator, M50367, on IgE production, eosinophilia, and airway hyperresponsiveness in mice. *J. Immunol.*, Vol. 162, No. 12, pp. 7470-7479

Khoruts A. & Fraser J.M. (2005). A causal link between lymphopenia and autoimmunity. *Immunol. Lett.*, Vol. 98, No. 1, pp. 23-31

Kim J., Park S., Kim H.-A., Jung D., Kim H.J., Choi H.-J., Cho H.R., & Kwon B. (2010). Roles of host nonhematopoietic cells in autoimmunity and donor cell engraftment in graft-versus-host disease. *Immune Netw.*, Vol. 10, No. 2, pp. 46-54

Kim Y.M., Bombeck C.A., & Billiar T.R. (1999). Nitric oxide as a bifunctional regulator of apoptosis. *Circ. Res.*, Vol. 84, No. 3, pp. 253-256

Kimura M. & Gleichmann E. (1987). Depressed antibody responses to exogenous antigens in mice with lupus-like graft-versus-host disease. *Clin. Immunol. Immunopathol., Vol.* 43, No. 1, pp. 97-109

Kimura K., Ida S., Shimada K., & Kanai Y. (1987). Specificity of anti-nuclear antibodies induced in F1 mice undergoing the graft versus host reaction: isotypes and cross-reactivities. *Clin. Exp. Immunol.*, Vol. 69, No. 2, 385-393

Klinman D., Yi A.-K., Beaucage S., Conover J., & Krieg A. (1996). CpG motifs present in bacterial DNA rapidly induce lymphocytes to secrete interleukin 6, interleukin 12, and interferon gamma. *Proc. Natl. Acad. Sci. USA*, Vol. 93, No. 7, pp. 2879-2883

Koide N., Sugiyama T., Mu M.M., Mori I., Yoshida T., Hamano T., & Yokochi T. (2003). Gamma interferon-induced nitric oxide production in mouse CD5+ B1-like cell line and its association with apoptotic cell death. *Microbiol. Immunol.*, Vol. 47, No. 9, pp. 669-679

Kolesnikova O.P., Kudaeva O.T., Loginov M.V., & Robinson M.V. (1991). Indicators of erythro- and immunopoiesis at the development of autoimmune disease induced by GVHR. *Vestnik AMN*, Vol. 12, No. 12, 13-16.

Kolesnikova O.P., Kudaeva O.T., Sukhenko T.G., Tuzova M.N., & Saphronova I.V. (2001). The correction of combined immuno- and hemopoiesis disordes induced by graft-versus-host reaction. *Russian J. Immunol.*, Vol. 6, No. 2, pp. 177-186

Kono D.H., Balomenos D., Park M.S., & Theofilopoulos A.N. (2000). Development of lupus in BXSB mice is independent of IL-4. *J. Immunol.*, Vol. 164, No. 1, pp. 38–42

Kootstra C.J., Sutmuller M., Baelde H.J., de Heer E., & Bruijn J.A. (1998). Association between leukocyte infiltration and development of glomerulosclerosis in experimental lupus nephritis. *J. Pathol.*, Vol. 184, No. 2, pp. 219-225

Koreth J. & Antin J.H. (2008). Current and future approaches for control of graft-versus-host disease. *Expert Rev. Hematol.*, Vol. 1, No. 1 : 111

Kozlov V.A., Kolesnikova O.P., Sukhenko T.G., Filimonov P.N., & Shklovskaya Ye.V. (1995). Erythropoiesis and interleukin-1 production in the mice with GVHR-induced immunodeficite and immune complex glomerulonephritis. *Immunologiia*, No. 1, pp. 36-38

Kozlov V.A., Kudaeva O.T., Kolesnikova O.P., Saphronova I.V., Lactionov P.V., Rykova E.U., & Obuchova L.A. (2002). Th1-and Th2-dependent variants of chronic graft-versus-host. *Immunologiia*, No. 3, pp. 143-146

Krenger W. & Ferrara J.L. (1996). Graft-versus-host disease and the Th1/Th2 paradigm. *Immunol. Res.*, Vol. 15, No. 1, pp. 50-73

Krenger, W., Rossi S., Piali L., & Hollander G.A. (2000). Thymic atrophy in murine acute graft-versus-host disease is effected by impaired cell cycle progression of host pro-T and pre-T cells. *Blood*, Vol. 96, No. 1, pp. 347-354

Krieg A. (1999). Direct immunologic activities of CpG DNA and implications for gene therapy. *J. Gene Med.*, Vol. 1, No. 1, pp. 56-63

Kudaeva O.T., Nenasheva E.V., & Kozlov V.A. (2005a). Determination of immunoglobulins in the whole blood. *Immunologiia*, No. 3, pp. 89-91

Kudaeva O.T., Goiman E.V., Lykov A.P., Kolesnikova O.P., & Kozlov V.A. (2005b). Effects of preparations modifying Th1/Th2 ratio on the incidence of clinical variants of chronic graft-versus-host reaction. *Bull. Exp. Biol. Med.*, Vol. 140, No. 3, pp. 338-340

Kudaeva O.T., Goiman E.V., Gavrilova E.D., Maiborodin I.V., & Kolesnikova O.P. (2009). Sex difference of autoimmune glomerulonephritis formation in the experimental model. *Vestnik Uralskoi meditsinskoi akademicheskoi nauki*, No. 2/1, pp. 42-43

Kudaeva O.T., Goiman E.V., Nenasheva E.V., Maiborodin I.V., Kolesnikova O.P., & Kozlov V.A. (2010a). Correction of autoimmune glomerulonephritis in experimental animals by lethal irradiation and cell transfer of syngeneic bone marrow. *Meditsinskaia immunologiia*, Vol. 12, No. 3, pp. 191-198

Kudaeva O.T., Gavrilova E.D., Goiman E.V., Nenasheva E.V., Kolesnikova O.P., & Kozlov V.A. (2010b). Features of immune response in chronic graft-versus-host disease. *Immunologiia*, No. 4, pp. 199-203

Kunzendorf U., Tran T., & Bulfone-Paus S. (1998). The Th1/Th2 paradigm in 1998: law of nature or rule with exception. *Nephrol. Dial. Transplant.*, Vol. 13, No. 10, pp. 2445-2448

Lang T.J., Nguyen P., Papadimitriou J.C., & Via C.S. (2003). Increased severity of murine lupus in female mice is due to enhanced expansion of pathogenic T cells. *J. Immunol.*, Vol. 171, No. 11, pp. 5795-5801

Lawman S., Mauri C., Jury E.C., Cook H.T., & Ehrenstein M.R. (2004). Atorvastatin inhibits autoreactive B cell activation and delays lupus development in New Zealand black/white F1 mice. *J. Immunol.*, Vol. 173, No. 12, pp. 7641-7646

Marleau A.M. & Sarvetnick N. (2005). T-cell homeostasis in tolerance and immunity. *J. Leukoc. Biol.*, Vol. 78, No. 3, pp. 575-584

Marques R., Antunes I., & Eksmond U. (2008). B lymphocyte activation by coinfection prevents immune control of Friend virus infection. *J. Immunol.*, Vol. 181, No. 5, 3432-3440

Martinez F.O., Sica A., Mantovani A., & Locati M. (2008). Macrophage activation and polarization. *Front. Biosci.*, Vol. 13, pp. 453-461

Martinez F.O., Helming L., & Gordon S. (2009). Alternative activation of macrophages: an immunologic functional perspective. *Annu. Rev. Immunol.*, Vol. 27, pp. 451-483

Matejuk A., Bakke A., Hopke C., Dwyer J., Vandenbark A., & Offner H. (2004). Estrogen treatment induces a novel population of regulatory cells, which suppresses experimental autoimmune encephalomyelitis. *J. Neurosci. Res.*, Vol. 77, No. 1, pp. 119-126

McMahon M. & Hahn B.H. (2007). Atherosclerosis and systemic lupus erythematosus: mechanistic basis of the association. *Curr. Opin. Immunol.*, Vol. 19, No. 6, pp. 633-639

Montes C.L., Acosta-Rodriguez E.V., Merino M.C., Bermejo D.A., & Gruppi A. (2007). Polyclonal B cell activation in infections: infectious agents' devilry or defense mechanism of the host. *J. Leukoc. Biol.*, Vol. 82, No. 5, pp. 1027-1032

Mori T., Nishimura T., Ikeda Y., Hotta T., Yagita H., & Ando K. (1998). Involvement of Fas-mediated apoptosis in the hematopoietic progenitor cells of graft-versus-host reaction-associated myelosuppression. *Blood*, Vol. 92, No.1, pp. 101-107

Morris S.C., Cheek R.L., Cohen P.L., & Eisenberg R.A. (1990). Autoantibodies in chronic graft versus host result from cognate T-B interactions. *J. Exp. Med.*, Vol. 171, No. 2, pp. 503-517

Morris S.C., Madden K.B., Adamovicz J.J., Gause W.C., Hubbard B.R., Gately M.K., & Finkelman F.D. (1994). Effects of IL-12 on in vivo cytokine gene expression and Ig isotype selection. *J. Immunol.*, Vol. 152, No. 3, pp. 1047-1056

Mosmann T., Cherwinsky H., Bond M., Giedlin M., & Coffman R. (1986). Two types of murine helper T cell clone. 1. Definition according to profile of lymphokine activities and secreted proteins. *J. Immunol., Vol. 136, No. 7, pp. 2348-2357*

Mosmann T. & Sad S. (1996). The expanding universe of T-cell subsets: Th1, Th2 and more. *Immunol. Today,* Vol. 17, No. 3, pp. 138-146

Mosmann T.R., Kobie J.J., Lee F.E-H., & Quataert S.A. (2009). T helper cytokine patterns: defined subsets, random expression, and external modulation. *Immunol. Res.*, Vol. 45, No. 2-3, pp. 173-184

Munder M., Eichmann K., & Modolell M. (1998). Alternative metabolic states in murine macrophages reflected by the nitric oxide synthase/arginase balance: competitive regulation by CD4+ T cells correlates with Th1/Th2 phenotype. *J. Immunol.*, Vol. 160, No. 11, pp. 5347-5354

Muracami M., Yoshioka H., Shirai T., Tsubata T., & Honjo T. (1995). Prevention of autoimmune symptoms in autoimmune-prone mice by elimination of B-1 cells. *Int. Immunol.*, Vol. 7, No. 5, pp. 877-882

O'Gor D., Rose N., & Greenspan N. (2003). Th1-Th2: a Procrustean paradigm. *Nature Immunol.*, Vol. 4, No. 6, pp. 503-505

Ogura A., Asano T., Matsuda J., Takano K., Nakagawa M., & Fukui M. (1989). Characteristics of mutant mice (ICGN) with spontaneous renal lesions: a new model for human nephrotic syndrome. *Lab. Anim.*, Vol. 23, No. 2, pp. 169-174

Okamoto I., Kohno K., Tanimoto T., Iwaki K., Ishihara T., Akamatsu S., Ikegami H., & Kurimoto M. (2000). IL-18 prevents the development of chronic graft-versus-host disease in mice. *J. Immunol.,* Vol. 164, No. 11, pp. 6067-6074

Okuda Y. & Sakoda S. (1996). Pentoxifylline delays the onset of experimental allergic encephalomyelitis in mice by modulating cytokine production in peripheral blood mononuclear cells. *Immunopharmacology,* Vol. 35, No. 2, pp. 141-148

Orlovskaya I. & Kozlov V. (2001). The interaction of hemopoiesis and immunogenesis in immunopathology development. *Russkii zhurnal immunologii,* Vol. 6, No. 2, pp. 167-176

Perminova O.M., Volsky N.N., Kudaeva O.T., Goiman E.V., & Kozlov V.A. (2009). Dyslipidemia and Th1/Th2 relationship at different stages of chronic graft-versus-host reaction. *Immunologiia,* No. 6, pp. 341-345

Philippe P. (2007). Autoimmune hemolytic anemia: diagnosis and management. *Presse Med.*, Vol. 36, No. 12, pp. 1959-1969

Piccinni M.-P., Giudizi M.-G., & Biagiotti R. (1995). Progesterone favors the development of human T helper cells producing Th2-type cytokines and promotes both IL-4 production and membrane CD30 expression in established Th1 cell clones. *J. Immunol.,* Vol. 155, No. 1, pp. 128-133

Poulsom R., Prodromidi E.I., Pusey C.D., & Cook H.T. (2006). Cell therapy for renal regeneration - time for some joined-up thinking. *Nephrol. Dial Transplant.*, Vol. 21, No. 12, pp. 3349-3353

Prodromidi E.I., Poulsom R., & Jeffery R. (2006). Bone marrow-derived cells contribute to podocyte regeneration and amelioration of renal disease in a mouse model of Alport syndrome. *Stem Cells*, Vol. 24, No. 11, pp. 2448-2455

Raj N., Cheung S., Rosztocry J., & Pitha P. (1992). Mouse genotype affects inducible expression of cytokine genes. *J. Immunol.,* Vol. 148, No. 6, pp. 1934-1940

Raz E. & Spiegelberg H.L. (1999). Deviation of the allergic IgE to an IgG response by gene immunotherapy. *Int. Rev. Immunol.*, Vol. 18, No. 3, pp. 271-289

Reddy P., Negrin R., & Hill G.R. (2008). Mouse models of bone marrow transplantation. *Biol. Blood Marrow Transplant.*, Vol. 14, No. 1, Suppl. 1, pp. 129-135

Reddy R. & Ferrara J.L.M. (2009). Mouse models of graft-versus-host disease. StemBook. Ed. The Stem Cell Research Community. StemBook, doi/10.3824/stembook.1.36.1, http://www.stembook.org

Reina-San-Martin B., Cosson A., & Minoprio P. (2000). Lymphocyte polyclonal activation: a pitfall for vaccine design against infectious agents. *Parasitol. Today*, Vol. 16, No. 2, pp. 62-67

Reiner S.L. (2005). Epigenetic control in the immune response. *Hum. Mol. Genet.*, Vol. 14, Spec. No. 1, pp. R41-R46

Reiss A.B., Awadallah N.W., Malhotra S., Montesinos M.C., Chan E.S.L., Javitt N.B. & Cronstein B.N. (2001) Immune complexes and IFN-γ decrease cholesterol 27-hydroxylase in human endothelium and macrophages. J. Lipid Res., Vol. 42, No. 11, pp. 1913-1922

Rolink A.G., Radaszkiewicz T., & Melchers F. (1987). The autoantigen-binding B cell repertoires of normal and of chronically graft-versus-host-diseased mice. (1987). J. Exp. Med., Vol. 165, No. 6, pp. 1675-1687

Rolink A., Thalmann P., Berger C., Radaszkiewicz T., & Melchers F. (1988). Autoreactive B cell repertoire in mice with chronic graft versus host disease. *Mol. Immunol.*, Vol. 25, No. 11, pp. 1217-1222

Rook G., Hernandez-Pamdo R., & Lightman S. (1994). Hormones, peripherally activated prohormones and regulation of the Th1/Th2 balance. *Immunol. Today*, Vol. 15, No. 7, pp. 301-303

Rozendaal L., Pals S.T., Gleichmann E., & Melief C.J. (1990). Persistence of allospecific helper T cells is required for maintaining autoantibody formation in lupus-like graft-versus-host disease. *Clin. Exp. Immunol.*, Vol. 82, No. 3, pp. 527-532

Sawai C., Anderson K., & Walser-Kuntz D. (2003). Effect of bisphenol A on murine immune function: modulation of interferon-g, IgG2a, and disease symptoms in NZBxNZW F1 mice. *Environ. Health Perspect.*, Vol. 111, No. 16, pp. 1883-1887

Schluns K.S., Kieper W.C., Jameson S.C., & Lefrancois L. (2000). Interleukin-7 mediates the homeostasis of naïve and memory CD8 T cells in vivo. *Nat. Immunol.*, Vol. 1, No. 5, 426-432

Serhan C.N. & Savill J. (2005). Resolution of inflammation: the beginning programs the end. *Nat. Immunol.*, Vol. 6, No. 12, pp. 1191-1197

Shearer G.C., Newman J.W., Hammock B.D., & Kaysen G.A. (2005). Graded effects of proteinuria on HDL structure in nephrotic rats. *J. Am. Soc. Nephrol.*, Vol. 16, No. 5, pp. 1309–1319

Shi Y., Yoshihara F., Nakahama H., Ichimaru N., Yazawa K., Sada M., Goto R., Kawano Y., Moriyama T., Takahara S., Okuyama A., & Kangawa K. (2005). A novel immunosuppressant FTY720 ameliorates proteinuria and alterations of intrarenal adrenomedullin in rats with autoimmune glomerulonephritis. *Regul. Pept.*, Vol. 127, No. 1-3, pp. 233-238

Shustov A., Luzina I., Nguyen P., & Papadimitriou J. (2000). Role of perforin in controlling B-cell hyperactivity and humoral autoimmunity. *J. Clin. Invest.*, Vol. 106, No. 6, pp. R39-R47

Snapper C. & Paul W. (1987). Interferon-gamma and B cell stimulatory factor-1 reciprocally regulate Ig isotype production. *Science*, Vol. 236, No. 4804, pp. 944-947

Soldan S., Retuerto A., Sicotte N., & Voskuhl R. (2003). Immune modulation in multiple sclerosis patients treated with the pregnancy hormone estriol. *J. Immunol.*, Vol. 171, No. 11, pp. 6267–6274

Souvannavong V., Brown S., & Adam A. (1990). Muramyl dipeptide (MDP) synergizes with interleukin 2 and interleukin 4 to stimulate, respectively, the differentiation and proliferation of B cells. *Cell Immunol.*, Vol. 126, No. 1, pp. 106-116

Spera J.M., Ugalde J.E., & Mucci J. (2006). A B lymphocyte mitogen is a Brucella abortus virulence factor required for persistent infection. *Proc. Natl. Acad. Sci. USA*, Vol. 103, No. 44, pp. 16514-16519

Stam W., Van Oosterhout A., & Nijkamp F. (1993). Pharmacologic modulation of Th1- and Th2-associated lymphokine production. *Life Sci.*, Vol. 53, No. 26, pp. 1921-1934

Subbaiah P.V. & Rodby R.A. (1994). Abnormal acyltransferase activities and accelerated cholesteryl ester transfer in patients with nephrotic syndrome. *Metabolism*, Vol. 43, No. 9, pp. 1126-1133

Sudo N., Yu X., & Kubo C. (2001). Dehydroepiandrosterone attenuates the spontaneous elevation of serum IgE level in NC/Nga mice. *Immunol. Lett.*, Vol. 79, No. 3, pp. 177-179

Sun Y., Tawara I., Toubai T., & Reddy P. (2007). Pathophysiology of acute graft-versus-host disease: recent advances. *Transl. Res.*, Vol. 150, No. 4, pp. 197-214

Surth C.D. & Sprent J. (2008). Homeostatic T cell proliferation: how far can T cells be activated to self-ligands. *Immunity*, Vol. 29, No. 6, pp. 848-862

Tipping P.G. & Kitching A.R. (2005). Glomerulonephritis, Th1and Th2: what's new? *Clin. Exp.Immunol.*, Vol. 142, No. 2, pp. 207-215

Tkachev V.O., Goiman E.V., Lykov A.P., Kudaeva O.T., & Kolesnikova O.P. (2006b). Indicators of hematopoiesis in the dynamics of development of chronic graft-versus-host reaction. *Immunologiia*, No. 3, pp. 168-171

Tkachev V.O., Volsky N.N., Kudaeva O.T., Kolesnikova O.P. & Kozlov V.A. (2009). Effect of the Th1/Th2-polarizing agents - dehydroepiandrosterone sulfate and muramyl dipeptide - on the metabolic state of macrophages, *Russkii immunologicheskii zhurnal*, Vol. 3, No. 2, pp. 158-163

Tschetter J., Mozes E., & Shearer G. (2000). Progression from acute to chronic disease in murine parent-into-F1 model of graft-versus-host disease. *J. Immunol.*, Vol. 165, No. 10, pp. 5987-5994

Umland S., Razac S., Nahrebne D., & Seymour B. (1992). Effect of in vivo administration of interferon-gamma, anti-IFN-gamma, or anti-IL-4 monoclonal antibodies in chronic autoimmune graft-versus-host disease. *Clin. Immunol. Immunopathol.*, Vol. 63, No. 1, pp. 66-73

Ushiyama C., Hirano T., Miyajima H., Okumura K., Ovary Z., & Hashimoto H. (1995). Anti-IL-4 antibody prevents graft-versus-host disease in mice after bone marrow transplantation. The IgE allotype is an important marker of graft-versus-host disease. *J. Immunol.*, Vol. 154, No. 6, pp. 2687-2696

Van Goor H., Ding G., Kees-Folts D., Grond J., Schreiner G.F., & Diamond J.R. (1994). Macrophages and renal disease. *Lab. Invest.*, Vol. 71, No. 4, pp. 456-464

Van Griensven M., Bergijk E., Baelde J., De Heer E., & Bruijn J. (1997). Differential effects of sex hormones on autoantibody production and proteinuria in chronic graft-versus-host disease-induced experimental lupus nephritis. *Clin. Exp. Immunol.*, Vol. 107, No. 2, pp. 254-260

Vaziri N.D. & Liang K. (2002). Up-regulation of acyl-coenzyme A:cholesterol acyltransferase (ACAT) in nephrotic syndrome. *Kidney Int.*, Vol. 61, No. 5, pp. 1769-1775

Vaziri N.D., Gollapudi P., Han S., Farahmand G., Yuan J., Rahimi A., & Moradi H. (2011). Nephrotic syndrome causes upregulation of HDL endocytic receptor and PDZK-1-dependent downregulation of HDL docking receptor. *Nephrol. Dial. Transplant.*, Mar 31. [Epub ahead of print]

Vercelli D. (2004). Genetics, epigenetics, and the environment: switching, buffering, releasing. *J. Allergy Clin. Immunol.*, Vol. 113, No. 3, pp. 381-386

Via C., Sharrow S., & Shearer G. (1987). Role of cytotoxic T lymphocytes in the prevention of lupus-like disease occurring in a murine model of graft-vs-host disease. *J. Immunol.*, Vol. 139, No. 6, pp. 1840-1849

Via C.S.& Shearer G.M. (1988). T cell interactions in autoimmunity: insights from a murine model of graft-versus-host disease. *Immunol. Today*, Vol. 9, No. 7-8, pp. 207-213

Vlasov V.V., Rykova E.Y., Safronova I.V., Lactionov P.P., Kudaeva O.T., & Kozlov V.A. (2002). Plasmid DNA modulates chronic graft-versus-host reaction. *Dokl. Biol. Sci.*, Vol. 382, pp. 75-77

Waddington S.N. (2002). Arginase in glomerulonephritis, *Kidney Int*, Vol. 61, No. 3, pp. 876-881

Wang Y., Rogers P.M., Su C., Varga G., Stayrook K.R., & Burris T.P. (2008). Regulation of cholesterologenesis by the oxysterol receptor, LXRalpha. *J. Biol. Chem.*, Vol. 283, No. 39, pp. 26332-26339

Whitacre C. (2001). Sex differences in autoimmune disease. *Nat. Immunol.*, Vol. 2, No. 9, pp. 777-780

Wilczynski J. (2005). Th1/Th2 cytokines balance - yin and yang of reproductive immunology. *Eur. J. Obstetrics Gynecol. Reprod. Biol.*, Vol. 122, No. 2, pp. 136-143

Williams T.M., Little M.H., & Ricardo S.D. (2010). Macrophages in renal development, injury, and repair. *Semin. Nephrol.*, Vol. 30, No. 3, pp. 255-267

Wilson Ch. & Makarb K. (2002). Epigenetic regulation of T cell fate and function. *J. Infect. Dis.*, Vol. 185, Suppl. 1, pp. S37-S45

Wilson Ch., Makarb K., Shnyreva M., & Fitzpatrick D. (2005). DNA methylation and the expanding epigenetics of T cell lineage commitment. *Sem. Immunol.*, Vol. 17, No. 2, pp. 105-119

Wong A., Gottesman I. & Petronis A. (2005). Phenotypic differences in genetically identical organisms: the epigenetic perspective. *Human Mol. Gen.*, Vol. 14, No. 1, pp. R11-R18

Wu C.C., Chen J.S., Lin S.H., Chen A., Sytwu H.K., & Lin Y.F. (2008). Experimental model of membranous nephropathy in mice: sequence of histological and biochemical events. *Lab. Anim.*, Vol. 42, No. 3, pp. 350-359

Xiao Z.Y., Zhou W.X., Zhang Y.X. Cheng J.P., He J.F., Yang R.F. & Yun L.H. (2007). Roquinimex-mediated protection effect on the development of chronic graft-versus-host disease in mice is associated with induction of Th1 cytokine production and inhibition of proinflammatory cytokine production. *Life Sci.,* Vol. 81, No. 19-20, pp. 1403-1410

Yoshioka H., Yoshida H., Doi T., Muso E., Ohshio G., Higuchi K., Inaba M., Miyake T., Kita T., Hamashima Y., & Takeda T. (1989). Autoimmune abnormalities in a murine model of accelerated senescence. *Clin. Exp. Immunol.*, Vol. 75, No. 1, pp. 129-135

Zhu L.-J., Yang X., Yu X.-Q. (2010). Anti-TNF-a therapies in systemic lupus erythematosus. *J. Biomed. Biotechnol.*, 2010 : 465898. Epub. 2010 Jun 22

5

Immunopathogenic Mechanism and Therapeutic Intervention in an Experimental Murine Model of Membranous Nephropathy

Chia-Chao Wu[1,2], Kuo-Cheng Lu[3], Jin-Shuen Chen[1], Yuh-Feng Lin[1,4] and Huey-Kang Sytwu[2]
[1]*Division of Nephrology, Department of Medicine, Tri-Service General Hospital*
[2]*Department of Microbiology and Immunology, National Defense Medical Center*
[3]*Department of Medicine, Cardinal Tien Hospital, School of Medicine, Fu Jen Catholic University*
[4]*Division of Nephrology, Department of Medicine, Shuang-Ho Hospital; Taipei Medical University, Taipei, Taiwan*

1. Introduction

Idiopathic membranous nephropathy (MN), an autoimmune-mediated glomerulonephritis (GN), is one of the most common causes of nephrotic syndrome in adults and may rarely lead to idiopathic nephrotic syndrome in childhood (Cattran, 2001; Chadban & Atkins, 2005; Ponticelli & Passerini, 1990). The clinical course in the majority of patients appears to be indolent and slowly, although some progress into end-stage renal failure. Spontaneous remissions of proteinuria occur in approximately one quarter of patients; approximately half will have stable renal function with or without persistent proteinuria (Rosen, 1971; Wasserstein, 1997). A minority of patients will demonstrate slowly decline in renal function, and a few will have rapidly decline leading to renal failure or death. Approximately 30%–40% of patients with MN develop progressive renal impairment, which results in end-stage renal failure after 10–15 years (Cattran, 2001; Chadban & Atkins, 2005; Honkanen et al., 1992). The etiology in the majority of cases is unknown (idiopathic or primary MN, 75%); MN can also be secondary to or associated with a variety of conditions, including systemic lupus erythematosus and other autoimmune disorders, chronic infections such as with hepatitis B virus, drugs such as penicillamine, and malignant neoplasms (Cattran, 2001; Chadban & Atkins, 2005; Honkanen et al., 1992; Ponticelli & Passerini, 1990; Rosen, 1971; Wasserstein, 1997). The characteristic finding in MN is the presence of *in situ* immune-complex deposition over the subepithelial space which presented with diffuse, discrete, granular glomerular capillary wall staining for immunoglobulins and complement on immunoflusrescence and subepithelial electron-dense deposits on electron microscopy. The deposited immune complexes sequentially induce the inflammatory response, complement activation, and oxidative injury, all of which participate in the pathogenesis of MN (Couser

& Abrass, 1988; Couser & Nangaku, 2006; Cunningham & Quigg, 2005; Kerjaschki, 2004; Nangaku et al., 2005; Ronco & Debiec, 2006).
However, the role of adaptive immunity in the mediation of glomerular injury in MN has not yet been fully elucidated (Couser & Abrass, 1988; Couser & Nangaku, 2006; Cunningham & Quigg, 2005; Kerjaschki, 2004; Nangaku et al., 2005; Ronco & Debiec, 2006). The prominent phenomenon of antigen and antibody immune-complex were observed in the process in the Heymann nephritis (HN), one of the most frequently used models of human MN in rat (Heymann et al., 1959; Salant et al., 1989). However, recent experiments with anti-T cell subset monoclonal antibody (mAb) therapies also suggested that T cells are central to the induction and glomerular injury of HN (Quiza et al., 1992). Indeed, the immunopathogenesis of MN, especially the role of T cell (including helper and cytotoxic T cells), is still not clear (Nangaku & Couser, 2005). The treatment of MN is controversial. Controlled trials of corticosteroids with or without cytotoxic or immunosuppressive agents have had variable results. Presently available immunosuppressive therapies are not always effective and often have many persistent side effects (Cattran, 2005; du Buf-Vereijken et al., 2005; Glassock, 2004; Perna et al., 2004; Piccoli et al., 1994; Polenakovik & Grcevska, 1999; Ponticelli et al., 1987; Ponticelli, 1987; Ponticelli & Passerini, 1991). The treatment of patients with MN is still up for debate. The current treatment of this disease remains inadequate and nonspecific. The purpose of this review is to bring together current informations concerning the roles of immunopathogenesis in the development and progression of MN. Specific emphasis is placed on the new murine MN model setup and the kinetics of adaptive immunity during MN. In addition, immuno-modulatory treatments using heme oxygenase-1 (HO-1) induction in the treatment of MN are also reviewed.

2. Immunopathogenic mechanism and therapeutic intervention in experimental murine model of MN

2.1 Experimental animal model of MN

MN is an important cause of nephrotic syndrome and end-stage renal disease in adults. For designing more rationale therapy, it would be useful if we really understood basic pathophysiology of disease. Since only limited information can be obtained from the direct study of diseased humans, animal models are very helpful for us to understand pathogenesis. Most results were obtained from HN. However, limited mouse models for study of human MN was well-characterized although mice offer the advantages of being cheaper, manipulate easily, and suitable for experimental applications.

2.1.1 Heymann Nephritis (HN)

HN is a rat model of autoimmune-mediated glomerulonephritis that is similar in histopathology to human idiopathic MN (Heymann et al., 1959; HEYMANN et al., 1962). In 1959, Heymann *et al.* (Heymann et al., 1959) first described a model of MN in rats induced by immunization with a tissue antigen fraction derived from proximal tubular brush borders (Fx1A) in complete Freund's adjuvant (CFA) (Kerjaschki & Farquhar, 1982; Kerjaschki & Farquhar, 1983). This model, subsequently referred to as HN, the morphology more closely resembled human MN because the deposits were exclusively subepithelial in location(Edgington et al., 1968; Edgington et al., 1967). The "active" HN model took several weeks to develop after immunization. Following, passive HN (PHN) model by passively transferring heterologous antibodies to the brush border (anti-Fx1A) into normal animals in which antibody deposition induced heavy proteinuria more rapidly within only 3 to 4 days, thus finally enabling studies to be conducted of the mediation of glomerular injury in MN (Dixon et al., 1961; Van Damme et al., 1978; Fleuren et al., 1978). Whether the immune complexes were formed *in situ* or passive trapping of small, soluble immune complexes formed in the circulation is an important issue. Within months, Van Damme *et al.* using *ex vivo* perfusion system, and Couser *et al.* using a physiologically intact isolated perfused kidney system established that the deposits in MN result not from circulating immune complex trapping but from direct, or *in situ*, binding of IgG antibody to native glomerular antigens, presumably expressed on the membrane of podocyte foot processes (Van Damme et al., 1978; Couser et al., 1978). The nature of the glomerular antigen involving in formation of subepithelial deposits in HN was systematically tracked down by Kerjaschki and Farquhar and demonstrated as a combination of megalin and a receptor-associated protein (RAP) in the podocyte membrane (and tubular brush border) (Kerjaschki & Farquhar, 1982; Makker & Singh, 1984; Farquhar et al., 1995). Megalin (gp330) has been identified as a pathogenic antigen in HN, but it has not been found in human or mice glomeruli. Hence, the precise nature of the idiopathic MN-initiating antigen is still unknown. (Ronco & Debiec, 2007b; Ronco & Debiec, 2007a; Ronco & Debiec, 2005).

2.1.2 Murine model of MN induced by cationic bovine serum albumin

The HN is a generalized model with morphological and functional aspects similar to those of human MN. However, it has rarely been applied to the mouse which have advantages of low cost, easily manipulation and the potential application of genetic and monoclonal antibody techniques (Quigg, 2003). Repeated doses of cationic bovine serum albumin (cBSA) are alternative methods to induce MN which had been applied in the dog, cat, rabbit and rat (Wright et al., 1985; Nash et al., 1990; Border et al., 1982; Bass et al., 1990). The purity of the cBSA antigen is an important factor to cause variants of MN. The heterogeneity of the antigenic charge distinctly affects its ability to cause damage: the more cationic the immunogen, the more nephritogenic it is and the greater its tendency to produce a typical MN pattern. Unlike the cBSA preparations previously used only characterized by polyacrylamide gel flat bed electrophoresis and fast protein liquid chromatography(Bass et al., 1990; Wright et al., 1985), which could not exclude the presence of native anionic and slightly cationic BSA, we used pH-dependent binding technique to purify a more homogenous cBSA preparation which made our model disclosing greater consistency (Chen et al., 2004; Wu et al., 2008a; Yang & Langer, 1985). Mice were immunized with 0.2 mg of cBSA emulsified in complete Freund's adjuvant (CFA), two weeks later, these mice received cBSA (13 mg/kg) intravenously three times per week, every other day, for six weeks to induce MN. There was a dose-related effect in the induction of MN and strain specificity because MN could be induced in BALB/c mice, but not in the C57BL/6 strain (Chen et al., 2004; Wu et al., 2008a). All cBSA-induced MN mice developed the characteristically clinical symptoms of proteinuria, hypoalbuminaemia, and hypercholesterolaemia. The MN induction rate did not differ between male and female mice reflecting the equal incidence of MN in men and women. Overt proteinuria appeared in week 4 and reached a plateau at week 8. Serum albumin concentration declined markedly after week 6 in the MN group and reached its nadir at week 8. However, serum cholesterol concentration showed a compensatory increase at week 6 and was maximal at week 8. The above presentations assemble like nephrotic syndrome in human MN. The blood urea nitrogen and serum creatinine concentrations did not change during MN induction. Urinalysis revealed no haematuria or leukocyturia during the study.

Histological findings revealed characteristically MN morphologic pattern, namely, diffuse thickening of the glomerular basement membrane (GBM) and no significant mesangial proliferation in light microscopy. (Figure 1A) Ultrastructural analysis identified severely irregular thickening of the basement membrane and subepithelial deposits in mice with cBSA-induced MN. (Figure 1D) Positive immunofluorescent staining for IgG was noted by progressively stronger granular fluorescence intensity along the glomerular capillary wall (GCW) with a discrete beaded appearance. Immunofluorescence staining for C3 revealed a similar time course and pattern to that of IgG. (Figure 1B and C) Loss of glomerular anions and the impairment of charge selectivity were noted evidenced by decreased the intensity of colloid iron staining progressively during the course of MN induction. We also found that the Th2 response was predominant: IgG1 concentration was significantly higher than IgG2a concentration. These data indicate that the MN mouse model is associated with a Th2 response. An important issue is to determine whether cBSA-induced MN in mice resembles the *in situ* immune-complex glomerulonephritis seen in humans. Immunofluorescence analysis revealed positive staining for both IgG and C3. Although a strong positive immunofluorescent staining of immune-complex deposition was concomitant with higher serum Ig concentrations, serum CIC concentration did not increase significantly before week 4. These observations suggest the *in situ* immune-complex formation in cBSA-induced MN, although we cannot exclude the possibility that the lower CIC concentration might have been generated in the earlier stages but was deposited rapidly in the kidney. Previous studies using both *in vitro* and *in vivo* approaches have demonstrated that cBSA binds directly to the glomerulus and then forms the *in situ* immune-complex deposition. BSA can induce *in situ* immune-complex formation in the isolated perfused rat kidney (Fleuren et al., 1980). Antigen quantity also seems to be a cofactor influencing MN induction and a threshold exposure to antigen is needed for induction (Breysse et al., 1994)]. Although the mechanisms responsible for this variable course remain unclear, our results suggest that lower antigen exposure might increase the chance of spontaneous remission. We speculate that the antigen source, dose and exposure duration are factors in the pathological and clinical diversity of MN.

We report the development of a new MN mouse model induced by cBSA. Clinically, the animals developed hypoalbuminaemia, hypercholesterolaemia and severe proteinuria. Morphologically, they exhibited diffuse GBM thickening, granular immunofluorescent staining, subepithelial deposits, and a lack of inflammatory cell infiltration and mesangial cells proliferation. Exogenous cBSA antigen had a dose-related influence on disease induction and may have induced *in situ* immune-complex GN. Moreover, this mouse MN model may display Th2 polarization and strain-specific dependence. Extending the MN model to the mouse has the advantages of lower cost, easy manipulation, and the potential benefits of using gene knockout and transgenic mice to investigate the mechanisms of disease initiation and progression. Thus, this model exhibits great similarity to human MN disease in clinical and pathological features over time. This murine model will provide a valuable tool to investigate the pathogenesis of MN and will help in the development of preventive and therapeutic strategies for MN, which is difficult to study in humans.

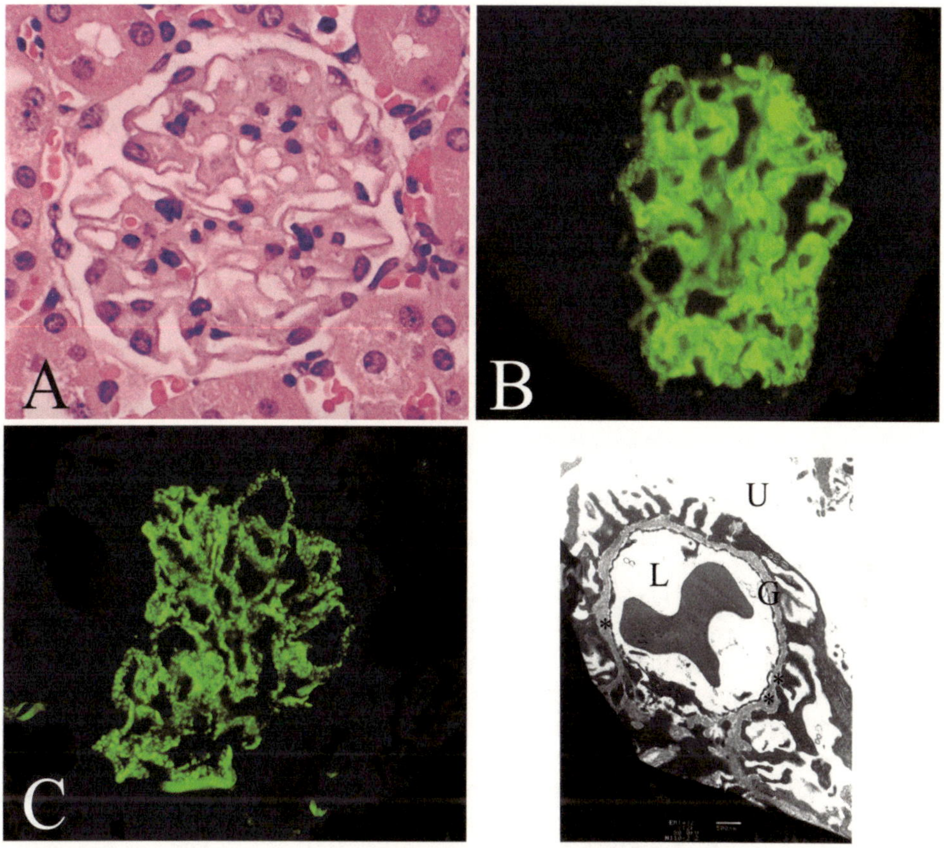

Fig. 1. Renal histopathology in mice with MN. Histopathology revealed characteristic findings of diffuse basement membrane thickening, as observed in the (A) hematoxylin and eosin staining, (B) positive granular immunofluorescent staining for IgG, (C) positive granular immunofluorescent staining for C3, and (D) subepithelial deposition (asterisk). NC, normal control; MN, membranous nephropathy; G, glomerular basement membrane; L, lumen of capillary; and U, urinary space.

2.2 Immunopathogenesis of cBSA-induced MN

MN has been recognized as an autoimmune-mediated GN and characterized by an *in situ* immune-complex disposition over the subepithelial space which caused physical disruption of the filtration barrier and triggered a cascade of events that contribute to the progression of the disease and result in glomerular injury and proteinuria (Ravnskov, 1998; Ronco & Debiec, 2005). The C-BSA binding to glomerular tuft anion site, then immunoglobulin and complement will be produced and aggregated to GBM and mesangial area. This results in glomerular epithelial cell injury and proteinuria in our cBSA-induced murine MN model. Mediation of glomerular injury in MN has been thought to be essentially leukocyte independent (Salant et al., 1985). Early studies using monoclonal antibodies to T cell subsets indicate that T cells are central to the induction and glomerular injury in HN, a rat model of idiopathic MN (Penny et al., 1997; Penny et al., 1998; Quiza et al., 1992). The T lymphocyte-derived cytokines also regulate the cellular and humoral immune responses to nephritogenic antigens and modulate inflammatory events (Holdsworth et al., 1999; Kelly et al., 1998). However, the role of adaptive immunity in the mediation of glomerular injury in MN has not yet been fully elucidated.

2.2.1 The role of T cells and their cytokines in MN

It is widely recognized that $CD4^+$ T cells can be differentiated into two subsets, Th1 and Th2, according to their cytokine profiles (Abbas et al., 1996; Mosmann & Sad, 1996). Th1 cells produce cytokines such as interleukin (IL) 2, interferon γ IFN- γ , and tumor necrosis factor α TNF- α to promote cell-mediated immunity. Th2 cells producing IL-4, IL-5, IL-10 and IL-13 can suppress Th1 cell activation and contribute to humoral immunity(Mosmann & Coffman, 1989). Th1 and Th2 subsets are regulated reciprocally to maintain a balance, which plays an important role in immune-mediated GN (Tipping & Kitching, 2005). Th1 and Th2 subsets direct diverging effector pathways and lead to different patterns of injury and outcomes in GN. Th1-predominant responses are strongly associated with proliferative and crescentic forms of GN while Th2 responses are associated with membranous patterns of injury (Schena, 1999; Ring & Lakkis, 1998). To our knowledge, the diversity of Th1/Th2 in MN is still controversial. Studies involving patients with idiopathic MN showed a consistently negative response for delay type hypersensitivity (DTH) effectors, an increase in IL-4 production by peripheral T helper cells; and a predominance of IgG4 (Th2-type subclass) as well as complement deposition in glomeruli; suggesting a Th2 response (Oliveira, 1998; Kuroki et al., 2005; Masutani et al., 2004; Hirayama et al., 2002; Doi et al., 1984; Doi et al., 1991; Haas, 1994; Imai et al., 1997; Iskandar et al., 1992; Roberts et al., 1983). The above findings favor Th2 response. However, Penny *et al* found that the progressive development of infiltrates of activated T cells—principally Th1 and cytotoxic effector cells—as well as macrophages identified within glomeruli of Lews rats with HN, coincides with the development of proteinuria (Penny et al., 1998). Early studies suggested that classical T cell effector responses are involved in HN, including passive transfer of HN to tolerant rats by lymphoid cells but not serum, and lymphoid cells in culture(Heymann et al., 1962; Hsieh et al., 2000). Furthermore, it has also been found that permanent $CD8^+$ T cell depletion both early and late in the course of disease prevents proteinuria in active Heymann Nephritis. It may indicate that $CD8^+$ cytotoxic T cells are essential to the mediation of glomerular injury in HN and may be relevant to the pathogenesis of MN (Penny et al., 1998). In addition,, Spicer et al found that IL-4 administration prior to the onset of protienuria, rather than the early rIL-4 treatment prevents the development of proteinuria in active Heymann Nephritis by inhibition of Tc1 cells (Spicer et al., 2001). All these results indicate the importance of CD8+ T cell in mediating the final effector phase of glomerular injury in HN (Penny et al., 1998; Spicer et al. 2001) and suggest that Th1 cells participate in the glomerular injury and proteinuria of MN (Penny et al., 1997).The conclusion of the diversity of Th1/Th2 in MN are not consistent.

2.2.2 The kinetics of adaptive immunity of cBSA-induced in MN

The kinetic distribution of different lymphocyte subsets, as well as the association between clinical manifestations and the complicated course of adaptive immune responses during MN is not well understood. To directly investigate immunoregulatory process and immunopathological mechanisms in cBSA-induced MN, we used TH1/TH2 double transgenic mouse (T1/T2 TG mice) which provides the best *in vivo* model to study the differentiation of helper T cell subsets during the Th process was used (Wu et al., 2007).

T1/T2 TG mice, originally in BALB/c background, bear two transgenes expressing two distinct cell surface markers, one is human Thy1 protein (human CD90) under the murine IFNγ promoter control, the other is murine Thy1.1 protein (murine CD90.1) under the murine IL-4 promoter control, designated as TH1/TH2 transgenes respectively(Hsieh et al., 2000; Hung et al., 2005).

T1/T2 TG MN mice showed overt proteinuria, hypoalbuminemia, and hypercholesterolemia characteristically. Renal histopathology revealed typical morphology of MN as glomerular basement membrane thickening, IgG granular deposition and subepithelial deposits seen in H & E, IF and EM sections. There were no significant differences between the MN mice of the BALB/c strain and the T1/T2 TG mice. The numbers of splenic lymphocytes increased progressively. The absolute numbers of $CD4^+$ and $CD8^+$ T cells showed reciprocal increased as total splenocytes despite relative consistent proportion. A progressive increase in the proportion and absolute numbers of $CD19^+$ B cells in the MN mice from week 2; this peaked at week 4 and persistent high throughout the MN process were also observed. Two weeks after immunization, the MN mice had a significant increase in splenic Th2 cells. This indicates an extended Th2 response at this point. We also noticed a trend of increase in the percentage of Th1 cells and most of the remaining $Th1^+$ cells is $CD8^+$ T cells. The percentage of $DX5^+$ cells, a marker for NK cell, in the MN mice did not differ from that in the controls and there were very few cells expressing hCD90 and DX5 markers simultaneously which suggested that most of the $Th1^+$ cells were T lymphocytes, but not IFN-γ producing NK cells. The expression levels of Th1 and Th2 cells among peripheral mononuclear blood cells from MN mice showed similar results. Whether what happening with the T cells in the spleen is also happening in the kidneys, we checked the expression of Th1/Th2 reporter in the kidneys by using quantitative RT-PCR at various time points. The Th1 reporter/Th2 reporter status of kidney revealed parallel changes with those in the spleen. Taken together, these results imply a progressive Th2 prone process of adaptive immunity during experimental MN. We also performed imunohistochemical staining for hCD90, mCD90.1 and CD4 in the kidneys to identify and localize the T-helper cells. The numbers of $CD4^+$ cells were very scanty in NC kidney and the numbers were increased in MN kidney. In contrast to hCD90, there were no $mCD90.1^+$ cells noted in NC kidney, but prominent $mCD90.1^+$ cells were noted in MN mice. The prominent and parallel expression between the $mCD90.1^+$ and $CD4^+$ cells may imply the Th2 polarization in renal T cell during MN.

The Th1 and Th2 subsets can be differentiated according to the production of individual cytokines, Th1 regulates Ig switching to the IgG2a subtype, whereas Th2 enhances IgG1 secretion. We found that the titers of anti-cBSA immunoglobulins—mostly IgG1—increased from week 2 and peaked at week 4. Serum level of immunoglobulins at week 6 and week 8 were lower than those at week 4. These findings may imply the development of tolerance and a Th2-predominant response. We further performed the immunofluorescent staining to investigate whether the isotype of antibodies deposited in the kidney parallels to the findings in sera, and the result revealed a prominent IgG1 antibody deposition in the kidney rather than IgG2a. A progressive increase in the proportion and absolute numbers of $CD19^+$ B cells in the MN mice during the early phase of MN combined with the production and deposition of IgG1 predominant anti-cBSA immunoglobulin in the serum and kidneys indicate that the initial immune response primarily involves the humoral-mediated mechanism. Recent studies have demonstrated that blocking the CD20-positive B cells by rituximab, and thereby, inhibiting B-cell differentiation and immunoglobulin secretion, can reduce proteinuria and prevent disease progression in patients with idiopathic MN. This further confirms the pathogenic role of B cells in MN (Cohen et al., 2005; Remuzzi et al., 2002; Ruggenenti et al., 2003). In our previous study, the cBSA-induced MN can be induced in Th2-prone BALB/c mice, but not in Th1-prone C57BL/6 mice(Chen et al., 2004). In this study, we further showed that the Th2 CD4+ response, and not the Th1 CD4+ response, significantly correlated with the progression of MN. All the results confirmed the relevant role of B cells participating in the process of MN.

We further investigated the secretion of IFN-γ and IL-4 from splenocytes to confirme whether cBSA is a specific antigen in this MN model by using antigen-specific stimulation test stimulated with or without cBSA. As compared to NC mice, levels of IL-4 were increased significantly in MN mice and cBSA restimulation may further enhance its secretion. We identified a significant increase in IL-4 producing cells in the MN group without specific antigen re-stimulation. However, Th1 cells were only slightly amplified. Interestingly, lymphocyte subsets from the MN group re-stimulated with specific antigens displayed a greater capacity to secrete IFN-γ and IL-4, especially among the IFN-γ-producing $CD8^+$ T cells and IL-4-producing $CD19^+$ B cells. Nevertheless, $CD8^+$ T cells contributed more to the augmented production of IFN-γ than did $CD4^+$ T cells; moreover, $CD19^+$ B cells also demonstrated greater IL-4 production than the $CD4^+$ T cells. Quantitative real-time PCR of renal cortex and splenocytes demonstrated a consistent change with slightly increased expression of proinflammatory (TNF-α and IL-6) and Th1 cytokines (IL-2, IFN-γ) and extremely high expression of Th2 (IL-4 and IL-10) cytokines. Finally, we found that the Th2 CD4+ response increased as the MN progression and showed that the number of Th2 cell not the Th1 cell significant correlated with serum cholesterol and proteinuria.

In the MN mice, production via cBSA re-stimulation and subsequent staining of intracellular cytokines from cultured splenocytes revealed a significant increase in IL-4-producing $CD4^+$ T cells, but only a slight increase in IFN-γ-producing $CD4^+$ T cells. This provides further evidence confirming the maintenance of Th2 cells post cBSA induction. Furthermore, data from intracellular cytokines post Ag-specific re-stimulation suggests that IFN-γ is secreted predominantly by $CD8^+$ T cells, while IL-4 is secreted by either $CD4^+$ T cells or B cells. These results may imply that $CD4^+$ T cells preserve their potential Th2 capacity after MN and that $CD8^+$ T cells function more effectively than $CD4^+$ T cells in the production of IFN-γ following re-exposure to antigens. In addition to assisting in antibody production, the T helper cell subsets also affect and direct cellular immune mechanisms in GN(Holdsworth et al. 1999). Interestingly, we found a latter increase in Th1 expression. The activation of CD8+ T cells appears to be much slower than that of the CD4+ T cell-dependent B cell response to cBSA. Previous studies have demonstrated that persistent depletion of CD8+ T cell both early and late in the course of disease prevented the development of proteinuria. In addition, it was also found that IL-4 administration prior to the onset of protienuria, rather than the early rIL-4 treatment prevented protienuria in HN, indicating the importance of CD8+ T cell in mediating the final effector phase of glomerular injury in HN(Penny et al., 1998; Spicer et al., 2001). This increase in Th1 cells may play a role in the counter-regulation of the Th2 response and implies an association between the characteristics of the disease process and the kinetics of the Th1/Th2 responses during MN. Taken together, these findings support that the functional dichotomy between the Th1 and Th2 lymphocyte subsets play a regulatory role in the disease and both the humoral and cell mediated immune responses may participate in the pathogenesis of MN.

T1/T2 TG mice still has advantages of stable and stronger signal expression, a wider time window for detection, lack of requirement of restimulation or permeabilization, and possible isolation of viable cells of given Th phenotypes. Thus, these T1/T2 TG mice are useful in providing a feasible and direct *in vivo* monitoring system for dissecting the changes in proportions of pathogenic T cells during the pathogenic or therapeutic processes using flow cytometry with surface immunofluorescent staining(Hsieh et al., 2000; Hung et al., 2005; Sung et al., 2004).

A progressive increase in Th2 cells were observed in splenocytes as well as in peripheral blood and kidney cells. In addition, the Th2 prone IgG1 immunoglobulin subclass was also noted in the serum and kidneys. Antigen-specific re-stimulation testing of cytokine production and intracellular cytokine staining revealed an IL-4 prominent immune response. Cytokine-related gene expression in the kidneys and splenocytes demonstrated enhancement of pro-inflammatory cytokines as well as Th1/Th2 cytokines. In conclusion, our data demonstrates that both peripheral and renal immune responses are strongly polarized toward the Th2 type immune response in the process of cBSA-induced MN. The T1/T2 double transgenic mice could provide an available model to dissect the complex kinetic changes of adaptive immunity in GN and promises a potential strategy for the development of immunotherapeutic strategies against MN in the future.

2.3 Immunomodulatory treatment using HO-1 induction for cBSA-induced MN

The central pathogenesis participating in MN involves the formation of subepithelial immune deposits and the subsequent production of glomerular injury through complement-dependent processes, oxidative stress, and inflammatory cytokines, resulting in the development of massive proteinuria (Nangaku et al. 2005). However, the appropriate treatment of patients with MN is still open to debate. Recently, HO-1 has been noted to have biological effects for protective and therapeutic use (Ryter et al., 2006; Kirkby & Adin, 2006). On the other hand, presently available immunosuppressive therapies are not always effective and often have many persistent side effects (Glassock, 2004). Therefore, whether HO-1 induction could be applied in MN treatment was discussed.

2.3.1 Heme oxygenase-1

Heme oxygenase (HO) is the rate-limiting enzyme that degrades heme into carbon monoxide (CO), ferritin, and biliverdin (Tracz et al., 2007a). Three distinct HO enzymes have been identified: HO-1, HO-2, and HO-3. The HO-1 identified as an enzyme in microsomes and was described as a new member of the cytochrome p450 family and later found to be a rapidly and transiently inducible mono-oxygenase. The inducible HO-1 is expressed in response to various stimuli, such as hydrogen peroxide, heat, heavy metal ions, hyperoxide, endotoxin, and inflammatory cytokines, whereas another isoenzyme of HO, HO-2, is constitutively expressed and abundant in testes, brain, liver and vasculature. HO-1 has been shown to have cytoprotective properties, as well as anti-inflammatory, anti-oxidant, anti-apoptotic, and possible immunomodulatory functions (Ryter et al., 2006; Kirkby & Adin, 2006; Nath, 2006). Using chemical inducers or genes, HO-1 has been shown to be expressed in various diseases, including respiratory diseases, cardiovascular diseases, renal disease, ocular diseases, liver injury and organ transplantation in animal models (Abraham & Kappas, 2005; Agarwal & Nick, 2000).

2.3.2 HO-1 induction for MN treatment

MN mice receiving HO-1 inducer, cobalt protoporphyrin (CoPP), treatment revealed a marked attenuation of proteinuria, hypoalbuminaemia and hypercholesterolaemia (Wu et al., 2008b). However, HO-1 inhibitor, tin protoporphyrin (SnPP), treatment did not have such therapeutic effects. The pathological severities of the kidney from MN mice receiving CoPP (MN-CoPP) were milder than those from the MN and MN receiving SnPP mice (MN-SnPP). All these three experimental groups showed positive immunofluorescent staining for IgG, with a discrete beaded appearance, along the glomerular capillary wall, but the immunofluorescence intensity in the MN-CoPP mice was lower than that in the MN-SnPP and MN mice. Immunofluorescent staining for C3 also presented as intense granular fluorescence along the glomerular capillary wall, with a similar pattern to that of IgG. Next, we checked the serum levels of anti-cBSA antibodies in mice to investigate whether the induction of HO-1 modulates the production of the immunoglobulins, causing the subsequent decrease in the immunofluorescence intensity of IgG and C3 during the course of experimental MN. Significantly elevated the levels of serum anti-cBSA antibodies were observed in the MN, MN-CoPP, and MN-SnPP groups compared with those of the control groups. Compared with control MN mice, CoPP treatment inhibited and SnPP treatment enhanced the production of immunoglobulins during MN course.

Oxidative stress plays an important pathogenic role in MN. We further assessed whether CoPP or SnPP treatment modulates the production of oxidative stress systemically in the serum and locally in kidneys. We checked the lipid peroxidation products, thiobarbituric acid reactive substances (TBARS), as markers of oxidative stress. The serum TBARS levels in MN mice were significantly higher than those in NC mice. CoPP treatment effectively attenuated the levels of TBARS to a level similar to that observed in NC mice. However, SnPP, which inhibits HO-1, did not reduce the level of oxidative stress, as indicated by the higher levels of serum TBARS observed in MN mice treated with SnPP. TBARS in the kidney displayed a similar pattern to that observed in serum. These findings suggest that HO-1 reciprocally affects both local and systemic oxidative stress. We also analyze *in situ* superoxide anion radical production by using DHE assay in fresh-frozen sections of renal tissue to more specifically and locally detect the ROS production in the kidney which revealed similar results as TBARS. Anti-apoptosis effect is another major cytoprotective function of HO-1. We then checked whether HO-1 induction alleviates cell apoptosis in MN. There were nearly undetectable TUNEL-positive cells, as an index of cell apoptosis, in normal mouse kidneys. However, increased numbers of apoptotic cells were detected in the glomeruli and surrounding tubules of MN mice. Compared with MN mice, little apoptosis was observed after MN mice were treated with CoPP, as indicated by a decrease in the number of TUNEL-positive nuclei. The administration of SnPP failed to reduce the apoptosis in kidney cells. Therefore, the anti-apoptotic effect induced by CoPP may also contribute to the therapeutic effect of HO-1 in MN mice.

In addition to its anti-oxidative and anti-apoptotic properties, HO-1 also displays well documented anti-inflammatory activity. We examined the mRNA expression of inflammation-associated cytokines in the renal cortex to answer the question of whether the induction of HO-1 modulates the inflammatory state. The expression of pro-inflammatory cytokines (IL-1β and TNF-α), Th1 cytokines (IFN-γ and IL-2), Th2 cytokines (IL-4 and IL-10), the fibrogenic cytokine transforming growth factor (TGF) β, and HO-1 were checked. Quantitative real-time PCR of the renal cortex demonstrated a consistent change in MN, with an increased expression of pro-inflammatory, Th1 cytokines and Th2 cytokines. CoPP treatment dramatically induced HO-1 expression in the kidneys, decreased the level of pro-inflammatory cytokines (IL-1β and TNF-α), and extremely increased the level of anti-inflammatory cytokine IL-10. SnPP also decreased the pro-inflammatory cytokines, but did not induce the anti-inflammatory cytokine IL-10.

Previous studies demonstrated that oxygen radical scavengers can dramatically reduce proteinuria in HN (Neale et al., 1994). In our study, MN mice treated with CoPP showed a dramatic reduction in the generation of highly reactive compounds of lipid peroxidation products, TBARS, and in proteinuria. These results indicate that oxidative stress may play a pathogenic role in damaging the glomerular filtration barrier, and could be causally related to proteinuria in experimental MN (Nangaku et al., 2005). The decrease in TUNEL-positive kidney cells after CoPP treatment observed in our study also demonstrates the anti-apoptotic properities of HO-1 (Ryter et al., 2006; Nath, 2006). The metabolic derivatives of heme produced by HO-1 (CO and biliverdin) have powerful anti-apoptotic and anti-oxidative properties. Whether the cytoprotective capacity of HO-1 in experimental MN is exerted via these byproducts requires further investigation. However, there was no prominent infiltration of inflammatory cells in our murine MN model. Therefore, we speculate that the resident kidney cells contribute to the induction of HO-1. Renal vascular and tubular structures express HO-1, particularly in response to injurious conditions (Abraham & Kappas, 2005). Glomeruli have also been reported to express HO-1 in the human kidney in various renal diseases (Morimoto et al., 2001). It seems that site-specific expression along the nephron or in the interstitium occurs due to the proximity of the stimulus. In our study, it was difficult to clarify whether the protective effect of HO-1 was mediated through systemic or local action, because both effects coexisted when the mice received CoPP treatment. Previous studies using either the exogenous administration of HO-1 by gene transfer specifically expressed in the kidney or chemical induction or transgenic mice, all demonstrated the therapeutic effects of HO-1 in different disease models (Kirkby & Adin, 2006; Agarwal & Nick, 2000). Therefore, we assume that both the systemic immunomodulatory effect, which decreases the production of immunoglobulins and subsequently or directly reduces inflammation, complement activation, oxidative stress, and apoptosis, and the local effect in the MN glomeruli contribute to the therapeutic effect of HO-1.

The HO-1 induction caused the effective attenuation of proteinuria via multiple mechanisms, including immunomodulatory, anti-oxidative, and anti-apoptotic effects. (Figure 2) CoPP-induced HO-1 suppressed the synthesis of pro-inflammatory cytokines such as IL-1β, IFN-γ and TNF-α. Furthermore, it stimulated the production of the anti-inflammatory cytokine, IL-10. It has been postulated that the degradation products of heme and its metabolic derivatives (CO in particular) might contribute to the anti-inflammatory functions of HO-1. The CO-mediated anti-inflammatory effect caused by the increasing production of IL-10 and the inhibition of TNF-α and IL-1β has been reported to be mediated through interactions with the MAPK signaling pathways (Ryter et al., 2006). In contrast, IL-10 mediates the immunosuppressive effect by an HO-1-dependent pathway (Lee & Chau, 2002). CoPP treatment also significantly reduced the production of serum anti-cBSA antibodies and glomerular immunodeposits in experimental MN mice. It has been demonstrated that the immunomodulatory effect of HO-1 is associated with regulatory T-cell *Foxp3* expression and T-cell proliferation via IL-2 (Brusko et al., 2005; Pae et al., 2004). However, the role of HO-1 in the reduction of immunoglobulin production remained unclear. The direct action of induced HO-1 against systemic inflammation, the concomitant decrease in the production of immunoglobulins, together with the subsequent decrease in immunodeposition, and other factors such as complement activation and inflammation, may all contribute to the attenuation of proteinuria. In our study, both CoPP and SnPP decreased the pro-inflammatory cytokines, but only CoPP increased the production of the anti-inflammatory cytokine IL-10. Apart from the regulation of pro-inflammatory and anti-inflammatory cytokines, CoPP also decreased the level of immunoglobulin production, complement activation, and oxidative stress, which have been proposed to be major pathogenic factors in MN. This may partially explain why only CoPP, and not SnPP, exerted a therapeutic effect in alleviating experimental MN in our study. In contrast, the deficiency of HO-1 impairs renal hemodynamics and exaggerates systemic inflammatory response in mice (Tracz et al., 2007c; Tracz et al., 2007b).

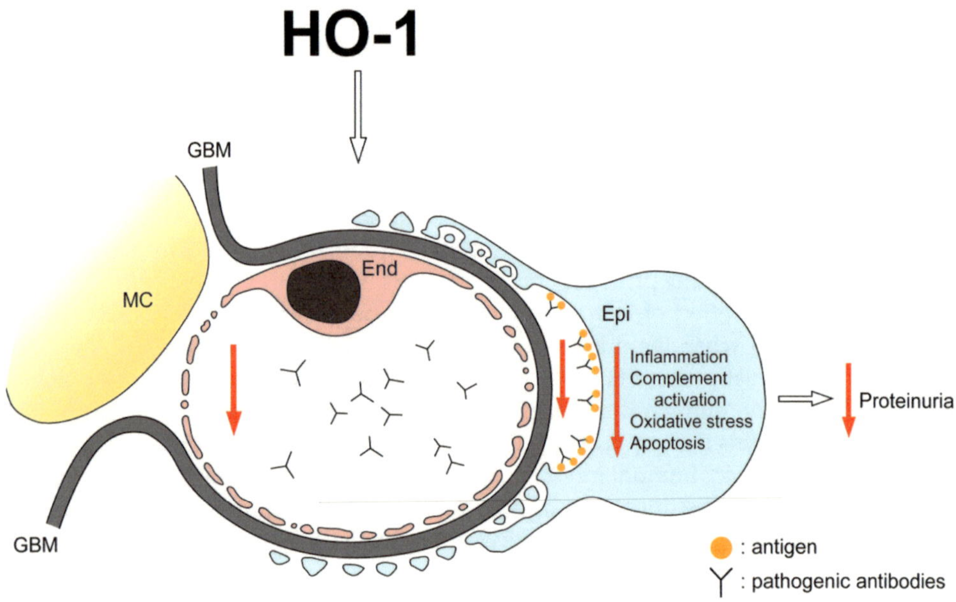

Fig. 2. Cytoprotection by HO-1 in experimental MN. HO-1 induction therapy decreased immunoglobulin production and subsequently or directly attenuated inflammation, complement activation, oxidative stress, and apoptosis in MN glomeruli, all of which contributed to the amelioration of disease severity in MN mice. End, glomerular endothelial cell; Epi, glomerular epithelial cell; GBM, glomerular basement membrane; MC, mesangial cell.

The development of ideal therapeutic agents that can effectively and specifically blunt the pathogenic pathway in MN is an important issue. This is the first study to demonstrate that the endogenous induction of HO-1 significantly ameliorates proteinuria and the severity of pathology in MN mice. The induction of HO-1 suppressed the production and deposition of immune complexes in the kidney. Both systemic and local oxidative stresses were reduced in the sera and kidneys of CoPP-treated MN mice compared with those of MN mice or SnPP-treated MN mice. Apoptosis in the kidney cells was also reduced after treatment with CoPP. Conversely, decreased pro-inflammatory cytokine expression and increased anti-inflammatory cytokine expression were observed in the kidneys after treatment with CoPP. The efficient administration of CoPP once weekly, which can significantly block the key inflammatory, oxidative, and immunomodulatory pathogenesis pathways of MN, make HO-1-inducing therapeutic regimens a plausible new option for future therapeutic interventions in MN. However, there are still no drugs available that have been specifically developed to induce HO-1 and can be applied to human clinical use. Although the therapeutic effects of HO-1 have been demonstrated in several diseases in animal models, including our experimental MN model, whether it can be applied to humans requires further investigation.

Our results suggest that HO-1 induction therapy ameliorates experimental MN via multiple pathways, including anti-oxidative, anti-apoptotic, and immunomodulatory effects. HO-1-inducing regimens will probably be considered a new therapeutic intervention for MN in the future.

3. Conclusion

Murine model of MN induced by cBSA exhibited great similarity in clinical and pathological features to human MN disease. This murine model will provide a valuable means to investigate the pathogenesis of MN and will help in the development of preventive and therapeutic strategies for MN. Both peripheral and renal immune responses are strongly polarized toward the Th2 type immune response in the process of cBSA-induced MN. The T1/T2 double transgenic mice could provide an available model to dissect the complex kinetic changes of adaptive immunity in GN and promises a potential strategy for the development of immunotherapeutic strategies against MN in the future. Finally, HO-1 induction therapy ameliorates experimental MN via multiple pathways, including anti-oxidative, anti-apoptotic, and immunomodulatory effects. HO-1-inducing regimens will probably be considered a new therapeutic intervention for MN in the future.

4. Acknowledgment

This work was supported by the National Science Council of Taiwan (NSC 97-2314-B-016-008-MY3) and a grant for C-C Wu by the Tri-Service General Hospital (TSGH-C100-031).

5. References

Abbas, A.K.; Murphy, K.M. & Sher, A. (1996) Functional diversity of helper T lymphocytes. *Nature*, 383, 787-793.

Abraham, N.G. & Kappas, A. (2005) Heme oxygenase and the cardiovascular-renal system. *Free Radic.Biol.Med.*, 39, 1-25.

Agarwal, A. & Nick, H.S. (2000) Renal response to tissue injury: lessons from heme oxygenase-1 GeneAblation and expression. *J.Am.Soc.Nephrol.*, 11, 965-973.

Bass, P.S.; Drake, A.F. & Wang, Y. et al. (1990) Cationization of bovine serum albumin alters its conformation as well as its charge. *Lab Invest*, 62, 185-188.

Border, W.A.; Ward, H.J. & Kamil, E.S. et al. (1982) Induction of membranous nephropathy in rabbits by administration of an exogenous cationic antigen. *J.Clin.Invest*, 69, 451-461.

Breysse, P.; Couser, W.G. & Alpers, C.E. et al. (1994) Membranous nephropathy and formaldehyde exposure. *Ann.Intern.Med.*, 120, 396-397.

Brusko, T.M.; Wasserfall, C.H., & Agarwal, A. et al. (2005) An integral role for heme oxygenase-1 and carbon monoxide in maintaining peripheral tolerance by CD4+CD25+ regulatory T cells. *J.Immunol.*, 174, 5181-5186.

Cattran, D. (2005) Management of membranous nephropathy: when and what for treatment. *J.Am.Soc.Nephrol.*, 16, 1188-1194.

Cattran, D.C. (2001) Idiopathic membranous glomerulonephritis. *Kidney Int.*, 59, 1983-1994.

Chadban, S.J. & Atkins, R.C. (2005) Glomerulonephritis. *Lancet*, 365, 1797-1806.

Chen, J.S.; Chen, A. & Chang, L.C. et al. (2004) Mouse model of membranous nephropathy induced by cationic bovine serum albumin: antigen dose-response relations and strain differences. *Nephrol.Dial.Transplant.*, 19, 2721-2728.

Cohen, C.D.; Calvaresi, N. & Armelloni, S. et al. (2005) CD20-positive infiltrates in human membranous glomerulonephritis. *J.Nephrol.*, 18, 328-333.

Couser, W.G. & Abrass, C.K. (1988) Pathogenesis of membranous nephropathy. *Annu.Rev.Med.*, 39, 517-530.

Couser, W.G. & Nangaku, M. (2006) Cellular and molecular biology of membranous nephropathy. *J.Nephrol.*, 19, 699-705.

Couser, W.G.; Steinmuller, D.R. & Stilmant, M.M. et al. (1978) Experimental glomerulonephritis in the isolated perfused rat kidney. *J.Clin.Invest*, 62, 1275-1287.

Cunningham, P.N. & Quigg, R.J. (2005) Contrasting roles of complement activation and its regulation in membranous nephropathy. *J.Am.Soc.Nephrol.*, 16, 1214-1222.

Dixon, F.J.; Feldman,J.D. & Vazquez,J.J. (1961) Experimental glomerulonephritis. The pathogenesis of a laboratory model resembling the spectrum of human glomerulonephritis. *J.Exp.Med.*, 113, 899-920.

Doi, T.; Kanatsu, K. & Mayumi, M. et al. (1991) Analysis of IgG immune complexes in sera from patients with membranous nephropathy: role of IgG4 subclass and low-avidity antibodies. *Nephron*, 57, 131-136.

Doi, T.; Mayumi, M. & Kanatsu, K. et al. (1984) Distribution of IgG subclasses in membranous nephropathy. *Clin.Exp.Immunol.*, 58, 57-62.

Dubuf-Vereijken, P.W.; Branten, A.J. & Wetzels, J.F. (2005) Idiopathic membranous nephropathy: outline and rationale of a treatment strategy. *Am.J.Kidney Dis.*, 46, 1012-1029.

Edgington, T.S.; Glassock, R.J. & Dixon, F.J. (1968) Autologous immune complex nephritis induced with renal tubular antigen. I. Identification and isolation of the pathogenetic antigen. *J.Exp.Med.*, 127, 555-572.

Edgington, T.S.; Glassock, R.J. & Dixon, F.J. (1967) Autologous immune-complex pathogenesis of experimental allergic glomerulonephritis. *Science*, 155, 1432-1434.

Farquhar, M.G.; Saito,A. & Kerjaschki, D. et al. (1995) The Heymann nephritis antigenic complex: megalin (gp330) and RAP. *J.Am.Soc.Nephrol.*, 6, 35-47.

Fleuren, G.; Grond, J. & Hoedemaeker, P.J. (1980) In situ formation of subepithelial glomerular immune complexes in passive serum sickness. *Kidney Int.*, 17, 631-637.

Fleuren, G.J.; Vd, L.R. & Greben, H.A. et al. (1978) Experimental glomerulonephritis in the rat induced by antibodies directed against tubular antigens. IV. Investigations into the pathogenesis of the model. *Lab Invest*, 38, 496-501.

Glassock, R.J. (2004) The treatment of idiopathic membranous nephropathy: a dilemma or a conundrum? *Am.J.Kidney Dis.*, 44, 562-566.

Haas, M. (1994) IgG subclass deposits in glomeruli of lupus and nonlupus membranous nephropathies. *Am.J.Kidney Dis.*, 23, 358-364.

Heymann, W.; Hackel,d. B. & Harwood,S. et al. (1959) Production of nephrotic syndrome in rats by Freund's adjuvants and rat kidney suspensions. *Proc.Soc.Exp.Biol.Med.*, 100, 660-664.

Heymann, W.; Hunter, J.L. & Hackel, D.B. (1962) Experimental auto-immune nephrosis in rats: III. *J.Immunol.*, 88, 135-141.

Hirayama, K.; Ebihara, I. & Yamamoto, S. et al. (2002) Predominance of type-2 immune response in idiopathic membranous nephropathy. Cytoplasmic cytokine analysis. *Nephron*, 91, 255-261.

Holdsworth, S.R.; Kitching, A.R. & Tipping, P.G. (1999) Th1 and Th2 T helper cell subsets affect patterns of injury and outcomes in glomerulonephritis. *Kidney Int.*, 55, 1198-1216.

Honkanen, E.; Tornroth, T. & Gronhagen-Riska, C. (1992) Natural history, clinical course and morphological evolution of membranous nephropathy. *Nephrol.Dial.Transplant.*, 7 Suppl 1, 35-41.

Hsieh, S.; Chen, N. & Tarbell, K. et al. (2000) Transgenic mice expressing surface markers for IFN-gamma and IL-4 producing cells. *Mol.Immunol.*, 37, 281-293.

Hung, J.T.; Liao, J.H. & Lin, Y.C. et al. (2005) Immunopathogenic role of TH1 cells in autoimmune diabetes: evidence from a T1 and T2 doubly transgenic non-obese diabetic mouse model. *J.Autoimmun.*, 25, 181-192.

Imai, H.; Hamai, K. & Komatsuda, A. et al. (1997) IgG subclasses in patients with membranoproliferative glomerulonephritis, membranous nephropathy, and lupus nephritis. *Kidney Int.*, 51, 270-276.

Iskandar, S.S.; Falk, R.J. & Jennette, J.C. (1992) Clinical and pathologic features of fibrillary glomerulonephritis. *Kidney Int.*, 42, 1401-1407.

Kelly, C.J.; Frishberg, Y. & Gold, D.P. (1998) An appraisal of T cell subsets and the potential for autoimmune injury. *Kidney Int.*, 53, 1574-1584.

Kerjaschki, D. (2004) Pathomechanisms and molecular basis of membranous glomerulopathy. *Lancet*, 364, 1194-1196.

Kerjaschki, D. & Farquhar, M.G. (1982) The pathogenic antigen of Heymann nephritis is a membrane glycoprotein of the renal proximal tubule brush border. *Proc.Natl.Acad.Sci.U.S.A*, 79, 5557-5561.

Kerjaschki, D. & Farquhar, M.G. (1983) Immunocytochemical localization of the Heymann nephritis antigen (GP330) in glomerular epithelial cells of normal Lewis rats. *J.Exp.Med.*, 157, 667-686.

Kirkby, K.A. & Adin, C.A. (2006) Products of heme oxygenase and their potential therapeutic applications. *Am.J.Physiol Renal Physiol*, 290, F563-F571.

Kuroki, A.; Iyoda, M. & Shibata, T. et al. (2005) Th2 cytokines increase and stimulate B cells to produce IgG4 in idiopathic membranous nephropathy. *Kidney Int.*, 68, 302-310.

Lee, T.S. & Chau, L.Y. (2002) Heme oxygenase-1 mediates the anti-inflammatory effect of interleukin-10 in mice. *Nat.Med.*, 8, 240-246.

Makker, S.P. & Singh, A.K. (1984) Characterization of the antigen (gp600) of Heymann nephritis. *Lab Invest*, 50, 287-293.

Masutani, K.; Taniguchi, M. & Nakashima, H. et al. (2004) Up-regulated interleukin-4 production by peripheral T-helper cells in idiopathic membranous nephropathy. *Nephrol.Dial.Transplant.*, 19, 580-586.

Morimoto, K.; Ohta, K. & Yachie, A. el al. (2001) Cytoprotective role of heme oxygenase (HO)-1 in human kidney with various renal diseases. *Kidney Int.*, 60, 1858-1866.

Mosmann, T.R. & Coffman, R.L. (1989) Heterogeneity of cytokine secretion patterns and functions of helper T cells. *Adv.Immunol.*, 46, 111-147.

Mosmann, T.R. & Sad, S. (1996) The expanding universe of T-cell subsets: Th1, Th2 and more. *Immunol.Today*, 17, 138-146.

Nangaku, M. & Couser, W.G. (2005) Mechanisms of immune-deposit formation and the mediation of immune renal injury. *Clin.Exp.Nephrol.*, 9, 183-191.

Nangaku, M.; Shankland, S.J. & Couser, W.G. (2005) Cellular response to injury in membranous nephropathy. *J.Am.Soc.Nephrol.*, 16, 1195-1204.

Nash, A.S.; Mohammed, N.A. & Wright, N.G. (1990) Experimental immune complex glomerulonephritis and the nephrotic syndrome in cats immunised with cationised bovine serum albumin. *Res.Vet.Sci.*, 49, 370-372.

Nath, K.A. (2006) Heme oxygenase-1: a provenance for cytoprotective pathways in the kidney and other tissues. *Kidney Int.*, 70, 432-443.

Neale, T.J.; Ojha, P.P. & Exner, M. el al. (1994) Proteinuria in passive Heymann nephritis is associated with lipid peroxidation and formation of adducts on type IV collagen. *J.Clin.Invest*, 94, 1577-1584.

Oliveira, D.B. (1998) Membranous nephropathy: an IgG4-mediated disease. *Lancet*, 351, 670-671.

Pae, H.O.; Oh, G.S. & Choi, B.M. el al. (2004) Carbon monoxide produced by heme oxygenase-1 suppresses T cell proliferation via inhibition of IL-2 production. *J.Immunol.*, 172, 4744-4751.

Penny, M.J.; Boyd, R.A. & Hall, B.M. (1997) Role of T cells in the mediation of Heymann nephritis. ii. Identification of Th1 and cytotoxic cells in glomeruli. *Kidney Int.*, 51, 1059-1068.

Penny, M.J.; Boyd, R.A. & Hall, B.M. (1998) Permanent CD8(+) T cell depletion prevents proteinuria in active Heymann nephritis. *J.Exp.Med.*, 188, 1775-1784.

Perna, A.; Schieppati, A. & Zamora, J. el al. (2004) Immunosuppressive treatment for idiopathic membranous nephropathy: a systematic review. *Am.J.Kidney Dis.*, 44, 385-401.

Piccoli, A.; Pillon, L., & Passerini, P. el al. (1994) Therapy for idiopathic membranous nephropathy: tailoring the choice by decision analysis. *Kidney Int.*, 45, 1193-1202.

Polenakovik, M.H. & Grcevska, L. (1999) Treatment and long-term follow-up of patients with stage II to III idiopathic membranous nephropathy. *Am.J.Kidney Dis.*, 34, 911-917.

Ponticelli, C. (1987) Treatment of idiopathic membranous nephropathy. *Nephron*, 46, 402-403.

Ponticelli, C. & Passerini, P. (1990) The natural history and therapy of idiopathic membranous nephropathy. *Nephrol.Dial.Transplant.*, 5 Suppl 1, 37-41.

Ponticelli, C. & Passerini, P. (1991) Conventional treatment of idiopathic nephrotic syndrome and membranous nephropathy in adults. *Clin.Nephrol.*, 35 Suppl 1, S16-S21.

Ponticelli, C.; Zucchelli, P. & Passerini, P. (1987) Therapy of idiopathic membranous nephropathy. *Springer Semin.Immunopathol.*, 9, 431-440.

Quigg, R.J. (2003) Why study membranous nephropathy in rats? *Kidney Int.*, 64, 2318-2319.

Quiza, C.G.; Leenaerts, P.L. & Hall, B.M. (1992) The role of T cells in the mediation of glomerular injury in Heymann's nephritis in the rat. *Int.Immunol.*, 4, 423-432.

Ravnskov, U. (1998) The subepithelial formation of immune complexes in membranous glomerulonephritis may be harmless and secondary to toxic or allergic factors. *Scand.J.Immunol.*, 48, 469-474.

Remuzzi, G.; Chiurchiu, C. & Abbate, M. el al. (2002) Rituximab for idiopathic membranous nephropathy. *Lancet*, 360, 923-924.

Ring, G.H. & Lakkis, F.G. (1998) T lymphocyte-derived cytokines in experimental glomerulonephritis: testing the Th1/Th2 hypothesis. *Nephrol.Dial.Transplant.*, 13, 1101-1103.

Roberts, J.L.; Wyatt, R.J. & Schwartz, M.M. el al. (1983) Differential characteristics of immune-bound antibodies in diffuse proliferative and membranous forms of lupus glomerulonephritis. *Clin.Immunol.Immunopathol.*, 29, 223-241.

Ronco, P. & Debiec, H. (2007a) Podocyte antigens and glomerular disease. *Nephron Exp.Nephrol.*, 107, e41-e46.

Ronco, P. & Debiec, H. (2007b) Target antigens and nephritogenic antibodies in membranous nephropathy: of rats and men. *Semin.Immunopathol.*, 29, 445-458.

Ronco, P. & Debiec, H. (2006) New insights into the pathogenesis of membranous glomerulonephritis. *Curr.Opin.Nephrol.Hypertens.*, 15, 258-263.

Ronco, P. & Debiec, H. (2005) Molecular pathomechanisms of membranous nephropathy: from Heymann nephritis to alloimmunization. *J.Am.Soc.Nephrol.*, 16, 1205-1213.

Rosen, S. (1971) Membranous glomerulonephritis: current status. *Hum.Pathol.*, 2, 209-231.

Ruggenenti, P.; Chiurchiu, C. & Brusegan, V. et al. (2003) Rituximab in idiopathic membranous nephropathy: a one-year prospective study. *J.Am.Soc.Nephrol.*, 14, 1851-1857.

Ryter, S.W.; Alam, J. & Choi, A.M. (2006) Heme oxygenase-1/carbon monoxide: from basic science to therapeutic applications. *Physiol Rev.*, 86, 583-650.

Salant, D.J.; Adler, S. & Darby, C. et al. (1985) Influence of antigen distribution on the mediation of immunological glomerular injury. *Kidney Int.*, 27, 938-950.

Salant, D.J.; Quigg, R.J. & Cybulsky, A.V. (1989) Heymann nephritis: mechanisms of renal injury. *Kidney Int.*, 35, 976-984.

Schena, F.P. (1999) Cytokine network and resident renal cells in glomerular diseases. *Nephrol.Dial.Transplant.*, 14 Suppl 1, 22-26.

Spicer, S.T.; Ha, H. & Boyd, R.A. et al. (2001) Il-4 therapy prevents the development of proteinuria in active Heymann nephritis by inhibition of Tc1 cells. *J.Immunol.*, 167, 3725-3733.

Sung, H.H.; Juang, J.H. & Lin, Y.C. et al. (2004) Transgenic expression of decoy receptor 3 protects islets from spontaneous and chemical-induced autoimmune destruction in nonobese diabetic mice. *J.Exp.Med.*, 199, 1143-1151.

Tipping, P.G. & Kitching, A.R. (2005) Glomerulonephritis, Th1 and Th2: what's new? *Clin.Exp.Immunol.*, 142, 207-215.

Tracz, M.J.; Alam, J. & Nath, K.A. (2007a) Physiology and pathophysiology of heme: implications for kidney disease. *J.Am.Soc.Nephrol.*, 18, 414-420.

Tracz, M.J.; Juncos, J.P. & Croatt, A.J. et al. (2007b) Deficiency of heme oxygenase-1 impairs renal hemodynamics and exaggerates systemic inflammatory responses to renal ischemia. *Kidney Int.*, 72, 1073-1080.

Tracz, M.J.; Juncos, J.P. & Grande, J.P. et al. (2007c) Renal hemodynamic, inflammatory, and apoptotic responses to lipopolysaccharide in HO-1-/- mice. *Am.J.Pathol.*, 170, 1820-1830.

Van Damme, B.J.; Fleuren, G.J. & Bakker, W.W. et al. (1978) Experimental glomerulonephritis in the rat induced by antibodies directed against tubular antigens. V. Fixed glomerular antigens in the pathogenesis of heterologous immune complex glomerulonephritis. *Lab Invest*, 38, 502-510.

Wasserstein, A.G. (1997) Membranous glomerulonephritis. *J.Am.Soc.Nephrol.*, 8, 664-674.

Wright, N.G.; Mohammed, N.A. & Eckersall, P.D. et al. (1985) Experimental immune complex glomerulonephritis in dogs receiving cationized bovine serum albumin. *Res.Vet.Sci.*, 38, 322-328.

Wu, C.C.; Chen, J.S. & Chen, S.J. et al. (2007) Kinetics of adaptive immunity to cationic bovine serum albumin-induced membranous nephropathy. *Kidney Int.*, 72, 831-840.

Wu, C.C.; Chen, J.S. & Lin, S.H. et al. (2008a) Experimental model of membranous nephropathy in mice: sequence of histological and biochemical events. *Lab Anim*, 42, 350-359.

Wu, C.C.; Lu, K.C. & Chen, J.S. et al. (2008b) HO-1 induction ameliorates experimental murine membranous nephropathy: anti-oxidative, anti-apoptotic and immunomodulatory effects. *Nephrol.Dial.Transplant.*, 23, 3082-3090.

Yang, V.C. & Langer, R. (1985) pH-dependent binding analysis, a new and rapid method for isoelectric point estimation. *Anal.Biochem.*, 147, 148-155.

6

Glomerular Injury in Domestic Cats and the Iberian Lynx (Lynx pardinus): A Comparative Review

María Ángeles Jiménez, Belén Sánchez and Laura Peña
Facultad de Veterinaria, Universidad Complutense de Madrid
Spain

1. Introduction

Glomerular lesions, in particular glomerulonephritis, were once considered rare in the domestic cat (Nash et al, 1979; Slawson & Lewis, 1979), but in the past decades, the diagnosis of these lesions has increased substantially possibly due to a better understanding and awareness of these diseases (DiBartola & Rutgers, 1994; Grant Maxie & Newman, 2007). Most of the feline glomerulonephritis reported to date are of immune-complex origin (Slawson & Lewis, 1979; Newman et al, 2007; Grant Maxie & Newman, 2007) although some fibrillary glomerulopathies such as glomerular amyloidosis (Boyce et al, 1984; DiBartola et al, 1985, 1986, Gruys 2004; Newman et al, 2007; Grant Maxie & Newman, 2007) and to lesser extent noncongophilic glomerulopathies (Nakamura et al, 1996; Cavana et al, 2008) are also described.

The etiology is frequently elusive, though many associations with infectious and other diseases have been identified (Newman et al, 2007; Grant Maxie & Newman, 2007). In particular, association between certain viral diseases such as feline leukemia, feline immunodeficiency virus and feline infectious peritonitis are known to course with some degree of glomerular injury (Glick et al, 1978; Hayasi et al, 1982; Newman et al, 2007). Several reports also relate certain neoplasms with the presence of glomerular injury (Hayasi et al, 1982; Newman et al, 2007).

Primary glomerular diseases severe enough to cause the nephrotic syndrome are relatively uncommon in the domestic cat (Schwartz, 2007, as cited in Cavana et al, 2008) and in general lack relevance in most non-domestic felids (Newkirk et al, 2010). However, once renal failure ensues, the outcome is fatal and treatment is only palliative (Nash et al, 1979; DiBartola & Rutgers, 1994). Knowledge on the pathogenesis, type of injury, origin and similarities to human counterparts enables a better understanding of the disease which may permit earlier detection or its prevention. This becomes of even greater importance when considering endangered species such as the Iberian lynx (*Lynx pardinus*), with less than 200 individuals remaining in the wild and captivity (Guzman et al, 2002). The survival of a single animal becomes crucial.

The Iberian lynx is a large felid that has inhabited the Iberian Peninsula for over centuries (Garcia et al, 1997; García & Arsuaga, 1998). Nowadays this species is rated as "critically endangered" (Nowel & Jackson, 1996) and remaining samples are confined to two isolated

populations in southwestern Spain (Palomares et al, 2000; Guzmán et al, 2002; Rodriguez & Delibes, 2002). The population decline was exacerbated towards the mid twentieth century mainly because of habitat loss (Palomares et al, 1991) and lack of adequate prey (Moreno & Villafuerte, 1995). Studies have also shown a serious compromise of genetic variability in this species mostly due to inbreeding (Johnson et al, 2004).
Recovery and conservation efforts are at hand and continuous research on the ecology, welfare, natural pathogens or diseases regarding these animals is crucial for survival efforts. With this in mind, a histopathological survey was conducted through 1998-2006 in which glomerular lesions in a high number of the surveyed population were detected. This led to a thorough investigation of these lesions and how they could affect the overall survival of the species (Jiménez et al, 2008).

2. Glomerular disease in the domestic cat

Several types of glomerular injury have been reported in cats, all of which correspond to a certain extent with a human counterpart of the disease. The most frequent are the immune-mediated glomerulonephritis (membranous glomerulonephritis and membranoproliferative glomerulonephritis) and rarely have some fibrillary glomerulopathies been described.
Immune-mediated mechanisms causing glomerulonephritis involve deposition of soluble immune complexes within glomeruli or the formation of antibodies directed against antigens within the glomerular basement membranes (Valaitis, 2002; Newman et al, 2007; Grant Maxie & Newman, 2007). The former is the most frequent mechanism described in the cat and in domestic animals in general (Nash, et al, 1979; DiBartola & Rutgers, 1994; Newman et al, 2007). Immune-complex glomerulonephritis is usually associated with situations of prolonged antigenemia such as infectious diseases or neoplastic processes (Newman et al, 2007).
Glomerular diseases are classified according to the histopathologic and ultrastructural morphology of the glomeruli. In most cases disease is progressive and may secondarily affect the entire nephron (Valaitis, 2002; Grant Maxie & Newman, 2007). Most progress to chronic interstitial nephritis. In chronic terminal stages, the morphological aspect of the lesions may overlap and determination of the primary injury is hindered (Valaitis, 2002; Grant Maxie & Newman et al, 2007).
The clinical presentation courses with the nephrotic syndrome, end-stage renal disease or both (DiBartola & Rutgers, 1994). The former is characterized by subcutaneous edema, ascites, proteinuria, hypercholesterolemia, and hypoalbuminemia. Mild azotemia may be present. Proteinuria and moderate to marked azotemia together with polydipsia, polyuria or oliguria, vomiting and anorexia are more common with end-stage renal disease (DiBartola & Rutgers, 1994).

2.1 Membranous glomerulonephritis

The most common glomerular lesion in the domestic cat is diffuse membranous glomerulonephritis (Nash et al, 1979; Slauson & Lewis, 1979; Newman et al, 2007; Grant Maxie & Newman, 2007). Numerous studies have related the presence of this disease with renal failure and the nephrotic syndrome (Nash et al, 1979; Slauson & Lewis, 1979; DiBartola & Rutgers, 1994). Membranous glomerulonephritis is characterized by a segmental to diffuse thickening of the glomerular capillary basement membranes caused by subepithelial and intramembranous immunoglobulin deposits. These deposits are eventually encompassed by the capillary basement membranes and reabsorbed (Valaitis, 2002; Newman et al, 2007). If antigenemia persists, glomerular capillary basement membranes are damaged beyond repair and undergo sclerosis. In this phase, renal basement membrane type IV collagen is replaced by abundant type III collagen (Martinez-Hernandez & Menta, 1983; Haralson et al, 1987). The membranes are no longer able to reabsorb immune deposits and the glomerulus terminally undergoes fibrosis with ultimate loss of the nephron (Valaitis, 2002). It is not uncommon to find various stages of membranous glomerular damage and sclerosis in a single case, particularly in those classified as most severe (Valaitis, 2002; Newman et al, 2007).

In the domestic cat, the immunoglobulin (Ig) deposits are frequently IgG or IgM and only rarely IgA (Newman et al, 2007). The location, composition and granular deposition of these deposits suggest that they are of immune-complex origin (DiBartola & Rutgers, 1994, Newman et al, 2007; Grant Maxie & Newman, 2007). However, in the majority of cases the type of antigen is not identified and therefore the disease is considered idiopathic and primary (Nash et al, 1979; Grant Maxie & Newman et al, 2007).

Membranous glomerulonephritis in the cat is usually progressive, age related and generally sufficiently slow for the animals to live a relatively normal life, even without treatment (Nash et al, 1979). Although, once renal failure ensues the outcome is fatal and treatment options are only palliative (Nash et al, 1979; DiBartola & Rutgers, 1994).

2.2 Membranoproliferative glomerulonephrits

Membranoproliferative glomerulonephritis is also a chronic, progressive renal disease, characterized by mesangial hypercellularity and diffuse thickening of capillary basement membranes and mesangium (Valaitis, 2002; Newman et al, 2007). According to the World Health Organization classifications of human glomerular diseases, there are three subtypes based on morphologic appearance. The changes that permit classification are not perceivable with light microscopy and have to be detected by immunofluorescence, immunohistochemistry or electron microscopy. Type I is characterized by subendothelial immune deposits in a granular pattern of immunogloulins and complement components such as C3. Type II is characterized by intramembranous dense deposits of unknown composition and smaller quantities of complement. This type is also known as "dense deposit disease" and is suspected to be associated with autoimmunity. Type III is characterized by subendothelial and subepithelial deposits (Newman et al, 2007).

All three subtypes have been reported in domestic animals including cats (Newman et al, 2007). Type I is rare in the cat (Asano et al, 2008) and type III has only been reported in the cat (Inoue et al, 2001). Asano and collaborators (2008) described a single case of type I membranoproliferative glomerulonephritis in a young male Japanese domestic cat with nephrotic syndrome. Histopathology of a biopsy sample revealed mesangial hypercellularity with increased matrix and thickening of glomerular capillary basement membranes consistent with membranoproliferative glomerulonephritis. Double contours of glomerular capillary walls were also observed. Subendothelial and rare intramembranous dense deposits were identified ultrastructurally. No underlying infectious or other diseases were identified in this case.

Type III membranous glomerulonephritis has not been reported in domestic animals except rarely in the cat. Inoue and collaborators (2001) described a case of atypical membranous glomerulonephritis consistent with the type III category of the human classification system.

The case involved a two year old Japanese domestic cat with clinical evidence of glomerular injury and renal failure. Granular deposits of IgG and C3 in capillary walls and mesangium were identified by immunohistochemistry and subepithelial, subendothelial and intramembranous depostis were noted by electron microscopy. Both antibodies against feline infectious peritonitis and feline immunodeficiency viruses were detected in this animal however the relationship between infection and the renal lesions was unclear (Inoue K et al, 2001). Additionally, in 1978 a case series of 63 domestic cats revealed that one third of animals had glomerulonephritis possibly related to feline leukemia virus infection and associated viral hematopoietic neoplasms (Glick et al, 1978). The authors did not give a morphologic classification of the type of glomerulonephritis but described diffuse mesangial proliferation on light microscopy and electron dense subendothelial, subepithelial and intramembranous deposits. This description would closely fit with a type III membranoproliferative glomerulonephritis.

2.3 Fibrillary glomerulopathies

Fibrillary glomerulopathies are a specific category of human glomerular disease in which pathologic fibrillary materials are observed in the glomerulus (Korbert et al, 1994; Schwartz, 2007). The first step for diagnosis is to differentiate amyloid from other fibrillary deposits with either specific stains such as Congo red or ultrastructural evaluation (Korbert et al, 1994). To date glomerular amyloidosis, collagenofibrotic glomerulopathy and noncongophilic fibrillary glomerulopathy have been described in the domestic cat (Boyce et al, 1984; DiBartola et al, 1986; Nakamura et al, 1996; Cavana et al, 2008).

2.3.1 Glomerular amyloidosis

Amyloidosis is a known cause of glomerular injury in cats (Boyce et al, 1984; DiBartola et al, 1986; Van der Linde-Sipman et al, 1996). Amyloid is an extracellular fibrillar proteinaceous substance produced after incomplete proteolysis of several soluble amyloidogenic proteins. This substance is not a distinct chemical entity despite its uniform appearance and staining properties. Ultrastructurally, amyloid is composed of continuous, nonbranching fibrils of approximately 7.5 to 10 nm in diameter. Protein fibrils have a beta-pleated sheet conformation which confers the distinctive coloration and birefringence with Congo red staining (Kumar et al, 2010).

Several clinical settings course with different types of amyloid deposition. Reactive systemic amiloidosis (or secondary amyloidosis) is the most common form in domestic animals, including the cat (Van der Linde-Sipman et al, 1997; Gruys, 2004). Amyloid is derived from serum protein AA (serum amyloid associated), and is produced in excess as a result of chronic antigenic stimulation (inflammatory, infectious or neoplastic conditions) (Obici et al, 2005; Kumar et al, 2010). Another form is immunoglobulin-derived amiloidosis (primary or AL), in which amyloid is produced from immunoglobulin light chains in plasma cell dyscrasias as a product of monoclonal B-cell proliferation (Obici et al, 2005; Merlini et al, 2011). This type of amyloidosis is uncommon in domestic animals but has been described in the dog, cat and horse (Platz et al, 1997; Kim et al, 2005).

Both AA and AL amyloidosis occur in systemic or localized forms (Merlini et al, 2011). In the cat, particularly in Siamese and Oriental breeds, systemic AA is the most frequent type of amyloid (van der Linde-Sipman et al, 1997). AA amyloid has been described in liver, spleen, lung, pancreas and kidney (van der Linde-Sipman et al, 1997; Zini et al, 2008). On the contrary, AL amyloidosis in the cat has been reported localized within neoplastic tissue of extramedullary plasmacytomas (Platz et al, 1997).

For the purpose of this chapter we will discuss only renal amyloidosis in cats. In the glomerulus, amyloid is first deposited in the mesangial area and subendothelium of glomerular capillaries and gradually accumulates compressing and obliterating endothelial and epithelial cells, and capillary loops. Amyloid is also deposited in the tubular basement membranes of the cortex and medulla. The physical presence of amyloid causes ischemia and pressure atrophy of the nephrons and susequently secondary scarring (Grant Maxie & Newman, 2007). The cat differs from other species in that amyloid is deposited predominantly in the renal papilla and outer medulla with lesser involvement of the glomeruli (Grant Maxie & Newman, 2007).

Familial secondary amyloidosis is a known entity in Abyssinian cats (Boyce et al, 1984). In these animals, amyloid can have a systemic distribution affecting organs such as thyroid glands, stomach and colon, however clinical lesions are usually only related to renal amyloidosis (DiBartola et al, 1985). Similar to other cases of secondary amyloidosis in the cat, the glomeruli are less affected than the medullary interstitium (DiBartola et al, 1985; Grant Maxie & Newman, 2007). The mode of inheritance is still undetermined but some studies suggest a likely autosomal dominant trait with incomplete penetrance (Niewold et al, 1999).

2.3.2 Collagenofibrotic glomerulonephropathy

In various human and animal renal diseases, collagen fibrils accumulate in the mesangium as a secondary change to various glomerular injuries, including chronic forms of any of the previously described glomerulonephritis (Valaitis, 2002). Fibrillar collagen such as type III collagen should not be present in the glomerulus. Glomerular capillary basement membranes contain type IV collagen which is arranged in sheets instead of fibrils. Only small amounts of type III collagen are found in the renal interstitium and interstitial capillary basement membranes (Martinez-Hernandez & Menta, 1983; Kumar et al, 2010).

Collagenofibrotic glomerulonephropathy or primary glomerular fibrosis, is a type of primary nephropathy in humans characterized by an abundant accumulation of type III collagen in the glomerular subendothelial spaces and mesangium and marked increase in serum of type III procollagen peptides (Alchi et al, 2007; Ikeda et al, 1990; Shirota et al, 1995; Nakamura et al, 1996). Collagen fibrils show characteristic structural abnormalities displaying frayed or spiral forms and marked disarray (Ikeda et al, 1990). The cause and pathogenesis are unknown and whether the disease is primary or secondary to systemic disease remains controversial (Alchi et al, 2007).

Spontaneous renal diseases with collagen fibril deposition are rare in domestic animals but some cases have been described in dogs, pigs and cats (Koeman et al, 1994; Shirota et al, 1995; Nakamura et al, 1996). Nakamura and collaborators (1996) reported a case of renal glomerular fibrosis in a young female Japanese domestic cat with clinical evidence of renal failure. Histopathology revealed that most glomeruli contained mesangial sclerosis and capillary collapse. Immunohistochemistry identified the matrix content as type III collagen. Collagen fibrils were also identified in mesangial and subendothelial areas by electron microscopy and the structural characteristics resembled human collagenofibrotic nephropathy. The cause for these collagenofibrotic glomerulopathy-like lesions was not identified and thus were considered of primary origin. This cat was serologically positive for feline leukemia virus, however the authors did not consider an association between infection and and the renal lesions. Serum concentrations of type III procollagen peptides were not evaluated in the feline case.

2.3.3 Noncongophilic fibrillary glomerulonephritis

Noncongophilic fibrillary glomerulonephritis is believed by some authors to represent a new entity among the primary glomerulonephritis (Alpers, 1992; Schwartz et al, 2002). This disease is characterized by randomly oriented, non-branching fibrils of approximately 10-22 nm diameter in the mesangial matrix and glomerular capillary basement membranes of glomeruli. Fibrils are heterogeneous and appear to be of immune complex origin. The exact chemical nature of the fibrils remains unknown (Alpers, 1992; Schwartz et al, 2002; Hvala et al, 2003).

A single case of noncongophilic fibrillary glomerulonephritis has been reported in an adult female European shorthair cat with clinical evidence of renal disease (Cavana et al, 2008). The renal lesions consisted of thickened glomerular capillary basement membranes and Bowman´s capsules. Capillary basement membranes were PAS positive and Congo red negative. Electron microscopy revealed subepithelial and subendothelial randomly scattered fibrillary deposits in the capillary basement membranes. Fibrils were larger than amyloid fibrils, measuring between 18-26 nm in diameter. Mesangial expression of IgG and IgM was detected by immunohistochemistry. The animal had a lymphoplasmacytic enteritis that was considered a possible source of immune stimulation. Concomitant systemic diseases, such as inflammatory, autoimmune or neoplastic processes, have been occasionally associated with this entity in humans (Ozawa et al, 1991; Masson et al, 1992; Hvala et al, 2003).

3. Glomerular injury in the Iberian lynx

Uncommon diseases are often described in non-domestic endangered animals, many times associated with deficient genetic diversity, captivity conditions or both. Little has been reported on health aspects of the Iberian lynx and research on this approach has become a priority for current conservation programs. There have been several cases reported of Mycobacterium bovis infection in the Iberian lynx (Briones et al, 2000; Aranaz et al, 2004). Disease was likely acquired by preying on infected animals (Briones et al, 2000). Our group also reported a generalized immune depletion apparently unrelated to infectious agents or other systemic diseases after evaluating lymphoid tissues in a representative portion of the population during the years 1998-2003 (Peña et al, 2006). A feline leukemia virus infection outbreak in the Doñana National Park population of Iberian lynxes was reported during a six month period between 2006 and 2007 (Meli et al, 2010, 2011). During this period, six animals died presumably due to the infection (Meli et al, 2011). Sequence analysis revealed homology with a strain originally identified in domestic cats suggesting co-infection between species (Meli et al, 2011; Geret et al, 2011). Prior to this time, the reported prevalence of feline leukemia virus in the same population was relatively low (Luaces et al, 2008) and evidence of lesions or death directly associated with the viral infection was unknown.

During the years 1998-2006, a thorough histopathological investigation on necropsied Iberian lynxes revealed the presence of glomerulonephritis in an important percentage of the surviving population, both free-ranging and captive (Jiménez et al, 2008). The disease was chronic, progressive and age related. None of the animals in this study died from renal disease nor was there evidence of clinical disease in the small percentage of animals with available urinalyses. Proteinuria and low urine specific gravity were detected in few of these animals which may suggest some degree of glomerular filtration impairment. However the quality and accuracy of the samples and obtainment methods were unaccounted for and thus interpretation of these results may be inexact.

Histopathology of the glomerular lesions revealed a focal, diffuse membranous glomerulonephritis of variable severity in all animals regardless of their age, sex and captivity or free-ranging conditions. The only exception was found in a 44 day old cub without any evidence of renal lesions. The number and severity of affected glomeruli varied within samples and these factors were used to evaluate the overall severity of the disease in each animal.

Glomerular changes included segmental to diffuse glomerular capillary basement membrane thickening, decreased glomerular tuft cellularity, diffusely enlarged Bowman´s epithelium, synechia between glomerular tufts and Bowman´s capsules and Bowman´s capsule fibrosis. In more severe cases the number of sclerotic glomeruli increased within the sample. Glomerular capillary basement membranes appeared thickened with PAS and silver stains (Fig.1 and Fig.2), and in sclerotic glomeruli, the mesangium stained blue with Masson´s trichromic stain revealing the presence of collagen (Fig.3). Additional changes in the renal parenchyma included interstitial lymphoplasmacytic aggregates and fibrosis (Fig.3), and intratubular mineralization and protein casts. Both fibrosis and inflammation were significantly associated with severity and together with the glomerular sclerosis, were considered secondary to the membranous glomerulonephritis and not primary changes.

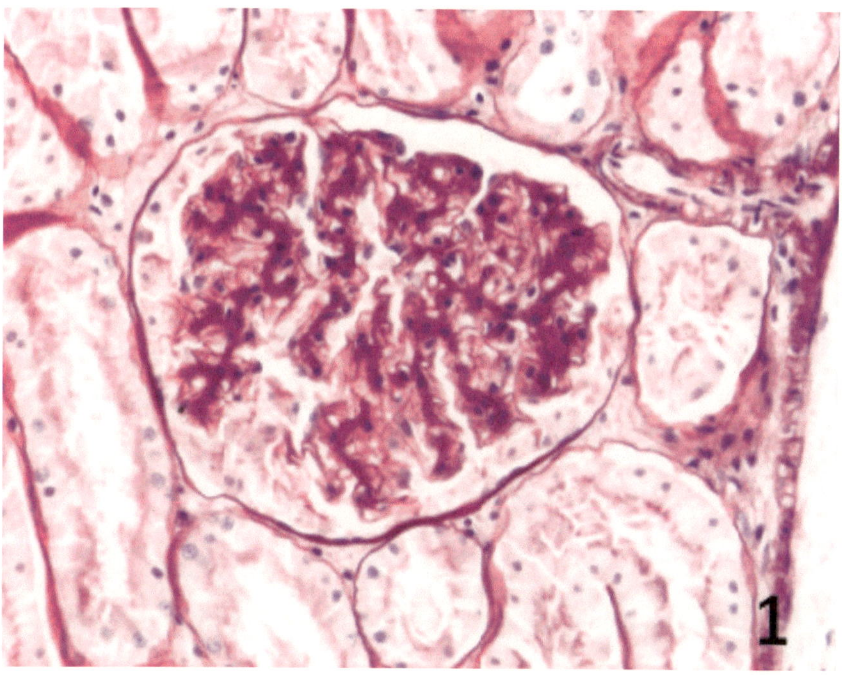

Fig. 1. Iberian Lynx. Kidney. PAS stain. Glomerulus with diffusely thickened capillary basement membranes, 20X

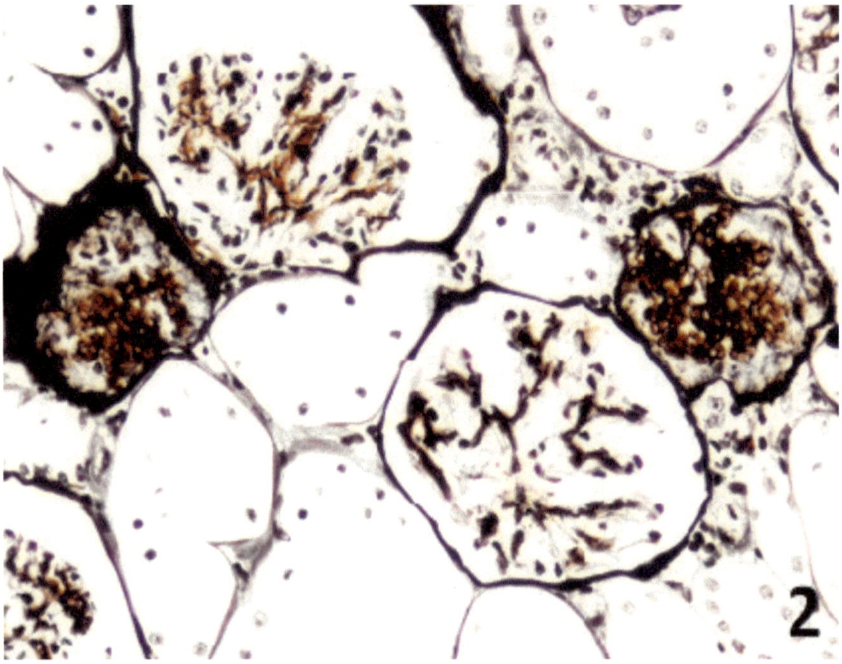

Fig. 2. Silver stain of glomeruli with membranous glomerulonephritis and glomerulosclerosis, 20X

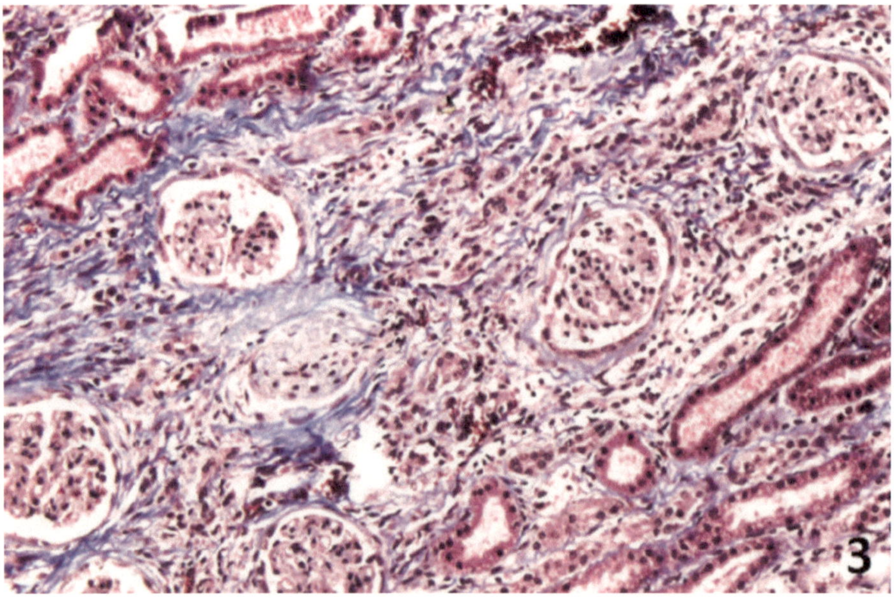

Fig. 3. Masson´s trichromic stain. Chronic interstitial nephritis with fibrosis and sclerotic glomeruli, 10X

Increased amounts of laminin, type IV collagen and fibronectin were identified in affected basement membranes. As the severity of the lesions increased, glomerular tufts contained higher amounts of laminin and the amount of type IV collagen decreased. IgG and IgM were identified in early lesions and expectedly were negative in sclerotic glomeruli. As was previously mentioned when describing membranous glomerulonephritis, immune complexes are present during initial stages and as severity progresses, the capacity of basement membranes to reabsorb these complexes is hindered. IgA was consistently negative. Readers are referred to Jimenez et al, 2008 for a more detailed discussion on these cases.

Electron microscopy of selected samples showed irregularly thickened up to twice normal width glomerular capillary basement membranes (Fig.4). Sparse intramembranous, large, scattered, irregular electron-dense deposits were noted, often surrounded by electron lucent spaces (Fig.5). Similarly, randomly distributed electron lucent areas in the capillary basement membranes were observed and interpreted as areas of immune deposit resorption. Foot processes in affected areas were variably blunted, fused or effaced. Degeneration of endothelial cells and rarely epithelial cells was also observed. The presence of IgG and IgM was corroborated within the electron dense deposits with immunogold labeling (Fig.6). Electron dense deposits were not observed in subepithelial or subendothelial areas (Jimenez et al, 2008).

No fibrillary deposits of any type were noted within the sampled areas, ruling out amyloidosis or other fibrillary glomerulopathies. Sclerotic glomeruli would have been expected to contain some amount of fibrillar collagen accumulation given the intensely blue staining with Masson´s trichromic stain, however only moderate membranous lesions were sampled for electron microscopy. The ultrastructure of sclerotic glomeruli was not evaluated.

The origin of the circulating immune-complexes is elusive and the membranous glomerulonephritis of the Iberian lynx remains idiopathic for the majority of cases. Hence this disease may be a primary affection in the Iberian lynx. Only a small number of animals showed evidence of systemic diseases such as mycobacteriosis or malignant neoplasms (cutaneous squamous cell carcinomas) (Jimenez et al, 2009). Both processes are chronic, course with debilitation and are known causes of persistent antigenemia that may be associated with immune-complex glomerulonephritis. Feline coronavirus and feline leukemia viruses were rarely detected by PCR in the animals during the 1998-2006 study period and never associated with histopathological evidence of disease. It is unlikely that in these instances the renal lesions were related with infection. However, even if an association between antigenemia in these cases and the membranous glomerulonephritis existed, there would still be an important number of animals in which the origin of the immune-complexes remained unaccounted for.

Immune deposits were also detected by immunohistochemistry and electron microscopy in approximately 76% of the spleens from animals during the 1998-2006 study period. Deposits were located in splenic arteriolar basement membranes. These basement membranes were also thickened, particularly in areas with the deposits. Similar electron-lucent spaces surrounded the electron dense deposits. Immunoglobulins were also identified as IgG and IgM (Fig.7). This finding conveys the possibility of a systemic immune-complex disease of uncertain etiology also responsible for the glomerular lesions. An autoimmune origin for this disease was speculated given the apparent lack of a defined cause for the lesions and that lesions do not appear to be secondary to tissue damage (Jimenez et al, 2009; Jacobson et al, 1997). An inherited cause for this disease has also been hypothesized. Given the low genetic diversity of the Iberian lynx (Johnson et al, 2004), an inherited trait or predisposing genetic condition could easily show in a high number of the population. These possibilities together with the identification of the circulating causative antigens are currently under study.

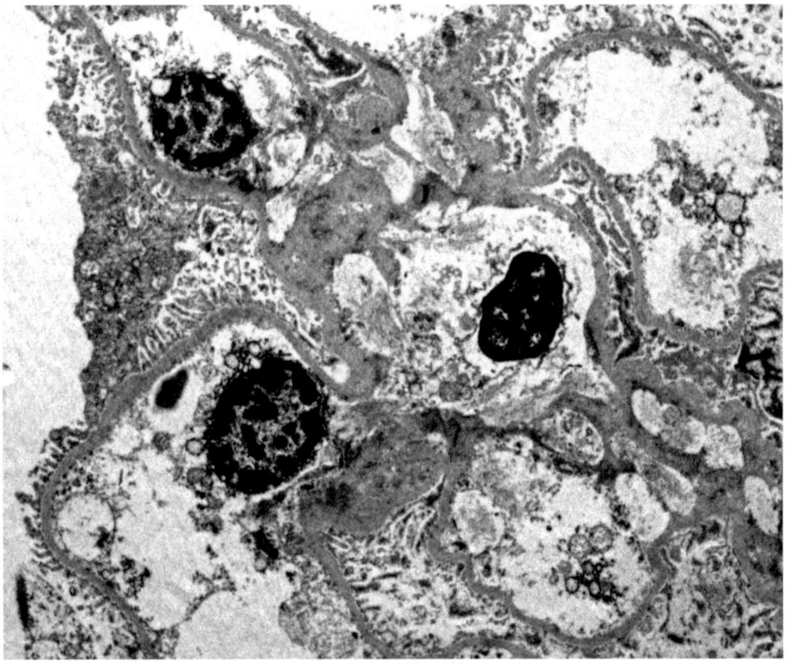

Fig. 4. Iberian lynx. Renal glomerulus. Electron microscopy. Multifocally and segmentally thickened capillary basement membranes with intramembranous electron dense deposits.

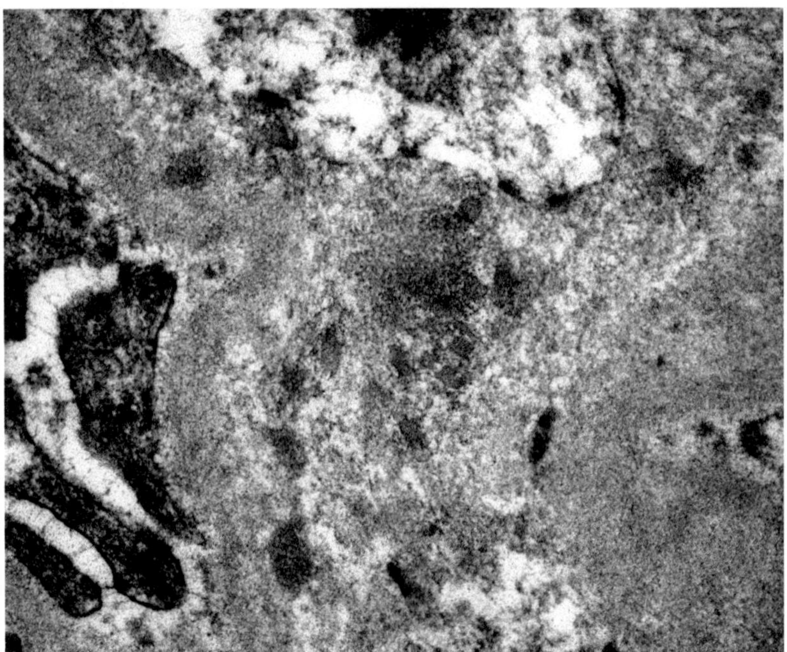

Fig. 5. Iberian lynx. Glomerular capillary basement membrane. Electron microscopy. Detail of intramembranous electron dense deposits and electron-lucent peripheral areas.

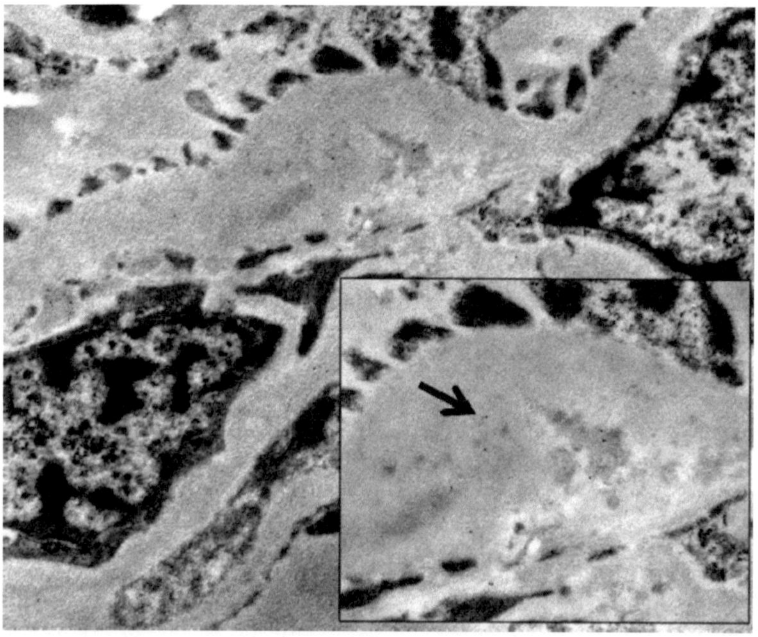

Fig. 6. Iberian lynx. Renal glomerulus. Immunogold labeling of IgM. Thickened capillary basement membranes with intramembranous electron dense deposits and colloid gold labeling of IgM. Inset: Detail of labeled gold particles

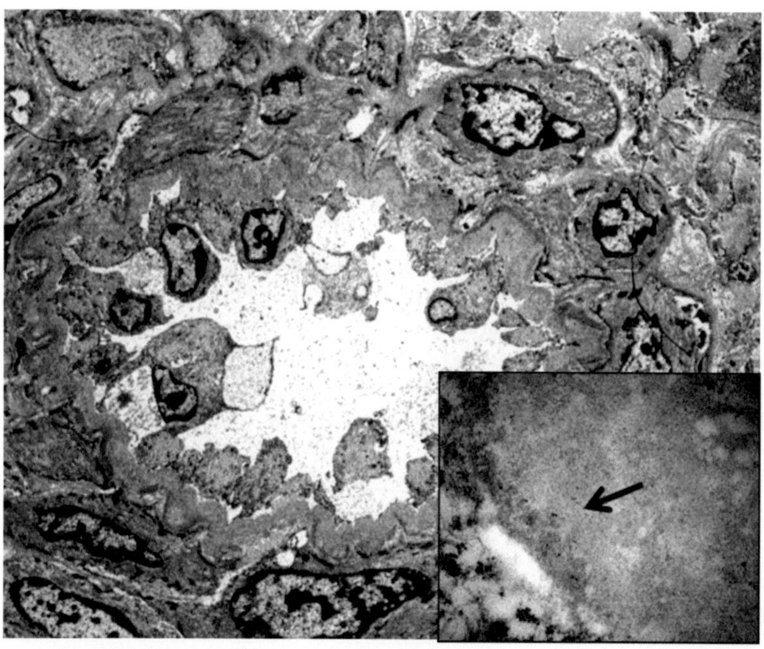

Fig. 7. Iberian lynx. Splenic follicular arteriole. Diffusely thickened capillary basement membrane with intramembranous linear electron dense deposits. Inset: Detail of positive labeling for IgG.

Despite the prevalence of these lesions within the population, the progress appeared to be slow. Animals seem to be able to live normally. This is similar to what is observed in domestic cats with membranous glomerulonephritis. However, the impact and consequences of this disease are yet far from known and caution on how this species will be able to confront overlapping renal injuries is warranted.

It is interesting to mention that glomerular lesions have also been described in other non-domestic felids. The most important have been secondary to systemic amyloidosis. Systemic AA amyloidosis has been described in black-footed cats (Felis nigripes) and cheetahs (Acinonyx jubatus) (Terio et al, 2008; Papendick et al, 1997). In both species, despite the systemic distribution, renal amyloidosis was the significant cause of morbidity and mortality. It is interesting to highlight that in the cheetah amyloidosis was associated with underlying systemic inflammatory diseases and was only observed in captive animals (Papendick et al, 1997). Contrarily, in the black footed cats amyloidosis was not associated with inflammatory conditions and was also detected in a young, free-ranging animal. Familial amyloidosis is suspected in this species (Terio et al, 2008). In both species, amyloidosis was more severe in the medulla than in glomeruli, similar to what is observed in domestic and Abyssinian cats.

Glomerulosclerosis has also been described in captive cheetahs. The lesion resembled human diabetic glomerulopathy. Hypertension, possibly associated with stress, dietary, and genetic factors, was speculated as a possible cause for the disease (Bolton & Munson, 1999).

Primary glomerular injury was considered a rare condition when surveying renal lesions of non-domestic felids of some zoological collections (Newkirk et al, 2010). Glomerular lesions similar to those described in the Iberian lynx with high prevalence in the free-ranging population as well as in captivity, and apparent primary origin, have not been described in other non-domestic felids.

4. Conclusions

The comparative study of diseases among different species often helps respond questions and elucidate unsolved enigmas of pathogenesis. The glomerular disease here reported appears to be unique for the Iberian lynx when considering non-domestic felids. The fact that this disease has not been reported previously in other non-domestic felids does not mean a similar entity may not exist. The study of these species is often difficult given the many interfering factors usually revolving these animals. Such factors include difficult access to wild-life populations, sample numbers compromised due to endangerment or limited access to captive populations among others. Often information is limited when encountering certain diseases or other situations regarding health and answers many times are sought in comparative pathology.

The purpose of this review was to compare the membranous glomerulonephritis of the Iberian lynx with the different types of glomerular injury reported, particularly in the domestic cat because of the close relationship and the extensive research available on the latter. Hopefully, the continuous study of these diseases will reveal new insights on pathogenesis, treatment or even prevention of these entities.

5. Acknowledgements

This research was supported by the Spanish Ministry of Environment, Research Project 90/2002, the Junta de Andalucia, Project CGL2004-00346/BOS, Red Nacional de Parques Nacionales, Project 17/2006, and TRAGSATEC, Project 244-2010.

6. References

Alpers C.E. (1992). Immunotactoid (microtubular) glomerulopathy: an entity distinct from fibrillary glomerulonephritis? *American Journal of Kidney Disease*, Vol.19, pp. 85-191

Aranaz, A.; De Juan, I.; Montero, N.; Sánchez, C.; Galka, M.; Delso, C.; Alvarez, J.; Romero, B.; Bezos, J.; Vela, A.I.; Briones, V.; Mateos, A. & Domínguez, L. (2004). Bovine tuberculosis (Mycobacterium bovis) in wildlife in Spain. *Journal of Clinical Microbiology*, Vol.42, No.6, pp. 2602-2608

Asano, T.; Tsukamoto, A.; Ohno, K.; Ogihara, K.; Kamiie, J. & Shirota, K. (2008). Membranoproliferative glomerulonephritis in a young cat. *Journal of Veterinary Medical Science*, Vol.70, No.12, pp. 1373-1375

Bolton, L.A. & Munson, L. (1999). Glomerulosclerosis in captive cheetahs (Acinonyx jubatus). *Veterinary Pathology*, Vol.36, pp. 14-22

Boyce, J.T.; DiBartola, S.P.; Chew, D.J. & Gasper, P.W. (1984). Familial renal amyloidosis in Abyssinian cats. *Veterinary Pathology*, Vol.21, No.1, (January), pp. 33-38

Briones, V.; De Juan, I.; Sánchez, C.; Vela, A.I.; Galka, M.; Montero, N.; Goyache, J.; Aranaz, A.; Mateos, A. & Domínguez, L. (2000). Bovine tuberculosis and the endangered Iberian lynx. *Emerging Infectious Diseases*, Vol.6, No.2, pp. 189-191

Cavana, P.; Capucchio, M.T.; Bovero, A.; Ripanti, D.; Catalano, D.; Scaglione, F.E.; Miller, J.; Blunden, T. & Farca, A.M. (2008). Noncongophilic fibrillary glomerulonephritis in a cat. Veterinary Pathology, Vol.45, pp. 347-351

DiBartola, S.P.; Benson, M.D.; Dwulet, F.E. & Cornacoff, J.B. (1985). Isolation and characterization of amyloid protein AA in the Abyssinian cat. *Laboratory Investigations*, Vol.52, No.5, (May), pp. 485-489

DiBartola, S.P.; Tarr, M.J. & Benson, M.D. (1986). Tissue distribution of amyloid deposits in abyssinian cats. *Journal of Comparative Pathology*, Vol.96, No.4, (July) pp.387-398

DiBartola, S.P. & Rutgers, H.C. (1994). Diseases of the kidney. In: *The cat, diseases and clinical management. 2nd Ed.*; Sherding, R.G.; pp. 1711-1717, Saunders, Philadelphia

Garcia, N.; Asuaga, J.L. & Torres, T. (1997). The carnivore remains from the Sima de los Huesos Middle Pleistocene Site (Sierra de Atapuerca, Spain). *Journal of Human Evolution*, Vol.33, pp.155-174

Garcia, N. & Asuaga, J.L. (1998). The carnivore remains from the hominid-bearing Trinchera-Galeria, Sierra de Atapuerca, Middle Pleistocene site (Spain). *Geobiosphere*, Vol.31, pp. 659-674

Geret, C.P.; Cattori, V.; Meli, M.L.; Riond, B.; López, G.; Vargas, A.; Simón, M.A.; López-Bao, J.V.; Hofmann-Lehmann, R. & Lutz, H. (2011). Feline leukemia virus outbreak in the critically endangered Iberian lynx (Lynx pardinus): high-throughput sequencing of envelope variable region A and experimental transmission. *Archive of Virology*, (February 8), Epub ahead of print

Glick, A.D.; Horn, R.G. & Holscher, M. (1978). Characterization of feline glomerulonephritis associated with viral-induced hematopoietic neoplasms. *American Journal of Pathology*, Vol.92, pp. 321-332

Grant Maxie, M. & Newman, S.J. (2007). The urinary system. In: *Pathology of Domestic Animals. 5th Ed.*; Jubb, K.V.F.; Kennedy, P.C. & Palmer, N.; pp. 425-522, Elsevier Saunders, Edinburgh,

Gruys, E. (2004). Protein folding pathology in domestic animals. *Journal of Zhejiang University Science*, Vol.5, No.10, pp. 1226-1238, ISSN 1009-3095

Guzman, J.N.; Garcia, F.J.; Garrote, G.; Perez de Ayala, R. & Iglesias, M.C. (2002): Iberian lynx (Lynx pardinus) distribution and current conservation status in Spain. In: *Proceedings of the International Seminar on the Iberian Lynx, Andujar, Spain,* (October), pp. 18-20

Haralson, M.A.; Jacobson, H.R. & Hoover, R.L. (1987). Collagen polymorphism in cultured rat kidney mesangial cells. *Laboratory Investigation,* Vol.57, pp. 513-523

Hayasi, T.; Ishida, T. & Fujiwara, K. (1982). Glomerulonephritis associated with feline infectious peritonitis. *Japanese Journal of Veterinary Science,* Vol.44, pp. 909-916

Hvala, A.; Ferluga, D.; Vizjak, A. & Koselj-Kajtna, M. (2003). Fibrillary noncongophilic renal and extrarenal deposits: a report on 10 cases. *Ultrastructural Pathology,* Vol.27, pp. 341-347

Ikeda, K.; Yokoyama, H.; Tomosugi, N.; Kida, H.; Ooshima, A. & Kobayashi, K. (1990). Primary glomerular fibrosis: a new nephropathy caused by diffuse intra-glomerular increase in atypical type III collagen fibers. *Clinical Nephrology,* Vol.33, pp. 155-159

Inoue, K.; Kami-Ie, J.; Ohtake, S.; Wakui, S.; Machida, S. & Shirota, K. (2001). Atypical membranoproliferative glomerulonephritis in a Cat. *Veterinary Pathology,* Vol.38, pp. 468-470

Jacobson, C.N.; Gange, S.L.; Rose, N.R. & Graham, N.M. (1997). Epidemiology and estimated population burden of selected autoimmune diseases in the United States. Clinical Immunology and Immunopathology, Vol.84, pp. 223-243

Johnson, W.E.; Godoy, A.; Palomares, F.; Delibes, M.; Fernández, M.; Revilla, E. & O´Brien, S.J. (2004). Phylogenetic and Phylographic analysis of Iberian lynx populations. *Journal of Heredity,* Vol.95, No.1, pp. 19-28

Jimenez, M.A.; Sanchez, B.; Perez-Alenza, M.D.; Garcia, P.; Lopez, J.V.; Rodriguez, A.; Muñoz, A.; Martinez, F.; Vargas, A. & Peña, L. (2008) Membranous glomerulonephritis in the Iberian lynx (Lynx pardinus). *Veterinary Immunology and Immunopathology,* Vol.121, pp. 34-43

Jimenez, M.A.; Sanchez, B.; García, P.; Pérez-Alenza, M.D.; Carrillo, E.; Moreno, F.J. & Peña, L. (2009). Diseases of the Iberian lynx: Histopathological survey, lymphoid depletion, glomerulonephritis and related clinical findings, In*: Iberian lynx ex situ conservation, an interdisciplinary approach.* Vargas, A.; Breitenmoser, C.; & Breitenmoser, U.; Fundación Biodiversidad, UICN Cat Specialist Group

Kim, D.Y.; Taylor, W.; Eades, S.C. & Cho, D.-Y. (2005). Systemic AL amyloidosis associated with multiple myeloma in a horse. *Veterinary Pathology,* Vol.42, pp. 81-84

Koeman, J.P.; Biewenga, W.J. & Gruys, E. (1994). Proteinuria associated with glomerulosclerosis and glomerular collagen formation in three Newfoundland dog littermates. *Veterinary Pathology,* Vol.31, pp. 188-193

Kumar, V.; Abbas, A.K.; Fausto, N. & Aster, J.C. (2010). Diseases of Immunity. In: *Robbins and Cotran Pathologic Basis of Disease, eighth Ed.*; Kumar, V.; Abbas, A.; Fausto, N. & Aster, J.C.; ISBN 978-1-4160-3121-5, Philadelphia, PA

Luaces, I.; Doménech, A.; García-Montijano, M.; Collado, V.M.; Sánchez, C.; German Tejerizo, J.; Galka, M.; Fernández, P. & Gómez-Lucía, E. (2008). Detection of Feline leukemia virus in the endangered Iberian lynx (Lynx pardinus). *Journal of Veterinary Diagnostic Investigation,* Vol.20, pp. 381-385

Martinez-Hernandez, A. & Menta, P.S. (1983). The basement membrane in pathology. *Laboratory Investigation*, Vol.48, pp. 656-677

Masson, R.G.; Rennke, H.G. & Gottlieb, M.N. (1992). Pulmonary hemorrhage in a patient with fibrillary glomerulonephritis. *New England Journal of Medicine*, Vol.326, pp. 36-39

Meli, M.L.; Cattori, V.; Martinez, F.; López, G.; Vargas, A.; Simón, M.A.; Zorrilla, I.; Muñoz, A.; Palomares, F.; López-Vao, J.V.; Pastor, J.; Tandon, R.; Willi, B.; Hofmann-Lehmann, R. & Lutz, H. (2009). Feline leukemia virus and other pathogens as important threats to the survival of the critically endangered Iberian lynx (Lynx pardinus). *PLoS One*, Vol.4, No.3, e4744

Meli, M.L.; Cattori, V.; Martinez, F.; López, G, Vargas, A.; Palomares, F.; Lopez-Bao, J.V.; Hofmann-Lehmann, R. & Lutz, H. (2010). Feline leukemia virus infection: a threat for the survival of the critically endangered Iberian lynx. *Veterinary Immunology and Immunopathology*, Vol.134, No.1-2, (March 15), pp.61-67

Merlini, G.; Seldin, D.C. & Gertz, M.A. (2011). Amyloidosis: Pathogenesis and new therapeutic options. *Journal of Clinical Oncology*, (April 11) Epub ahead of print

Moreno, S. & Villafuerte, R. (1995). Traditional management of scrubland for the conservation of rabbits Oryctolagus cuniculus and their predators in the Doñana National Park, Spain. *Biological Conservation*, Vol.118, pp. 183-193

Nakamura, S.; Shibata, S.; Shirota, K.; Abe, K.; Uetsuka, K.; Nakayama, H.; Goto, N. & Doi, K. (1996) Renal glomerular fibrosis in a cat. *Veterinary Pathology*, Vol.33, pp. 696-699

Nash, A.S.; Wright, N.G.; Spencer, A.J.; Thompson, H. & Fisher, E.W. (1979). Membranous nephropathy in the cat: a clinical and pathological study. *Veterinary Records*, Vol.105, No.4, (July 28), pp. 71-77

Newkirk, K.M.; Newman, S.J.; White, L.A.; Rohrbach, B.W.; Ramsay, E.C. (2010). Renal lesions in nondomestic felids. *Veterinary Pathology*, Vol.

Newman, S.J.; Confer, A.W. & Panciera, R.J. (2007). Urinary System. In: *Pathologic Basis of Veterinary Disease.* 4th Ed.; McGavin, M.D.; Zachary, J.F.; pp. 613-692, Mosby Elsevier, St Louis

Niewold, T.A.; van der Linde-Sipman, J.S.; Murphy, C.; Tooten, P.C. & Gruys, E. (1999). Familial amiloidosis in cats: Siamese and Abyssinian AA proteins differe in primary sequence and pattern of deposition. *Amyloid*, Vol.6, No.3, (September), pp. 205-209

Nowel & Jackson, (1996). Wildcats-status survey and conservation action plan. IUCN/SS Gland, Switzerland

Obici, L.; Perfetti, V.; Palladini, G.; Moratti, R. & Merlini, G. (2005). Clinical aspects of systemic amyloid. *Biochemistry and Biophysics Acta*, Vol.1753, No.1, pp. 11-22

Ozawa, K.; Yamabe, H.; Fukushi, K.; Osawa, H; Chiba, N.; Miyata, M.; Seino, S.; Inuma H.; Sasaki, T.; Yoshikawa, T. (1991). Case report of amyloidosis-like glomerulopathy with hepatic involvement. *Nephron*, Vol.58, pp. 347-350

Palomares, F.; Rodriguez, A.; Laffite, R. & Delibes, M. (1991). The status and distribution of the Iberian lynx (Felis pardina, Temminck) in Coto de Doñana area, SW Spain. *Biological Conservation*, Vol.57, pp. 159-169

Palomares, F.; Delibes, M.; Revilla, E. (2000). Iberian lynx in a fragmented landscape: predispersal, dispersal and postdispersal hábitats. *Conservation Biology*, Vol.14, No.13, pp. 809-818

Papendick, R.E.; Munson, L.; O´Brien, T.D. & Johnson, K.H. (1997). Systemic AA amiloidosis in captive cheetahs (Acinonyx jubatus). *Veterinary Pathology*, Vol.34, No.6, pp. 549-556

Peña, L.; García, P.; Jiménez, M.A.; Benito, A.; Pérez Alenza, M.D. & Sánchez, B. (2006). Histopathological and immunohistochemical findings in lymphoid tissues of the endangered Iberian lynx (Lynx pardinus). *Comparative Immunologic and Microbiologic Infectious Disease*, Vol.29, No.2-3, pp. 114-126

Platz, S.J.; Breuer, W.; Geisel, O.; Linke, R.P. & Hermanns, W. (1997). Identification of lambda light chain amyloid in eight canine and two feline extramedullary plasmacytomas. *Journal of Comparative Pathology*, Vol.116, pp. 45-54

Poli, A.; Falcone, M.L.; Bigalli, L.; Massi, C.; Hofmann-Lehmann, R.; Lombardi, S. & Bendinelli, M. (1995). Circulating immune complexes and analysis of renal immune deposits in feline immunodeficiency virus-infected cats. *Clinical Experimental Immunology*, Vol.101, pp. 254-258

Rodríguez, A. & Delibes, M. (2002). Internal structure and patterns of contraction in the geographic range of the Iberian lynx. *Ecography*, Vol.25, No.3, pp. 314-328

Schwartz, M.M. 2007. Glomerular diseases with organized deposits. In: *Heptinstall´s pathology of the kidney. 6th Ed.*; Jennette, J.C.; Olson, J.L.; Schwartz, M.M. & Silva, F.G.; Lippincott Williams & Wilkins, Philadelphia

Schwartz, M.M.; Korbert, S.M. & Lewis, E.J. (2002). Immunotactoid glomerulopathy. *Journal of the American Society of Nephrology*, Vol.13, pp. 1390-1397

Shirota, K.; Masaki, T.; Kitada, H.; Yanagi, M.; Ikeda, Y.; Une, Y.; Nomura, Y. & Jothy, S. (1995). Renal glomerular fibrosis in two pigs. *Veterinary Pathology*, Vol.32, pp.236-241

Slauson, D.O. & Lewis, R.M. (1979). Comparative pathology of glomerulonephritis in animals. *Veterinary Pathology*, Vol.16, pp.135-164

Terio, K.A.; O´Brien, T.; Lamberski, N.; Famula, T.R. & Munson, L. (2008). Amyloidosis in black-footed cats (Felis nigripes). *Veterinary Pathology*, Vol.45, No.3, pp. 393-400

Valaitis, J. (2002). Renal glomerular disease. In: *Atlas of electron microscopy with histopathological bases and immunofluoresence findings*, p. 99, ASCP Press, Chicago,

Van der Linde-Sipman, J.S.; Niewold, T.A.; Tooten, P.C.J.; de Neijs-Backer, M. & Gruys, E. (1997). Generalized AA-amyloidosis in Siamese and Oriental cats. *Veterinary Immunology and Immunopathology*, Vol.56, pp.1-10

Zini, E.; Hauser, B.; Meli, M.L. & Glaus, T. M. (2008). Transient laboratory changes in a cat with repeated hepatic hemorrhages due to amyloidosis. *Veterinary Record*, Vol.162, pp. 24-26

Part 3

Cytokines and Signalling Pathways

7

Role of TGF-ß in Mesangial Matrix Accumulation in Chronic Progressive Glomerular Disease

Hyun Soon Lee
Department of Pathology, Seoul National University College of Medicine, Seoul, Korea

1. Introduction

Lesions of focal segmental glomerulosclerosis (FSGS) are a pathological hallmark of progressive glomerular injury. Glomerulosclerosis frequently complicates most renal diseases, and is characterized by the collapse of the glomerular tuft with the accumulation of mesangial matrix. Transforming growth factor-ß (TGF-ß) is a key regulator of extracellular matrix (ECM) protein synthesis in renal cells. TGF-ß is secreted as latent complexes, which are stored in the ECM to provide stability to the active molecule and a readily activable source of it (Lawrence 2001). Overexpression of active TGF-ß1 in transgenic mice causes mesangial expansion and thickened capillary loops in the glomeruli (Kopp et al. 1996), while monoclonal antibody to TGF-ß reduces the glomerulosclerosis in experimental proliferative glomerulonephritis (GN) (Yu et al. 2004) and diabetic nephropathy (Benigni et al. 2003; Ziyadeh et al. 2000).

Cultured mesangial cells secrete TGF-ß and ECM proteins in response to various fibrogenic stimuli (Kim et al. 2001; Lee et al. 2004; Lee and Song 2009a; Ziyadeh et al. 1994, 1998). In chronic mesangial diseases, such as IgA nephropathy (IgAN) and diabetic nephropathy, TGF-ß1 mRNA expression by mesangial cells is increased, yet mesangial immunostaining for active TGF-ß1 is frequently negative (Kim et al. 2002; Stein-Oakley et al. 1997; Wahab et al. 2005). Only podocytes covering the sclerotic segments exhibit increased expression of TGF-ß1 protein (Kim et al. 2002; Wahab et al. 2005). These findings suggest that mesangial cells secrete latent TGF-ß in chronic mesangial disease, which may be localized to the podocyte surface to be activated (Lee and Song 2009b).

Podocytes are the target of injury in most glomerular diseases. Expression of TGF-ß mRNA and/or protein by podocytes is increased in progressive podocyte diseases, such as primary FSGS, membranous nephropathy, Alport syndrome and Denys-Drash syndrome (Kim et al. 2003; Kim et al. 1999; Patek et al. 2003; Sayers et al. 1999; Shankland et al. 1996). In addition, mesangial matrix is frequently increased in association with glomerulosclerosis (Gregory et al. 1996; Lee and Koh 1993; Lee and Lim 1995; Kim et al. 1995; Patek et al. 2003). Thus, TGF-ß, that is expressed and/or activated by podocytes, may contribute to mesangial matrix oversynthesis in both chronic mesangial disease and podocyte disease (Lee 2011).

This review will discuss the recent findings on the mechanisms and consequences of latent TGF-ß activation and TGF-ß-induced mesangial matrix accumulation in chronic progressive glomerular disease.

2. Structure of mesangial cells

Glomerular mesangial cells together with their surrounding matrix constitute the mesangium, a structure that is separated from the capillary lumen by the endothelium. The mesangial cells are surrounded by mesangial matrix, that is similar but not identical to the peripheral glomerular basement membrane (GBM). The mesangial matrix contains type IV collagen, sulfated glycosaminoglycans, fibronectin and laminin. The mesangial cells are often compared with vascular smooth muscle cells, and are able to proliferate and produce excessive matrix proteins when stimulated.

3. Chronic progressive glomerular diseases with TGF-ß overexpression in podocytes

3.1 IgAN

The diagnosis of IgAN is based on the demonstration of predominant or codominant IgA deposition in the mesangium. The glomerular histopathology mainly represents the mesangial lesions showing cell proliferation and/or matrix expansion. In addition, focal abnormalities of the GBM are sometimes present, with reticulation, thinning and thickening, as well as subepithelial deposits (Lee et al. 1987, 1989). Up to 30% of patients with IgAN eventually progress to end-stage renal disease (ESRD) after a follow-up of 25 years (Ibels and Györy 1994). The more severe glomerular lesions, which have higher percentage of glomerulosclerosis and crescents, are significantly related to progressive IgAN (El Karoui et al. 2011; Lee et al. 2005). Other glomerular lesions, such as mesangial hyperplasia and endocapillary lesions, also contribute to worse prognosis (Working Group of the International IgA Nephropathy Network 2010).

The intensity of immunostaining for platelet-derived growth factor, type IV collagen, laminin, and fibronectin is increased in the mesangium in renal biopsies with IgAN (Kim et al. 2002). In the early stage of IgAN with mesangial cell proliferation, some mesangial cells show immunoreactivity for TGF-ß1 (Stein-Oakley et al. 1997). Mesangial immunostaining for active TGF-ß1, however, is very weak or almost negligible in most human IgAN, despite increased mesangial TGF-ß1 mRNA levels. Instead, hyperplastic podocytes covering the sclerotic segments exhibit increased expression of TGF-ß1 protein (Kim et al. 2002).

Mesangial expression of TGF-ß isoforms is transiently upregulated in acute anti-Thy1.1 nephritis, a rodent model of mesangial proliferative GN (Hartner et al. 2003; Ito et al. 2001; Liu et al. 2004), in which TGF-ß1 expression is only segmentally and weakly distributed (Ito et al. 2001).

3.2 Primary FSGS

Primary FSGS is a clinicopathologic entity characterized by nephrotic syndrome and progression to ESRD. Intrarenal transcription of TGF-ß1 is increased in children with FSGS compared to those with minimal lesion, suggesting that TGF-ß1 gene transcription is indicative of progressive renal damage typical of FSGS (Strehlau et al. 2002). Expression of TGF-ß1 is increased in patients with primary FSGS, particularly in podocytes of sclerotic segments (Kim et al. 2003). Volume density of mesangial matrix is significantly greater in the FSGS patients than in minimal lesion cases. In patients with FSGS, the percent glomerulosclerosis correlates directly with mesangial volume per glomerulus (Lee and Lim 1995).

3.3 The significance of FSGS formation in chronic glomerular disease

Some authors regarded FSGS as a nonspecific heterogeneous form of renal injury (Whitworth et al. 1978). The lesions of FSGS following primary glomerular diseases, such as IgAN and membranous nephropathy, have often been excluded in the category of secondary FSGS, because they were regarded as the nonspecific chronic scarred phase of the disease (D'Agati et al. 2004). Nonetheless, the lesions of FSGS in IgAN show immunohistochemical changes, which are basically identical to those described in primary FSGS, with loss of podocyte markers (Hill et al. 2011). Furthermore, podocytes covering the sclerotic segments exhibit enhanced expression of TGF-ß1 in IgAN and advanced diabetic nephropathy similar to those observed in primary FSGS. Thus, common podocyte lesions may contribute to the development of FSGS in both primary FSGS and other chronic glomerular diseases.

3.4 Membranous nephropathy

Membranous nephropathy is a well-characterized histological entity with a highly variable clinical course. Overall, approximately 30-40% of patients develop significant renal failure 10-15 years after the diagnosis of nephropathy (Perna et al. 2004). New genomwide association study suggests that sequence variations within HLA and receptor for phospholipase A2 are responsible in part for the development of idiopathic membranous nephropathy (Stanescu et al. 2011). The hallmark of membranous nephropathy is the presence of glomerular subepithelial deposits that typically contain immunoglobulin and complement component. Between and around these deposits, the GBM is thickened due to the accumulation of GBM material, forming subepithelial projections or spikes. Complement membrane attack complex (C5b-C9) plays an important role in the development of podocyte injury and proteinuria in passive Heymann nephritis (PHN), an experimental model of human membranous nephropathy (Couser and Nangaku 2006). Upregulation of TGF-ß1 and GBM protein mRNAs by podocytes is shown in patients with membranous nephropathy (Kim et al. 1999). Expression of TGF-ß2 is also markedly increased in podocytes in experimental membranous nephropathy, together with upregulation of TGF-ß receptors (Shankland et al. 1996).

Lesions of FSGS are observed in 43% of the membranous nephropathty patients, in whom the degree of mesangial expansion and GBM thickening is significantly greater than the remaining cases without FSGS (Lee and Koh 1993). In PHN, mesangial volume was also significantly elevated, together with GBM thickening (Remuzzi et al. 1999).

3.5 Diabetic nephropathy

Diabetic nephropathy remains the most common cause for ESRD as the burden of diabetes increases worldwide. Nearly one-third of patients with diabetes develop nephropathy (Choudhury et al. 2010). Mesangial matrix expansion and thickening of the GBM are hallmarks of diabetic nephropathy, which occur even within a few years after the onset of type 1 diabetes (Drummond and Mauer 2002). If left untreated, 20-40% of patients with type 2 diabetes show progression to renal failure (Adler et al. 2003; Remuzzi et al. 2002).

In the early stage of human diabetic nephropathy, some mesangial cells show immunoreactivity for TGF-ß1. Yet mesangial immunostaining for active TGF-ß1 is very weak or almost negligible in most human diabetic nodular glomerulosclerosis, despite increased mesangial TGF-ß1 mRNA levels. Rather, podocytes covering the sclerotic segments show increased expression of TGF-ß1 mRNA and protein (Wahab et al. 2005). In the glomeruli of experimental diabetic nephropathy, only a few cells show positive immunostaining for TGF-ß1 (Hill et al. 2000). Enhanced expression of glomerular TGF-ß1 is observed mainly in podocytes of diabetic animals (Baba et al. 2005; Okada et al. 2006).

3.6 Alport renal disease

Collagen type IV is the main component of the GBM, which includes six genetically distinct isoforms named α1(IV) to α6(IV). The α3-α5(IV) chains originate solely from podocytes in both the developing and mature glomerulus (Abrahamson et al. 2009). The α1/α2(IV) collagen network, by contrast, seems to originate mainly from glomerular endothelial cells (Lee et al. 1993), and is localized predominantly at the endothelial aspect of human GBM (Zhang and Lee 1997).

Alport syndrome is primary genetic disease of the basement membrane. In the kidney, this disorder is characterized by an absence of collagen α3α4α5(IV) in the GBM, progressive thickening and multilamination of the GBM, proteinuria, and renal failure. Yet collagen α1/α2(IV) is retained throughout the GBM (Abrahamson et al. 2003; Kashtan et al. 2001). In podocytes of α3(IV) collagen-knockout mice with Alport renal disease, mRNA expression of TGF-ß1 is increased (Sayers et al. 1999). With disease progression, mesangial matrix and cells are increased, followed by the development of glomerulosclerosis (Gregory et al. 1996; Kim et al. 1995).

3.7 Denys-Drash syndrome

Wilms' tumour suppressor gene, WT1, is essential for normal podocyte function. Mutations of WT1 induce Denys-Drash syndrome (DDS) characterized by diffuse mesangial sclerosis. In DDS mice, the development of glomerulosclerosis is preceded by de novo TGF-ß1 expression in podocytes, while TGF-ß1 expression is absent in the mesangium (Patek et al. 2003).

In summary, expression of TGF-ß1 by podocytes is increased not only in progressive podocyte disease but also in chronic mesangial disease. Despite mesangial matrix expansion in association with glomerulosclerosis in both types of disease, immunohistochemical antigen detection for mesangial TGF-ß1 seems to be difficult even in chronic mesangial disease.

4. Activation of latent TGF-ß

TGF-ß is secreted as latent complexes associated with a latency-associated peptide (LAP). TGF-ß/LAP complex is referred to as the small latent complex. Most cells secrete TGF-ß as part of a large latent complex, in which latent TGF-ß binding protein (LTBP) is linked to the small latent complex. LTBP has a role in targeting the transport of latent TGF-ß complex into the ECM (Hyytiäinen et al. 2004; Koli et al. 2008).

The large latent complex is susceptible to proteolysis, within which LTBP is first cleaved at the protease sensitive hinge region. The soluble large latent complex is then released from the ECM and is activated by another proteolytic event that releases TGF-ß from LAP (Koli et al. 2001). The TGF-ß released then binds to its receptor and exerts its cellular functions.

Under in vitro conditions, latent TGF-ß is activated by heating, acid or alkaline treatment, irradiation, reactive oxygen species (ROS), proteases including plasmin, cathepsin, calpain, matrix metalloproteinase (MMP)-2 and MMP-9, some integrins, or thrombospondin-1 (TSP-1) (for review, see Koli et al. 2001).

Several activation mechanisms may exist in vivo as reviewed below (Table 1).

4.1 TGF-ß activation by proteolysis

Plasmin could function as an in vivo activator of TGF-ß (Lyons et al. 1990; Edgtton et al. 2004). Plasmin can release the large latent TGF-ß complex from the ECM by cleaving LTBP at the amino terminal hinge region (Taipale et al. 1992). Furthermore, it can cleave LAP that releases active TGF-ß dimer from the large latent TGF-ß1 complex (Annes et al. 2003; George et al. 2005; Lyons et al. 1990).

MMP-2 and MMP–9 have also been implicated in the cleavage of LAP and the release of mature TGF-ß at the cell surface (Yu and Stamenkovic 2000).

4.2 TSP-1-mediated activation of TGF-ß

TSP-1 is known to be a major physiologic activator of latent TGF-ß (Crawford et al. 1998). A specific peptide sequence within TSP-1, KRFK, binds to the LSKL sequence in LAP, and releases mature TGF-ß by inducing conformational changes in the protein (Crawford et al. 1998; Lawrence 2001; Koli et al. 2008). However, it is not clear whether TSP-1 alone could directly activate latent TGF-ß (Abdelouahed et al. 2000; Grainger and Frow 2000; Otsuka et al. 2007).

Overexpression of both TSP-1 and active TGF-ß occurs in podocytes in patients with FSGS (Kim et al. 2003) and diabetic nephropathy (Wahab et al. 2005). In various experimental renal disease models, TSP-1 is co-localized with TGF-ß and predicts the development of tissue fibrosis (Hugo et al. 1998).

4.3 ROS-mediated activation of TGF-ß

ROS produced by ionizing radiation was found to induce rapid TGF-ß activation in vivo (Barcellos-Hoff and Dix 1996). ROS can activate TGF-ß directly through oxidation-induced conformational change in LAP, in which the unique methionine residue in the TGF-ß1/LAP functions as a redox switch center (Jobling et al. 2006), or indirectly through the activation of proteolytic enzymes (Koli et al. 2008).

4.4 Integrins in TGF-ß binding and activation

Integrins can bind to the RGD recognition domain in the LAP of TGF-ß1 and TGF-ß3. Particularly, αvß6 and αvß8 are known to activate the TGF-ß complex (Munger et al. 1999; Mu et al. 2002), leading to release of TGF-ß either by tractional force (αvß6) or by membrane type-1 MMP (MT1-MMP)-dependent proteolytic activity (αvß8) (Koli et al. 2008). By cell movement, an αvß6–integrin-expressing cell causes sufficient traction for the release of mature TGF-ß from the ECM-anchored large latent complex (Annes et al. 2004).

Activators	Mechanisms of action	1st author
Plasmin	- Proteolytic nicking of LTBP releasing large latent TGF-ß complex from the ECM - Proteolytic nicking of the LAP	Taipale (1992); Lyons (1990); Annes (2003); George (2005)
TSP-1	- Induction of conformational changes in LAP	Crawford(1998); Lawrence (2001); Koli (2008)
ROS	- Induction of conformational changes in LAP - Inducing activation of proteolytic enzymes	Jobling (2006); Koli (2008)
Integrin, αvß6	- Release of TGF-ß from LAP by tractional force	Annes (2004)

TGF-ß, transforming growth factor-ß; LTBP, latent TGF-ß binding protein; ECM, extracellular matrix; TSP-1, thrombospondin-1; LAP, latency-associated peptide; ROS, reactive oxygen species.

Table 1. Proposed mechanisms for latent TGF-ß activation in chronic glomerular disease

αvß6 integrin is expressed in the diseased kidneys confined to the distal tubules and collecting ducts (Trevillian et al. 2004). Deleting TGF-ß type II receptor in collecting duct cells in vitro resulted in increased integrin αvß6-dependent TGF-ß activation, that increased collagen synthesis in co-cultured renal interstitial fibroblasts (Gewin et al. 2010).

5. Mechanism of TGF-ß overexpression by podocytes in chronic glomerular disease

5.1 Incomplete activation of mesangial TGF-ß in chronic mesangial disease

Intense mesangial immunostaining for LTBP-1 is observed in anti-Thy1.1 nephritis associated with severe but transient mesangial matrix accumulation (Porst et al. 2006). In rats with anti-Thy1.1 nephritis, active TGF-ß1-positive area/glomerulus was 18%, while treatment with antisense TSP-1 oligodeoxynucleotides reduced it to 9% (Daniel et al. 2003). In wild-type and TSP-1 deficient diabetic mice, the TGF-ß1-positive area in the glomerulus was 5% and 3%, respectively (Daniel et al. 2007). Thus, TSP-1 seems to activate mesangial TGF-ß1 more actively in acute mesangial proliferative GN than in chronic mesangial disease.

Plasmin can release the large latent TGF-ß complex from the mesangial matrix by cleaving LTBP at the amino terminal hinge region (Taipale et al. 1992) (Fig. 1). The plasmin-mediated

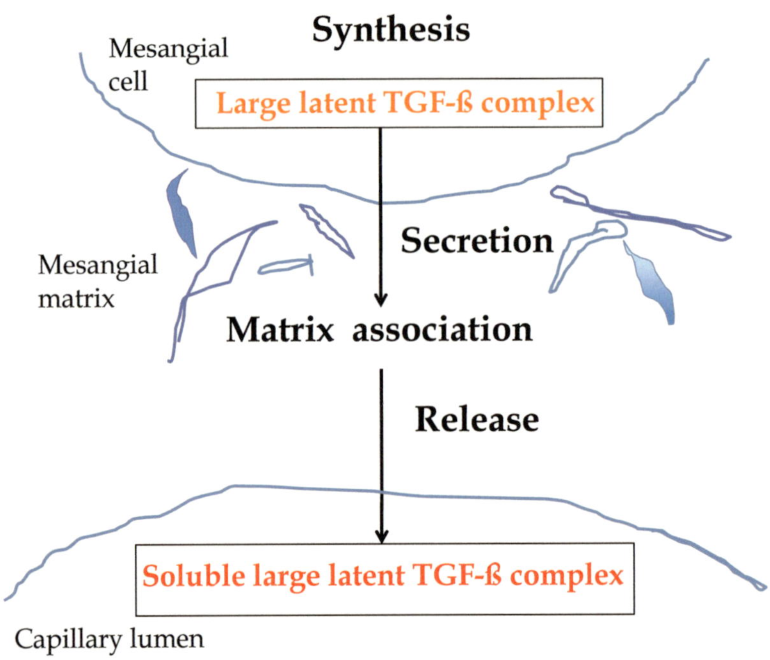

Fig. 1. Incomplete activation of mesangial TGF-ß in chronic mesangial disease. Upon fibrogenic stimuli, large latent TGF-ß complex in association with latent TGF-ß binding protein (LTBP) is synthesized and secreted from mesangial cells. It is then associated with mesangial matrix via N-terminus of LTBP. In protease-mediated activation of TGF-ß, LTBP is first cleaved at the protease sensitive amino terminal hinge region, and soluble large latent complex is released.

TGF-ß activation, however, may be neutralized via feedback inhibition, since TGF-ß-induced production of plasminogen activator inhibitor-1 decreases the active plasmin formation in mesangial cells (Baricos et al. 2003). Furthermore, accumulation of mesangial matrix progressed in association with enhanced mesangial fibrin deposition in rats with anti-Thy 1.1 nephritis (Liu et al. 2004). Thus, the mesangial cell surface surrounded by an enlarged matrix may not express sufficient plasmin to further cleave LAP that liberates active TGF-ß dimer from the large latent TGF-ß1 complex.

In view of the enhanced expression of TGF-ß1 in podocytes in human IgAN (Kim et al. 2002) and end-stage diabetic nephropathy (Wahab et al. 2005), podocytes seem to respond to paracrine TGF-ß coming from the mesangium. Even though free active TGF-ß is liberated from the mesangium, it has a very short half-life in plasma (2-3 min) (Coffey et al. 1987), in contrast to the latent TGF-ß complex with a significantly longer half-life (>100 min) (Wakefield et al. 1990). Thus, soluble forms of large latent TGF-ß complex, rather than active TGF-ß, may be localized to the podocyte surface after its release from the mesangial matrix (Fig. 1 and 2).

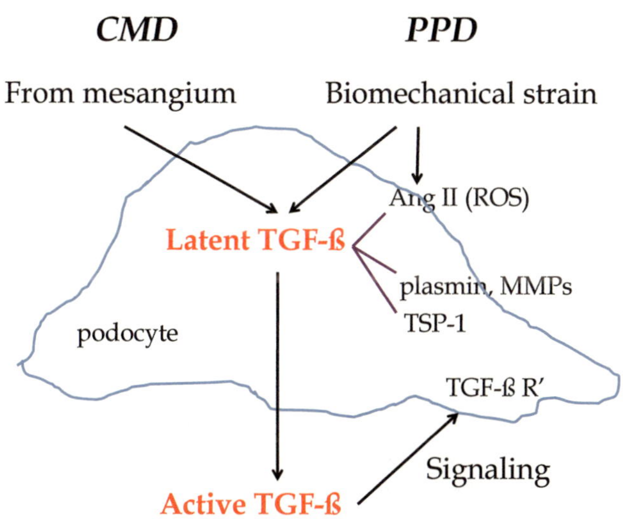

Fig. 2. Hypothetical pathway for TGF-ß activation by podocytes in the diseased glomeruli. Soluble large latent TGF-ß complex coming from the mesangium in chronic mesangial disease (CMD) and biomechanical strain-induced TGF-ß in progressive podocyte disease (PPD) may be the source of latent TGF-ß complex in podocytes. It is then activated by angiotensin II (Ang II)/reactive oxygen species (ROS), plasmin, matrix metalloproteinases (MMPs) and thrombospondin-1 (TSP-1). Active TGF-ß, which is released from latency-associated peptide, is able to associate with the signaling receptors (TGF-ß R'), and signal transduction pathway is activated.

5.2 Induction of podocyte TGF-ß by glomerular hypertension or biomechanical strain in progressive podocyte disease

In progressive podocyte diseases, TGF-ß expression is increased in podocytes (Kim et al. 1999, 2003; Patek et al. 2003; Sayers et al. 1999; Shankland et al. 1996; Wahab et al. 2005). Unlike mesangial cells, podocytes do not overexpress TGF-ß1 in response to common in vitro metabolic stimuli, such as high glucose (Iglesias-de la Cruz et al. 2002) and angiotensin II (Ang II) (Chen et al. 2005). Yet albumin load or mechanical strain increases the levels of TGF-ß1 and Ang II, as well as TGF-ß type I, II and III receptors in cultured podocytes (Abbatte et al. 2002; Dessapt et al. 2009; Durvasula et al. 2004).

Increased intraglomerular pressure results in cellular strain and perpetuates further damage to the podocytes in progressive glomerular disease, eventually leading to glomerulosclerosis (Kriz et al. 1998). The less cross-linked and possibly more elastic physical properties of the GBM in some podocyte diseases may subject the podocytes to elevated biomechanical strain even under normal glomerular blood pressure. As the disease progresses and nephron mass is lost, glomerular hypertension develops, further exacerbating the biomechanical strain and the effector functions influenced by it (Meehan et al. 2009). In the remnant kidney model of glomerular capillary hypertension, TGF-ß1 (Abbate et al. 2002) and Ang II type I receptor (Durvasula et al. 2004) are upregulated by podocytes.

Together, an increase in glomerular capillary pressure may stimulate Ang II and TGF-ß1 expression in podocytes through mechanical force injury in progressive podocyte diseases (Lee 2011) (Fig. 2).

5.3 Activation of latent TGF-ß by podocytes in chronic glomerular disease

In podocyte diseases, Ang II-induced oxidative stress may activate the latent TGF-ß and, subsequently, the TGF-ß signaling system in podocytes (Lee 2011) (Fig. 2). Indeed, diabetic podocytopathy seems to be mediated by Ang II (Ziyadeh and Wolf 2008) and oxidative damage (Zheng et al. 2008).

Osteopontin expression strongly correlates with glomerular disease, and is increased specifically in podocytes. Treatment of podocytes with recombinant osteopontin activated the NF-κB pathway, increased the expression of urokinase-type plasminogen activator (uPA) and MMP-2 and -9, and increased podocyte motility (Lorenzen et al. 2008). Strong expression of uPA protein and mRNA is sometimes observed within crescents (Lee et al. 2001). These observations suggest that damaged podocytes in the diseased glomeruli may release plasmin, MMP-2 and -9 to activate latent TGF-ß (Fig. 2).

In human FSGS, expression levels of TGF-ß1, TSP-1 and TGF-ß type II receptor mRNAs and proteins as with phosphorylated Smad2/Smad3 are increased by podocytes (Kim et al. 2003), suggesting that TSP-1 may activate TGF-ß in podocytes (Fig. 2). In addition, diabetic mediators upregulate the TGF-ß type II receptor that both binds the ligand and initiates the signaling cascade, suggesting that the podocyte is primed to respond to TGF-ß (Iglesias-de la Cruz et al. 2002; Wolf et al. 2005).

Altogether, podocyte-derived plasmin, MMPs and TSP-1, and particularly Ang II-induced oxidative stress may activate the latent TGF-ß in podocytes in diseased glomeruli. The activated TGF-ß may bind to its receptor on podocytes, activating the TGF-ß/Smad signaling pathway to induce the expression of its target genes, such as connective tissue growth factor (CTGF) and vascular endothelial growth factor (VEGF) (Fig. 2 and 3).

6. Paracrine effector mechanism of CTGF and VEGF for TGF-ß to act on mesangial cells

The podocyte TGF-ß, the active form of which has a very short half-life in plasma, is unlikely to traverse the GBM to promote sclerosis in the adjacent mesangium. Instead, some TGF-ß-induced humoral factors produced by podocytes seem to have fibrogenic effects on mesangial cells (Lee and Song 2009b).

CTGF is a major autocrine growth factor induced by TGF-ß. TGF-ß1 induces CTGF mRNA and protein expression in podocytes (Ito et al. 2001) and mesangial cells (Riser et al. 2000). Expression of CTGF mRNA and/or protein in the mesangium and podocytes is upregulated in human chronic glomerular disease (Ito et al. 1998; Wahab et al. 2005). It is increased particularly in the glomeruli of patients with mesangial matrix expansion (Suzuki et al. 2003). Treatment with the CTGF antisense oligonucleotides significantly reduced the mesangial matrix expansion in diabetic mice (Guha et al. 2007). Furthermore, induction of diabetes in podocyte-specific CTGF-transgenic mice results in an increased mesangial CTGF expression with more severe mesangial expansion than diabetic wild-type mice (Yokoi et al. 2008).
TGF-ß1 stimulates VEGF expression in podocytes (Iglesias-de la Cruz et al. 2002). VEGF is a potent angiogenic molecule and is detected predominantly in podocytes (Bailey et al. 1999; Wendt et al. 2003). Yet glomeruli are not sites of angiogenesis, possibly because podocytes mainly express $VEGF_{165}b$ protein, which inhibits $VEGF_{165}$-mediated angiogenesis (Cui et al. 2004). VEGF may play an important role in TGF-ß1-induced glomerular fibrosis (Chen et al. 2004, 2005). VEGF overexpression by podocytes led to mesangial expansion (Veron et al. 2010; Zhang et al. 2010). Furthermore, anti-VEGF attenuates the mesangial matrix expansion in diabetic mice (Flyvbjerg et al. 2002).
The dominant production of VEGF-A by podocytes and the localization of its receptor, VEGFR-2, on glomerular endothelial cells suggest that VEGF-A moves across the GBM, opposing the ultrafiltration gradient to move water and solutes from the capillaries into the Bowman's space (Satchell et al. 2006). In fact, about one third of VEGF secreted from

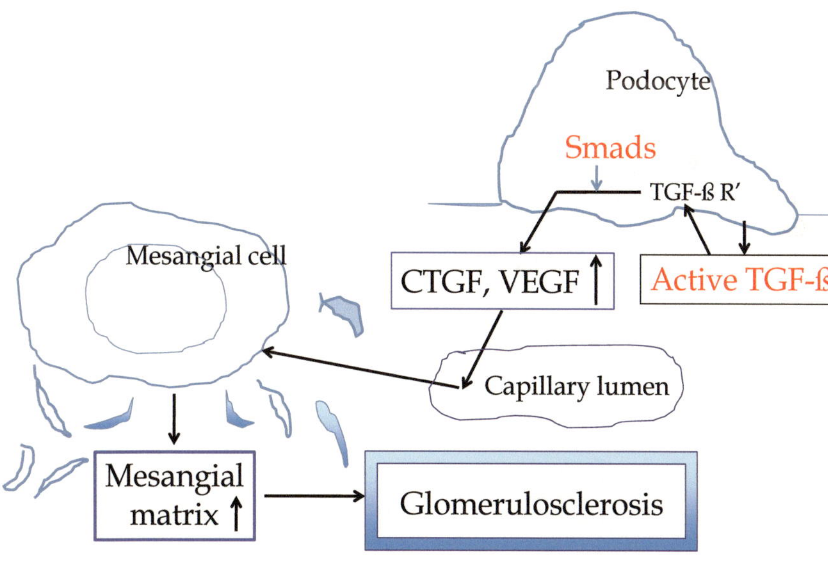

Fig. 3. Hypothetical pathway for mesangial matrix accumulation via activation of TGF-ß by podocytes in chronic glomerular disease. The activated TGF-ß may bind to its receptor (TGF-ß R') on podocytes, activating TGF-ß/Smad signaling pathway to induce the overexpression of its target genes, connective tissue growth factor (CTGF) and vascular endothelial growth factor (VEGF). The CTGF and VEGF secreted from podocytes may reach the capillary lumen and stimulate mesagial cells to produce excessive matrix proteins, culminating in the development of glomerulosclerosis.

podocytes would reach the capillary lumen and accumulate there, supporting the view that VEGF can move against the flow of glomerular filtration (Katavetin and Katavetin 2008). Although it is not clear whether this is also the case for CTGF, the experiments performed by Yokoi et al. (2008) support that possibility.

In summary, TGF-ß-induced CTGF and VEGF secretion by podocytes may act as an effector mechanism, necessary for mesangial matrix accumulation in chronic glomerular disease, culminating in the development of glomerulosclerosis (Fig. 3).

7. Conclusions

In chronic mesangial disease, large latent TGF-ß complexes secreted by mesangial cells may be stored in the mesangial matrix, from which soluble large latent TGF-ß complexes may be released and localized to the podocyte surface. In progressive podocyte disease, by contrast, mechanical pressure or biomechanical strain may upregulate Ang II and TGF-ß expression in podocytes. In both chronic mesangial disease and progressive podocyte disease, podocyte-derived plasmin, TSP-1 and ROS, particularly Ang II-induced oxidative stress, seem to be involved in TGF-ß activation. Active TGF-ß may induce CTGF and VEGF overexpression in podocytes, which may act as a paracrine effector mechanism on mesangial cells to stimulate mesangial matrix synthesis culminating in the development of glomerulosclerosis. In summary, this review provides new mechanistic insights into the role of TGF-ß in mesangial matrix synthesis in chronic progressive glomerular disease. Better understanding of the activation of TGF-ß signaling and its downstream effectors, CTGF and VEGF, may provide novel tools for the prevention of glomerulosclerosis.

8. References

Abbate M, Zoja C, Morigi M, Rottoli D, Angioletti S, Tomasoni S, Zanchi C, Longaretti L, Donadelli R, Remuzzi G (2002) Transforming growth factor-ß1 is up-regulated by podocytes in response to excess intraglomerular passage of proteins: a central pathway in progressive glomerulosclerosis. Am J Pathol 161:2179-2193

Abdelouahed M, Ludlow A, Brunner G, Lawler J (2000) Activation of platelet transforming growth factor ß-1 in the absence of thrombospondin-1. J Biol Chem 275:17933-17936

Abrahamson DR, Hudson BG, Stroganova L, Borza D-B, St. John PL (2009) Cellular origins of type IV collagen networks in developing glomeruli. J Am Soc Nephrol 20:1471-1479

Abrahamson DR, Prettyman AC, Robert B, St John PL (2003) Laminin-1 reexpression in Alport mouse glomerular basement membranes. Kidney Int 63:826-834

Adler AI, Stevens RJ, Manley SE, Bilous RW, Cull CA, Holman RR; UKPDS GROUP (2003) Development and progression of nephropathy in type 2 diabetes: the United Kingdom Prospective Diabetes Study (UKPDS 64). Kidney Int 63:225-232

Annes JP, Chen Y, Munger JS, Rifkin DB (2004) Integrin αvß6-mediated activation of latent TGF-ß requires the latent TGF-ß- binding protein-1. J Cell Biol 165:723-734

Annes JP, Munger JS, Rifkin DB (2003) Making sense of latent TGFß activation. J Cell Sci 116:217-224

Baba M, Wada J, Eguchi J, Hashimoto I, Okada T, Yasuhara A, Shikata K, Kanwar YS, Makino H (2005) Galectin-9 inhibits glomerular hypertrophy in db/db diabetic mice via cell-cycle-dependent mechanisms. J Am Soc Nephrol 16:3222-3234

Bailey E, Bottomley MJ, Westwell S, Pringle JH, Furness PN, Feehally J, Brenchley PEC, Harper SJ (1999) Vascular endothelial growth factor mRNA expression in minimal change, membranous, and diabetic nephropathy demonstrated by nonisotopic in situ hybridization. J Clin Pathol 52:735-738

Barcellos-Hoff MH, Dix TA (1996) Redox-mediated activation of latent transforming growth factor-ß1. Mol Endocrinol 10:1077- 1083

Baricos WH, Reed JC, Cortez SL (2003) Extracellular matrix degradation by cultured mesangial cells: mediators and modulators. Exp Biol Med. 228:1018-1022

Benigni A, Zoja C, Corna D, Zatelli C, Conti S, Campana M, Gagliardini E, Rottoli D, Zanchi C, Abbate M, Ledbetter S, Remuzzi G (2003) Add-on anti-TGF-ß antibody to ACE inhibitor arrests progressive diabetic nephropathy in the rat. J Am Soc Nephrol 14:1816-1824

Chen S, Kasama Y, Lee JS, Jim B, Marin M, Ziyadeh FN (2004) Podocyte-derived vascular endothelial growth factor mediates the stimulation of α3(IV) collagen production by transforming growth factor-ß1 in mouse podocytes. Diabetes 53:2939-2949

Chen S, Lee JS, Iglesias-de la Cruz MC, Wang A, Izquierdo-Lahuerta A, Gandhi NK, Danesh FR, Wolf G, Ziyadeh FN (2005) Angiotensin II stimulates α3(IV) collagen production in mouse podocytes via TGF-ß and VEGF signaling: implications for diabetic glomerulopathy. Nephrol Dial Transplant 20:1320-1328

Choudhury D, Tuncel M, Levi M (2010) Diabetic nephropathy--a multifaceted target of new therapies. Discov Med 10:406-415

Coffey RJ Jr, Kost LJ, Lyons RM, Moses HL, LaRusso NE (1987) Hepatic processing of transforming growth factor ß in the rat. Uptake, metabolism, and biliary excretion. J Clin Invest 80:750- 757

Couser WG, Nangaku M (2006) Cellular and molecular biology of membranous nephropathy. J Nephrol 19:699-705

Crawford SE, Stellmach V, Murphy-Ullrich JE, Ribeiro SM, Lawler J, Hynes RO, Boivin GP, Bouck N (1998) Thrombospondin-1 is a major activator of TGF-ß1 in vivo. Cell 93:1159-1170

Cui T-G, Foster RR, Saleem M, Mathieson PW, Gillatt DA, Bates DO, Harper SJ (2004) Differentiated human podocytes endogenously express an inhibitory isoform of vascular endothelial growth factor (VEGF165b) mRNA and protein. Am J Physiol Renal Physiol 286:F767-773

D'Agati VD, Fogo AB, Bruijn JA, Jennette JC (2004) Pathologic classification of focal segmental glomerulosclerosis: a working proposal. Am J Kidney Dis 43:368–382

Daniel C, Schaub K, Amann K, Lawler J, Hugo C (2007) Thrombospondin-1 is an endogenous activator of TGF-ß in experimental diabetic nephropathy in vivo. Diabetes 56:2982-2989

Daniel C, Takabatake Y, Mizui M, Isaka Y, Kawashi H, Rupprecht H, Imai E, Hugo C (2003) Antisense oligonucleotides against thrombospondin-1 inhibit activation of TGF-ß in fibrotic renal disease in the rat in vivo. Am J Pathol 163:1185-1192

Dessapt C, Baradez MO, Hayward A, Dei Cas A, Thomas SM, Viverti G, Gnudi L (2009) Mechanical forces and TGFß1 reduce podocyte adhesion through α3ß1 integrin downregulation. Nephrol Dial Transplant 24:2645-2655

Drummond K, Mauer M (2002) The early natural history of nephropathy in type 1 diabetes. II. Early renal structural changes in type 1 diabetes. Diabetes 51:1580-1587

Durvasula RV, Pettermann AT, Hiromura K, Blonski M, Pippin J, Mundel P, Pichler R, Griffin S, Couser WG, Shankland SJ (2004) Activation of a local tissue angiotensin system in podocytes by mechanical strain. Kidney Int 65:30-39

Edgtton KL, Gow RM, Kelly DJ, Carmeliet P, Kitching AR (2004) Plasmin is not protective in experimental renal interstitial fibrosis. Kidney Int 66:68-76

El Karoui K, Hill GS, Karras A, Moulonguet L, Caudwell V, Loupy A, Bruneval P, Jacquot C, Nochy D (2011) Focal segmental glomerulosclerosis plays a major role in the progression of IgA nephropathy. II. Light microscopic and clinical studies. Kidney Int 79:643-654

Flyvbjerg A, Dagnaes-Hansen F, De Vriese AS, Schrijvers BF, Tilton RG, Rasch R (2002) Amelioration of long-term renal changes in obese type 2 diabetic mice by a neutralizing vascular endothelial growth factor antibody. Diabetes 51:3090-3094

George SJ, Johnson JL, Smith MA, Angelini GD, Jackson CL (2005) Transforming growth factor-ß is activated by plasmin and inhibits smooth muscle cell death in human saphenous vein. J Vasc Res 42:247-254

Gewin L, Bulus N, Mernaugh G, Moeckel G, Harris RC, Moses HL, Pozzi A, Zent R (2010) TGF-ß receptor deletion in the renal collecting system exacerbates fibrosis. J Am Soc Nephrol 21:1334-1343

Grainger DJ, Frow EK (2000) Thrombospondin 1 does not activate transforming growth factor-ß 1 in a chemically defined system or in smooth muscle-cell cultures. Biochem J 350:291-298

Gregory MC, Terreros DA, Barker DF, Fain PN, Denison JC, Atkin CL (1996) Alport syndrome-clinical phenotypes, incidence, and pathology. Contrib Nephrol 117:1-28

Guha M, Xu Z-G, Tung D, Lanting L, Natarajan R (2007) Specific down-regulation of connective tissue growth factor attenuates progression of nephropathy in mouse models of type 1 and type 2 diabetes. FASEB J 21:3355–3368

Hartner A, Hilgers KF, Bitzer M, Veelken R, Schöcklmann HO (2003) Dynamic expression patterns of transforming growth factor-ß(2) and transforming growth factor-ß receptors in experimental glomerulonephritis. J Mol Med 81:32-42

Hill C, Flyvbjerg A, Gronbaek H, Petrik H, Hill DJ, Thomas CR, Sheppard MC, Logan A (2000) The renal expression of transforming growth factor-ß isoforms and their receptors in acute and chronic experimental diabetes in rats. Endocrinology 141:1196- 1208

Hill GS, El Karoui K, Karras A, Mandet C, Van Huyen J-P D, Nochy D, Bruneval P (2011) Focal segmental glomerulosclerosis plays a major role in the progression of IgA nephropathy. I. Immunohistochemical studies. Kidney Int 79:635-642

Hugo C, Shankland SJ, Pichler RH, Couser WG, Johnson RJ (1998) Thrombospondin-1 precedes and predicts the development of tubulointerstitial fibrosis in glomerular disease in the rat. Kidney Int 53:302-311

Hyytiäinen M, Penttinen C, Keski-Oja J (2004) Latent TGF-ß binding proteins: extracellular matrix association and roles in TGF-ß activation. Crit Rev Clin Lab Sci 41:233-264

Ibels LS, Györy AZ (1994) IgA nephropahy: analysis of the natural history, important factors in the progression of renal disease, and a review of the literature. Medicine 73:79-102

Iglesias-de la Cruz MC, Ziyadeh FN, Isono M, Kouahou M, Han DC, Kalluri R, Mundel P, Chen S (2002) Effects of high glucose and TGF-ß1 on the expression of collagen IV and vascular endothelial growth factor in mouse podocytes. Kidney Int 62:901-913

Ito Y, Aten J, Bende RJ, Oemar BS, Rabelink TJ, Weening JJ, Goldschmeding R (1998) Expression of connective tissue growth factor in human renal fibrosis. Kidney Int 53:853-861

Ito Y, Goldschmeding R, Bende RJ, Claessen N, Chand MA, Kleij L, Rabelink TJ, Weening JJ, Aten J (2001) Kinectics of connective tissue growth factor expression during experimental proliferative glomerulonephritis. J Am Soc Nephrol 12:472-484

Jobling MF, Mott JD, Finnegan MT, Jurukovski V, Erickson AC, Walian PJ, Taylor SE, Ledbetter S, Lawrence CM, Rifkin DB, Barcellos-Hoff MH (2006) Isoform-specific activation of latent transforming growth factor-ß (LTGF-ß) by reactive oxygen species. Radiat Res 166:839-848

Kashtan C, Kim Y, Lees GE, Thorner PS, Virtanen I, Miner JH (2001) Abnormal glomerular basement membrane laminins in murine, canine and human Alport syndrome: aberrant laminin α2 deposition is species independent. J Am Soc Nephrol 12:252-260

Katavetin P, Katavetin P (2008) VEGF inhibition and renal thrombotic microangiopathy. N Engl J Med 359:205-206

Kim HW, Moon KC, Park SY, Hong HK, Lee HS (2002) Differential expression of platelet-derived growth factor and transforming growth factor-ß in relation to progression of IgA nephropathy. Nephrology 7:S131-S139

Kim JH, Kim BK, Moon KC, Hong HK, Lee HS (2003) Activation of the TGF-ß/Smad signaling pathway in focal segmental glomerulosclerosis. Kidney Int 64:1715-1721

Kim KH, Kim Y, Gubler MC, Steffes MW, Lane PH, Kashtan CE, Crosson JT, Mauer SM (1995) Structural-functional relationships in Alport syndrome. J Am Soc Nephrol 5:1659-1668

Kim TS, Kim JY, Hong HK, Lee HS (1999) mRNA expression of glomerular basement membrane proteins and TGF-ß1 in human membranous nephropathy. J Pathol 189:425-430

Kim YS, Kim BC, Song CY, Hong HK, Moon KC, Lee HS (2001) Advanced glycosylation end products stimulate collagen mRNA synthesis in mesangial cells mediated by protein kinase C and transforming growth factor-beta. J Lab Clin Med 138:59-68

Koli K, Myllärniemi M, Keski-Oja J, Kinnula VL (2008) Transforming growth factor-ß activation in the lung: focus on fibrosis and reactive oxygen species. Antioxid Redox Signal 10:333-342

Koli K, Saharinen J, Hyytiäinen M, Penttinen C, Keski-Oja J (2001) Latency, activation, and binding proteins of TGF-ß. Microsc Res Tech 52:354-362

Kopp JB, Factor VM, Mozes M, Nagy P, Sanderson N, Boettinger EP, Klotman PE, Thorgeirsson SS (1996) Transgenic mice with increased plasma levels of TGF-ß1 develop progressive renal disease. Lab Invest 74: 991-1003

Kriz W, Gretz N, Lemley KV (1998) Progression of glomerular diseases: Is the podocyte the culprit? Kidney Int 54:687-697

Lawrence DA (2001) Latent TGF-ß: An overview. Mol Cell Biochem 219:163-170

Lee HS (2011) Pathogenic role of TGF-ß in the progression of podocyte diseases. Histol Histopathol 26:107-116

Lee HS, Choi Y, Lee JS, Yu BH, Koh HI (1989) Ultrastructural changes in IgA nephropathy in relation to histologic and clinical data. Kidney Int 35:880-886

Lee HS, Koh HI (1993) Nature of progressive glomerulosclerosis in human membranous nephropathy. Clin Nephrol 39:7-16

Lee HS, Koh HI, Lee HB, Park HC (1987) IgA nephropathy in Korea: a morphological and clinical study. Clin Nephrol 27:131-140

Lee HS, Lee MS, Lee SM, Lee SY, Lee ES, Lee EY, Park SY, Han JS, Kim S, Lee JS (2005) Histological grading of IgA nephropathy predicting renal outcome: revisiting HS Lee's glomerular grading system. Nephrol Dial Transplant 20:342-348

Lee HS, Lim SD (1995) The significance of glomerular hypertrophy in focal segmental glomerulosclerosis. Clin Nephrol 44:349-355

Lee HS, Moon KC, Song CY, Kim BC, Hong HK (2004) Glycated albumin activates PAI-1 transcription through Smad DNA binding sites in mesangial cells. Am J Physiol Renal Physiol 287:F665-F672

Lee HS, Park SY, Moon KC, Hong HK, Song CY, Hong SY (2001) mRNA expression of urokinase and plasminogen activator inhibitor-1 in human crescentic glomerulonephritis. Histopathology 39:203-209

Lee HS, Song CY (2009a) Oxidized low-density lipoprotein and oxidative stress in the development of glomerulosclerosis. Am J Nephrol 29:62-70

Lee HS, Song CY (2009b) Differential role of mesangial cells and podocytes in TGF-ß-induced mesangial matrix synthesis in chronic glomerular disease. Histol Histopathol 24:901-908

Lee LK, Pollock AS, Lovett DH (1993) Asymmetric origins of the mature glomerular basement membrane. J Cell Physiol 157:169-177

Liu N, Makino T, Nogaki F, Kusano H, Suyama K, Muso E, Honda G, Kita T, Ono T (2004) Coagulation in the mesangial area promotes ECM accumulation through factor V expression in MsPGN in rats. Am J Physiol Renal Physiol 287:F612-F620

Lorenzen J, Shah R, Biser A, Staicu SA, Niranjan T, Garcia AM, Gruenwald A, Thomas DB, Shatat IF, Supe K, Woroniecki RP, Susztak K (2008) The role of osteopontin in the development of albuminuria. J Am Soc Nephrol 19:884-890

Lyons R, Gentry LE, Purchio AF, Moses HL (1990) Mechanism of activation of latent recombinant transforming growth factor-ß1 by plasmin. J Cell Biol 110:1361-1367

Meehan DT, Delimont D, Cheung L, Zallocchi M, Sansom SC, Holzclaw JD, Rao V, Cosgrove D (2009) Biomechanical strain causes maladaptive gene regulation, contributing to Alport glomerular disease. Kidney Int 76:968-976

Mu D, Cambier S, Fjellbirkeland L, Baron JL, Munger JS, Kawakatsu H, Sheppard D, Broaddus VC, Nishimura SL (2002) The integrin αvß8 mediates epithelial homeostasis through MT1-MMP-dependent activation of TGF-ß1. J Cell Biol 157:493- 507

Munger JS, Huang X, Kawakatsu H, Griffiths MJ, Dalton SL, Wu J, Pittet JF, Kaminski N, Garat C, Matthay MA, Rifkin DB, Sheppard D (1999) The integrin αvß6 binds and activates latent TGFß 1: a mechanism for regulating pulmonary inflammation and fibrosis. Cell 96:319-328

Okada T, Wada J, Hida K, Eguchi J, Hashimoto I, Baba M, Yasuhara A, Shikata K, Makino H (2006) Thiazolidinediones ameliorate diabetic nephropathy via cell cycle-dependent mechanisms. Diabetes 55:1666-1677

Otsuka G, Stempien-Otero A, Frutkin AD, Dichek DA (2007) Mechanisms of TGF-ß1-induced intimal growth. Plasminogen-independent activities of plasminogen activator inhibitor-1 and heterogeneous origin of intimal cells. Circ Res 100:1300-1307

Patek CE, Fleming S, Miles CG, Bellamy CO, Ladomery M, Spraggon L, Mullins J, Hastie ND, Hooper ML (2003) Murine Denys-Drash syndrome: evidence of podocyte dedifferentiation and systemic mediation of glomerulosclerosis. Hum Mol Genet 12:2379-2394

Perna A, Schieppati A, Zamora J, Giuliano GA, Braun N, Remuzzi G (2004) Immunosuppressive treatment for idiopathic membranous nephropathy: a systematic review. Am J Kidney Dis 44:385-401

Porst M, Daniel C, Plank C, Schocklmann HO, Reinhardt DP, Hartner A (2006) Induction and coexpression of latent transforming growth factor ß-binding protein-1 and fibrillin-1 in experimental glomerulonephritis. Nephron Exp Nephrol 102:e99-e104

Remuzzi A, Monaci N, Bonassi ME, Corna D, Zoja C, Mohammed EI, Remuzzi G (1999) Angiotensin-converting enzyme inhibition prevents loss of glomerular hydraulic permeability in passive Heymann nephritis. Lab Invest 79:1501-1510

Remuzzi G, Schieppati A, Ruggenenti P (2002) Clinical practice. Nephropathy in patients with type 2 diabetes. N Engl J Med 346:1145-1151

Riser BL, Denichilo M, Cortes P, Baker C, Grondin JM, Yee J, Narins RG (2000) Regulation of connective tissue growth factor activity in cultured rat mesangial cells and its expression in experimental diabetic glomerulosclerosis. J Am Soc Nephrol 11:25–38

Satchell SC, Tasman CH, Singh A, Ni L, Geelen J, von Ruhland CJ, O'Hare MJ, Saleem MA, van den Heuvel LP, Mathieson PW (2006) Conditionally immortalized human glomerular endothelial cells expressing fenestrations in response to VEGF. Kidney Int 69:1633-1640

Sayers R, Kalluri R, Rodgers KD, Shield III CF, Meehan DT, Cosgrove D (1999) Role for transforming growth factor-ß1 in Alport renal disease progression. Kidney Int 56:1662-1673

Shankland SJ, Pippin J, Pichler RH, Gordon KL, Friedman S, Gold LI, Johnson RJ, Couser WG (1996) Differential expression of transforming growth factor-ß isoforms and receptors in experimental membranous nephropathy. Kidney Int 50:116-124

Stanescu HC, Arcos-Burgos M, Medlar A, Bockenhauer D, Kottgen A, Dragomirescu L, Voinescu C, Patel N, Pearce K, Hubank M, Stephens HA, Laundy V, Padmanabhan S, Zawadzka A, Hofstra JM, Coenen MJ, den Heijer M, Kiemeney LA, Bacq-Daian D, Stengel B, Powis SH, Brenchley P, Feehally J, Rees AJ, Debiec H, Wetzels JF, Ronco P, Mathieson PW, Kleta R (2011) Risk HLA-DQA1 and PLA_2R1 alleles in idiopathic membranous nephropathy. N Engl J Med 364:616-626

Stein-Oakley AN, Maguire JA, Dowling J, Perry G, Thomson NM (1997) Altered expression of fibrogenic growth factors in IgA nephropathy and focal and segmental glomerulosclerosis. Kidney Int 51:195-204

Strehlau J, Schachter AD, Pavlakis M, Singh A, Tejani A, Strom TB (2002) Activated intrarenal transcription of CTL-effectors and TGF-ß1 in children with focal segmental glomerulosclerosis. Kidney Int 61:90-95

Suzuki D, Toyoda M, Umezono T, Uehara G, Zhang S-Y, Sakai T, Nishina M, Suga T, Endoh M, Yagame M, Sakai H (2003) Glomerular expression of connective tissue growth factor mRNA in various renal diseases. Nephrology 8:92-97

Taipale J, Koli K, Keski-Oja J (1992) Release of transforming growth factor-ß1 from the pericellular matrix of cultured fibroblasts and fibrosarcoma cells by plasmin and thrombin. J Biol Chem 267:25378-25384

Trevillian P, Paul H, Millar E, Hibberd A, Agrez MV (2004) αvß6 integrin expression in diseased and transplanted kidneys. Kidney Int 66:1423-1433

Veron D, Reidy KJ, Bertuccio C, Teichman J, Villegas G, Jimenez J, Shen W, Kopp JB, Thomas DB, Tufro A (2010) Overexpression of VEGF-A in podocytes of adult mice causes glomerular disease. Kidney Int 77:989-999

Wahab NA, Schaefer L, Weston BS, Yiannikouris O, Wright A, Babelova A, Schaefer R, Mason RM (2005) Glomerular expression of thrombospondin-1, transforming growth factor beta and connective tissue growth factor at different stages of diabetic nephropathy and their interdependent roles in mesangial response to diabetic stimuli. Diabetologia 48:2650-2660

Wakefield LM, Winokur TS, Hollands RS, Christopherson K, Levinson AD, Sporn MB (1990) Recombinant latent transforming growth factor ß1 has a longer plasma half-life in rats than active transforming growth factor ß1, and a different tissue distribution. J Clin Invest 86:1976-1984

Wendt TM, Tanji N, Guo J, Kislinger TR, Qu W, Lu Y, Bucciarelli LG, Rong LL, Moser B, Markowitz GS, Stein G, Bierhaus A, Liliensiek B, Arnold B, Nawroth PP, Stern DM, D'Agati VD, Schmidt AM (2003) RAGE drives the develolpment of glomerulosclerosis and implicates podocyte activation in the pathogenesis of diabetic nephropathy. Am J Pathol 162:1123-1137

Whitworth JA, Turner DR, Leibowitz S, Cameron JS (1978) Focal segmental sclerosis or scarred focal proliferative glomerulonephritis? Clin Nephrol 9:229–235

Wolf G, Chen S, Ziyadeh FN (2005) From the periphery of the glomerular capillary wall toward the center of disease: podocyte injury comes of age in diabetic nephropathy. Diabetes 54:1626-1634

Working Group of the International IgA Nephropathy Network and the Renal Pathology Society, Coppo R, Troyanov S, Camilla R, Hogg RJ, Cattran DC, Cook HT, Feehally J, Roberts IS, Amore A, Alpers CE, Barratt J, Berthoux F, Bonsib S, Bruijn JA, D'Agati V, D'Amico G, Emancipator SN, Emma F, Ferrario F, Fervenza FC, Florquin S, Fogo AB, Geddes CC, Groene HJ, Haas M, Herzenberg AM, Hill PA, Hsu SI, Jennette JC, Joh K, Julian BA, Kawamura T, Lai FM, Li LS, Li PK, Liu ZH, Mezzano S, Schena FP, Tomino Y, Walker PD, Wang H, Weening JJ, Yoshikawa N, Zhang H (2010) The Oxford IgA nephropathy clinicopathological classification is valid for children as well as adults. Kidney Int 77:921-927

Yokoi H, Mukoyama M, Mori K, Kasahara M, Suganami T, Sawai K, Yoshioka T, Saito Y, Ogawa Y, Kuwabara T, Sugawara A, Nakao K (2008) Overexpression of connective tissue growth factor in podocytes worsens diabetic nephropathy in mice. Kidney Int 73:446-455

Yu L, Border WA, Anderson I, McCourt M, Huang Y, Noble NA (2004) Combining TGF-ß inhibition and angiotensin II blockade results in enhanced antifibrotic effect. Kidney Int 66:1774-1784

Yu Q, Stamenkovic I (2000) Cell surface-localized matrix metalloproteinase-9 proteolytically activates TGF-ß and promotes tumor invasion and angiogenesis. Genes Dev 14:163-176

Zhang H, Schin M, Saha J, Burke K, Holzman LB, Filipiak W, Saunders T, Xiang M, Heilig CW, Brosius FC 3rd (2010) Podocyte-specific overexpression of GLUT1 surprisingly reduces mesangial matrix expansion in diabetic nephropathy in mice. Am J Physiol Renal Physiol 299: F91-98

Zhang YZ, Lee HS (1997) Quantitative changes in the glomerular basement membrane components in human membranous nephropathy. J Pathol 183:8-15

Zheng S, Carlson EC, Yang L, Kralik PM, Huang Y, Epstein PN (2008) Podocyte-specific overexpression of the antioxidant metallothionein reduces diabetic nephropathy. J Am Soc Nephrol 19:2077-2085

Ziyadeh FN, Han DC, Cohen JA, Guo J, Cohen MP (1998) Glycated albumin stimulates fibronectin gene expression in glomerular mesangial cells: involvement of the transforming growth factor-ß sytstem. Kidney Int 53:631-638

Ziyadeh FN, Hoffman BB, Han DC, Iglesias-de la Cruz MC, Hong SW, Isono M, Chen S, McGowan TA, Sharma K (2000) Long-term prevention of renal insufficiency, excess matrix gene expression, and glomerular mesangial matrix expansion by treatment with monoclonal antitransforming growth factor-ß antibody in db/db diabetic mice. Proc Natl Acad Sci USA 97:8015-8020

Ziyadeh FN, Sharma K, Ericksen M, Wolf G (1994) Stimulation of collagen gene expression and protein synthesis in murine mesangial cells by high glucose is mediated by autocrine activation of transforming growth factor-ß. J Clin Invest 93:536-542

Ziyadeh FN, Wolf G (2008) Pathogenesis of the podocytopathy and proteinuria in diabetic glomerulopathy. Curr Diabetes Rev 4:39-45

8

Glomerulonephritis and Cellular Regulation of Prostaglandin Synthesis

Andrey Sorokin
Medical College of Wisconsin, USA

1. Introduction

Prostaglandins, hormone-like substances initially isolated from human semen in 1930, got their name from the presumption that they predominately come from the prostate gland (von Euler 1936). In fact, prostaglandins are lipid mediators generated by a wide variety of cell types and tissues. Being derivatives of 20 carbon fatty acids, their common feature is 20-carbon skeleton which includes 5-member carbon ring. Prostaglandins are major players in human physiology in both healthiness and illness and are key molecules in the generation of the inflammatory response (Miller 2006). Their synthesis is drastically increased in inflamed tissue and prostaglandin-mediated signaling contributes to the development of acute inflammation (Ricciotti and Fitzgerald 2011). Prostaglandins regulate a number of principal signal transduction pathways that modulate progression of renal diseases: cellular adhesion, growth, and differentiation. Cyclooxygenases (also termed PGH_2 synthases) are key enzymes in the production of prostaglandins from arachidonic acid and an immediate product of cyclooxygenase activity, prostaglandin H_2 (PGH_2), is used as a substrate by a number of terminal prostaglandin- and thromboxane synthases to produce a whole series of potent bioactive prostanoids. Multiple extracellular mitogens, including PDGF and endothelins, are involved in the pathogenesis of proliferative forms of glomerulonephritis. They share ability to induce Cox-2 expression in glomerular cells resulting in the release of prostanoids, with PGE_2 being a major prostaglandin produced by renal cells. Selective Cox-2 inhibitors have an anti-inflammation effect and reduce manifestation of experimental membranous glomerulonephritis. This chapter will discuss the role of prostaglandin synthesis and signaling via specific prostaglandin receptors in the progression of different types of glomerulonephritis.

2. Cellular synthesis of prostaglandins

Arachidonic acid is released from membrane glycerophospholipids by phospholipase A_2 and is converted to PGH_2 by cyclooxygenases in two steps. Firstly, it is catalyzed to the cyclic endoperoxidase, prostaglandin G_2 (PGG_2), via an intermediate radical. After that PGG_2 is further transformed to PGH_2 by a peroxidase reaction (Fig.1). Remarkably, cyclooxygenase molecule possesses two distinct active sites which are responsible for both steps (Marnett *et al.* 1999; Smith *et al.* 2000). The cyclooxygenase active site appears to be an L-shaped hydrophobic channel which contains active-site Tyr-385 shown to be directly involved in catalysis, whereas other residues in the active-site are controlling arachidonic acid positioning to ensure that PGG_2 is produced, not hydroperoxide side products (Thuresson *et al.* 2001). Both radical abstraction by a tyrosyl radical and combined radical/carbocationic models have been proposed for this reaction, but a combined radical/carbocation mechanism seems to be less likely (Silva *et al.* 2007). Generation of tyrosyl radical at Tyr-385 at cyclooxygenase active site is a consequence of oxidation of the heme group at the peroxidase active site by a hydroperoxide. The peroxidase site activity catalyzes the two-electron reduction of the hydroperoxide bond of PGG_2 to produce the PGG_2 and as indicated by site-directed mutagenesis the conserved cationic pocket is involved in enzyme-substrate binding (Chubb *et al.* 2006). Since cyclooxygenases function as homodimers and each monomer contains its own cyclooxygenase and peroxidase active sites, one would expect to have four total active sites per functional unit (dimer) of enzyme. On the contrary, it was shown, that while enzyme monomers comprising a dimer are identical in the resting enzyme, they differ from one another during catalysis: the nonfunctioning subunit provides structural support enabling its partner monomer to catalyze the cyclooxygenase reaction (Yuan *et al.* 2006). Each monomer of the functional

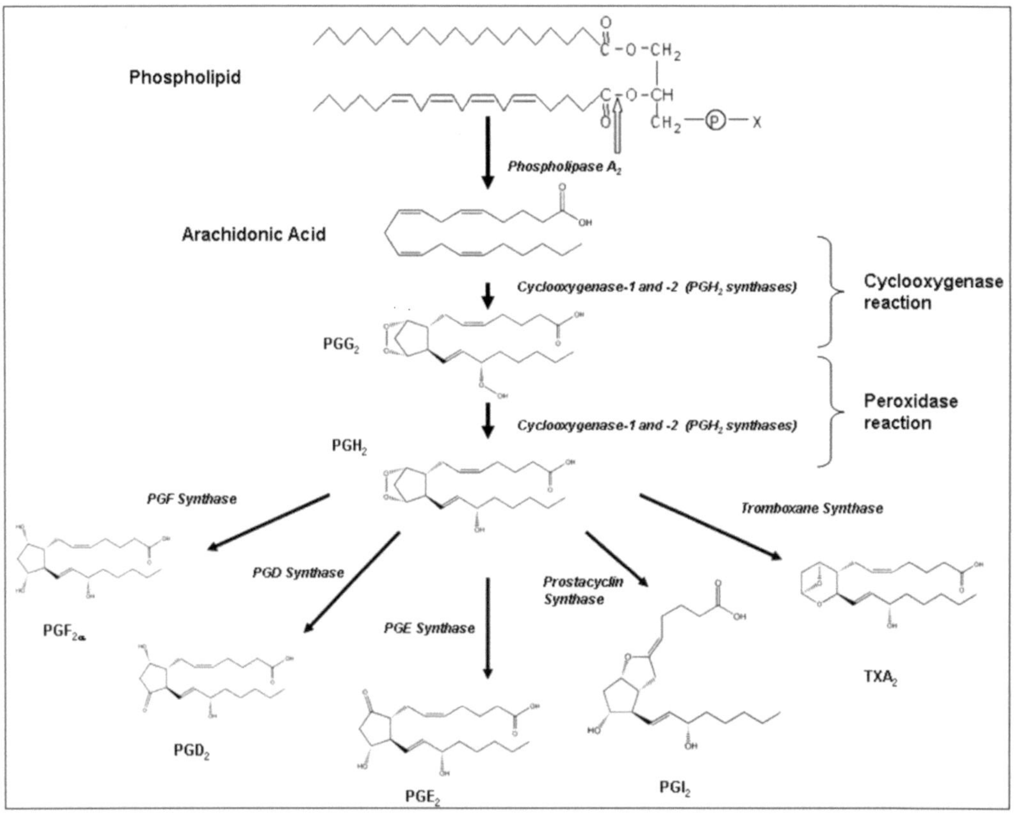

Fig. 1. Synthesis of prostanoids from arachidonic acid. Arachidonic acid is liberated from phospholipid by phospholipase A_2 which acts at the sn-2 position of glycerophospholipid (site shown by blank arrow). Both cyclooxygenase and peroxidase reactions catalyzed by cyclooxygenases are shown. Further conversion of cyclooxygenase products by terminal prostaglandin synthases is also depicted.

cyclooxygenase homodimer attaches to the endoplasmic reticulum or nuclear envelope membrane through membrane binding domain which contains the main route of substrate entry into the cyclooxygenase active site (Menter *et al.* 2010; Spencer *et al.* 1999; Chandrasekharan and Simmons 2004). Being a relatively unstable intermediate, PGH_2 is rapidly converted to distinct prostanoids by corresponding terminal prostaglandin synthases (Helliwell *et al.* 2004). Five major active prostanoids produced in vivo are $PGF_{2\alpha}$, PGD_2, PGE_2, prostacyclin (PGI_2) and thromboxane (TXA_2) (Fig.1). J-series prostaglandins including PGJ_2, Δ12-PGJ_2, and 15-deoxy-Δ12,14- PGJ_2 (15d-PGJ_2) are naturally occurring metabolites of PGD_2. In addition to prostaglandin synthase mediated conversion to prostanoids, PGH_2 can undergo spontaneously non-enzymatically decomposition, resulting in production of γ-keto aldehydes - levuglandins (Salomon and Miller 1985). Since PGI_2 contains an oxygen bridge between carbons 6 and 9, whereas TXA_2 is characterized by unstable bicyclic oxygenated ring, they are structurally different from prostaglandins and considered to be separate groups of lipid mediators. In this chapter we will discuss the cellular regulation and signaling of only three true prostaglandins $PGF_{2\alpha}$, PGD_2 and PGE_2.

There are two isoforms of cyclooxygenses: Cyclooxygenase 1 (Cox-1) and Cyclooxygenase 2 (Cox-2) which differ remarkably in the mode of expression (Smith *et al.* 2000). Cox-1 is characterized by constitutive expression in most tissues, whereas Cox-2 is the inducible form of the enzyme, which is expressed upon stimulation with a wide variety of growth factors and cytokines (DuBois *et al.* 1998; Smith *et al.* 2000). Both Cox-1 and Cox-2 catalyze the same enzymatic reaction and segregated utilization of Cox-1 and Cox-2 (even whey they are expressed in same cell) is believed to occur in the distinct prostaglandin biosynthetic pathways (Kudo and Murakami 2005). Even though Cox-2 expression is often a part of the complex biological response (such as inflammation) to harmful stimulus or pathogens, the constitutive expression of Cox-2 is observed in restricted subpopulations of cells (Harris and Breyer 2001). In renal cortex Cox-2 expression was localized to the macula densa of the juxtaglomerular apparatus and to adjacent epithelial cells of the cortical thick ascending limb of Henle (Harris *et al.* 1994). Since macula densa cells are constantly exposed to varying levels of luminal salt concentrations and stress-inducing variability in osmolarity (Bell *et al.* 2003) the constitutive activation of Cox-2 in these cells could be explained by resulting steady activation of intracellular signaling pathways known to regulate Cox-2 expression. Given that enforced activation of three major mammalian MAPK (ERK, SAPK and p38 MAPK) leads to the induction of Cox-2 mRNA and protein (McGinty *et al.* 2000) it is possible that constitutive activation of any of these MAPK in macula densa cells is the cause of Cox-2 up-regulation. The transcriptional regulation of Cox-2 is studied in sufficient details. Overall, expression of Cox-2 mRNA is regulated by several transcription factors including the cyclic-AMP response element binding protein (CREB), nuclear factor kappa B (NFkB) and the CCAAT-enhancer binding protein (C/EBP) (Tsatsanis *et al.* 2006). Another example of cells constitutively expressing Cox-2 is offered by tumor cells of different origin. Not only tumor progression is frequently accompanied by enlarged Cox-2 expression, but also selective Cox-2 inhibitors shield against the formation of numerous tumor types in experimental animals (Dannenberg *et al.* 2005). It is likely, that increased expression of Cox-2 in tumor cells can be in part caused by constitutively active signaling cascades set off by activating mutations in signaling molecules which happen in carcinogenesis. It is generally accepted that Cox-2-mediated resistance to apoptosis of cancer cells is amongst mechanisms of Cox-2 related tumor promotion (Riedl *et al.* 2004; Arun and Goss 2004). Since anticancer drugs typically act through induction of apoptotic cell death in cancer cells (Jendrossek and Handrick 2003; Kawanishi and Hiraku 2004), Cox-2 expression antagonizes anticancer treatment making cells resistant to apoptosis and therefore decreases the efficiency of therapy.

Traditional nonsteroidal anti-inflammatory drugs (NSAIDs) inhibit both cyclooxygenase isoforms and act as competitive active site inhibitors (Ricciotti and Fitzgerald 2011). It is believed, however, that NSAIDs have their anti-inflammatory, analgesic and antipyretic effects due to inhibition of Cox-2. There is a lot of interest in NSAIDs as possible accessories to cancer chemotherapy (Moore and Simmons 2000; Subbaramaiah *et al.* 1997; Thun *et al.* 2002) and they were shown to reduce incidence of colon cancer (DuBois *et al.* 1998). Still their undesirable side effects such as gastrointestinal ulceration, bleeding and platelet dysfunctions (due to inhibition of Cox-1) drastically limited enthusiasm about them as anti-cancer drugs. Since a new class of Cox-2 selective inhibitors (COXIBs) which preferentially inhibit the Cox-2 with significantly reduced side effects became available, these compounds have emerged as an important therapeutic tool for treatment of pain and arthritis (3). Again, the initial excitement about Cox-2 selective inhibitors has diminished in recent times because it became clear that their use is associated with an increased cardiovascular risk (Fitzgerald 2004; Furberg *et al.* 2005). Furthermore, COXIBs can probably act independently of their effect upon Cox-2 (Hanif *et al.* 1996) leaving physicians uncertain about mechanism of their action.

Biologically active prostaglandins regulate various physiological functions outside kidney which are of principal significance for embryo development, performance of cardiovascular and nervous systems and multiple other biological processes not necessarily connected with renal pathologies. The aim of current chapter is to evaluate the role of Cox-2 activity in the progression of glomerulonephritis and analyze contribution of signaling pathways initiated by particular prostaglandins to the manifestation of the disease. We will also discuss regulation of glomerular prostaglandin synthesis both by regulation of Cox-2 expression and by interaction of Cox-2 with specific proteins spatially co-localized with the enzyme in its natural environment. The significance of the discussed issues is that this cellular regulation of prostaglandin synthesis is an important contributor to the progression of glomerular renal diseases.

3. Renal effects of prostaglandins

3.1 Signaling by prostaglandins

Newly synthesized prostaglandins are crossing the membrane two times: first they are secreted into the extracellular space and later on operate as local hormones in the locality of their production site and again enter the cell prior to inactivation. The efflux could be maintained by simple diffusion, but often is facilitated by several prostaglandin carriers – transporters, which maintain energy-dependent prostaglandin transport across the plasma membrane (Schuster 2002). The common feature of all extracellular prostaglandins is that they accomplish their biological task via binding and activation of seven transmembrane domain G-protein coupled receptors (GPCR), of which eight types and subtypes (FP, DP, IP, TP and $EP_{1\text{-}4}$) are known (Narumiya *et al.* 1999). The rank order of affinity of prostaglandin ligands to their receptors is known and roles of individual receptors were established in individual mice knockdown systems (Kobayashi and Narumiya 2002). The mouse FP receptor binds $PGF_{2\alpha}$ with high affinity, IP receptor binds prostacyclin analogs, thromboxane is a ligand for TP receptor. Likewise, mouse DP receptor binds PGD_2, but PGD_2 can also interact and signal via chemoattractant receptor named CRTH2 (chemoattractant receptor homologous molecule expressed on Th2 cells), a seven-transmembrane G protein–coupled receptor selectively expressed in Th2 cells, T cytotoxic type 2 cells, eosinophils, and basophils (Satoh *et al.* 2006). DP receptor and CRTH2 receptor are named DP1 and DP2 receptors. PGE_2 is the most versatile prostaglandin because it has four types of receptors (Milatovic *et al.* 2011). All four EP receptors bind PGE_2 albeit with different affinity. The EP_1 receptor couples with the G_q protein and activates phospholipase C inducing mobilization of intracellular Ca^{2+}. The EP_2 and EP_4 receptors are coupled with the G_s protein, so they signal through elevation of intracellular cAMP levels and stimulate protein kinase A. On the contrary, the EP_3 receptor is coupled with the G_i protein causing the decrease of intracellular cAMP levels. Additionally to exerting their actions via G-protein coupled receptors, prostaglandins can activate peroxisome proliferator-activated receptors (PPAR), the superfamily of nuclear receptors that function as ligand-activated transcription factors (Rizzo and Fiorucci 2006). While three PPAR isoforms were described (PPAR-α, PPAR-β/δ, and PPAR-γ), PPAR-γ appears to be an intracellular target of 15d-PGJ_2 (Scher and Pillinger 2005).

3.2 Renal expression of prostaglandin receptors

Since focus of our attention is renal action of prostaglandins, intra-renal distribution of only prostaglandin receptors FP, $EP_{1\text{-}4}$ and DP will be discussed. For information about thromboxane TP and prostacyclin IP receptors please look at the excellent review by Breyer and Breyer (Breyer and Breyer 2001) and recent update by Nasralla and co-authors (Nasrallah *et al.* 2007). Using RT-PCR analysis and immunohistochemistry intra-renal distribution was established for the majority of prostaglandin receptors and transporters (Fig.2).

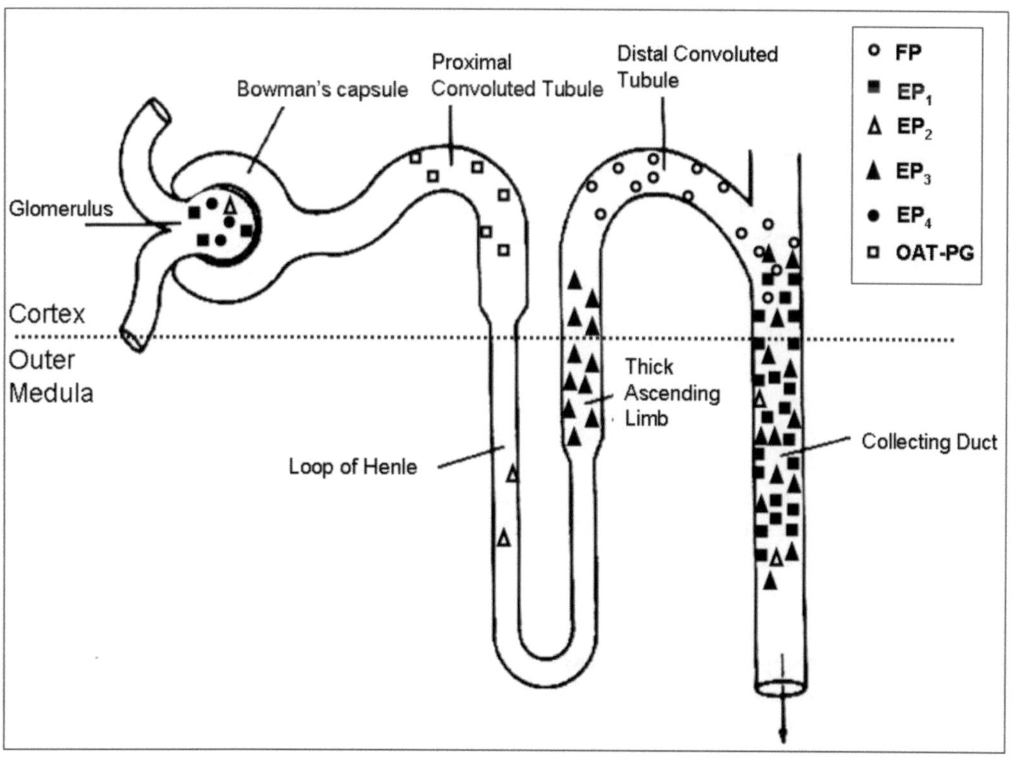

Fig. 2. Intra-renal distribution of selected prostaglandin receptors and transporters.

3.2.1 EP_1 receptors

EP_1 is expressed in glomerulus, collecting duct and vasculature (Breyer and Breyer 2001). Northern blotting indicated EP_1 expression in glomerular mesangial cells (Ishibashi *et al.* 1999). In reverse transcription-PCR studies, podocyte mRNA for the EP_1 could be amplified (Bek *et al.* 1999). In a mouse model of accelerated antiglomerular basement membrane (anti-GBM) nephrotoxic serum (NTS) nephritis EP_1 knockout resulted in stronger impairment of renal function (Rahal *et al.* 2006). EP_1 receptor immunoreactiviy is found in human renal tissue mainly in connecting segments, cortical and medullary collecting ducts, as well as in the media of arteries and afferent and efferent arterioles (Morath *et al.* 1999). It is not found in either proximal tubules, or thin limbs, thick ascending limbs of Henle's loop or distal convoluted tubules (Morath *et al.* 1999). It is able to mediate pain perception and regulate blood flow (Stock *et al.* 2001).

3.2.2 EP_2 receptors

The exact intra-renal distribution of EP_2 receptors is not entirely defined. Northern blot analysis of EP_2 mRNA distribution suggested diffuse expression with no specific increased localization in any particular segments of nephron (Breyer and Breyer 2001). RT-PCR analysis of microdissected rat nephron segments implied EP_2 expression in Henle's loop and in vasa recta of the outer medulla (Jensen *et al.* 2001). Immunolocalization data demonstrated prominent staining of EP_2 receptor only in the media of human arteries and of glomerular arterioles whereas staining of other structures of renal cortex or medulla was negative (Morath *et al.* 1999). It is interesting, that whereas EP_2 receptor is hard to detect in normal human kidney, EP_2 receptor expression was prominent in cystic epithelial cells lining cysts in polycystic kidney tissue from patients with autosomal-dominant polycystic kidney disease (Elberg *et al.* 2007).

3.2.3 EP_3 receptors

There are more than six alternatively spliced variants of EP_3 receptor in humans which differ by unique COOH-terminal intracellular tails (Breyer and Breyer 2000). By in situ hybridization and reverse-transcription PCR the intra-renal location of EP_3 receptor was shown to be the thick ascending limb (TAL) and collecting duct. Immunohistochemistry confirmed expression of EP_3 receptor in late distal convoluted tubules and in cortical and medullary collecting ducts (Morath *et al.* 1999).

3.2.4 EP_4 receptors

EP_4 receptor mRNA is found predominately in glomerulus. Like EP_2 receptors, EP_4 signals through increase of cAMP production, but it is much more abundant (Breyer and Breyer 2000). The strongest expression of the human protein was detected in smooth muscle cells of arteria, vasa recta and in glomerulus (Morath *et al.* 1999). In glomerulus EP_4 is detected in mesangial cells and podocytes (Ishibashi *et al.* 1999; Bek *et al.* 1999).

3.2.5 FP receptors

Studies using FP receptor promoter driving a β-galactosidase reporter indicated that these receptors are expressed in distal convoluted tubule (Breyer and Breyer 2001). Expression of gene encoding FP receptor in distal convoluted tubule and cortical collected duct was further confirmed by in situ hybridization, whereas glomeruli, proximal tubules, or thick ascending limbs showed no expression (Saito *et al.* 2003; Hebert *et al.* 2005a).

3.2.6 DP receptors

Even though DP receptor renal localization has not been shown for any species (Breyer and Breyer 2001), indirect evidence (altered tubular transport and haemodynamic effects of infused PGD_2) suggest the presence of renal DP receptors (Nasrallah *et al.* 2007).

3.3 Renal effect of PGE_2

3.3.1 Non-glomerular renal effect of PGE_2

It is sometimes difficult to distinguish glomerular and non-glomerular effects of prostaglandins, since even when the target cells are located outside the glomerulus, prostaglandin-mediated signaling events could be still relevant for the maintenance of glomerular function. For example changes in vascular tone could contribute to hypertension, which affects glomerular filtration rate. For the purposes of this review we consider effects of prostaglandins to be non-glomerular, if target cells are localized outside the glomeruli. PGE_2 is indisputably the most abundant kidney prostaglandin and since, in addition, it signals via four distinct subtypes of EP receptors, the renal effects of PGE_2 are multiple and complex. Furthermore, some of non-renal PGE_2 effects were abolished by inhibitors of EGF receptor tyrosine kinase indicating that transactivation of EGF receptor is part of the complex response to PGE_2 (Buchanan *et al.* 2003; Ding *et al.* 2005; Han *et al.* 2006). PGE_2-mediated transactivation of EGF receptor can't be ruled out for renal effects of PGE_2 either. Adding additional level of complexity, heterodimerization of EP1 with β2-adrenergic receptors was reported (McGraw *et al.* 2006). Probably the most important renal non-glomerular roles of PGE_2 are regulation of tubular transport processes along the nephron and regulation of vascular tone (Nasrallah *et al.* 2007). Availability of knockout mice deficient in each EP subtype facilitated understanding the role of each receptor subtype in renal and non-renal effects of PGE_2 (Sugimoto and Narumiya 2007; Kobayashi and Narumiya 2002). Thus, studies of mice deficient in each EP subtypes demonstrated that EP_4 receptor mediates renin secretion and that signaling via EP_1, EP_3, and EP_4 receptors contributes to increased PGE_2-mediated salt and water excretion in the model of hyperprostaglandin E syndrome/antenatal Bartter syndrome, a renal disease which is characterized by NaCl wasting, water loss, and hyperreninism (Nusing *et al.* 2005). In another study on isolated perfused kidneys from knockout mice both EP_2 and EP_4 stimulated renin secretion and all four subtypes were controlling renal vascular tone: EP_1 and EP_3 receptors were increasing it, whereas EP_2 and EP_4 were decreasing it (Schweda *et al.* 2004). Afferent arteriole diameter responses to vasoconstrictor peptide Endothelin-1 were enhanced in mice deficient in EP_2 receptor, indicating that PGE_2 vasodilative activity is handled at least partially through EP_2 (Imig *et al.* 2002). Similar data was obtained using mice deficient in microsomal PG synthase-1 (PGE synthase), enzyme responsible for converting PGH_2 into PGE_2. In these mice a 7 day AngII infusion at 0.35 mg/kg per day via osmotic minipump induced marked hypertensive response, which did not occur in wild type mice, suggesting that PGE_2 attenuates Ang II-induced vasoconstriction, probably because of inhibition of NADPH oxidase-dependent ROS production (Jia *et al.* 2008). Basal renal hemodynamics was not affected by EP_2 deficiency, but absence of EP_3 caused significant increase in basal renal blood flow. EP_3 receptor mediates vasoconstriction in the kidney, controls renal blood flow in basal state and buffers PGE_2-mediated renal vasodilation (Audoly *et al.* 2001).

Sodium reabsorption by epithelial Na+ channels (ENaC) located on the apical membrane of kidney distal and collecting duct plays central role in the maintenance of the extracellular fluid volume. Two classes of arachidonic acid metabolites, those produced by cytochrome P 450 enzymes (HETEs and EETs) and those generated by cyclooxygenases (prostaglandins) have opposite effect upon ENaC activity (Wang *et al.* 2009). 11,12-EET, 8,9-EET and 14,15-EET significantly inhibited ENaC NPo (probably due to direct and very fast interaction between EETs and ENaC) whereas PGE_2 had stimulatory effect and acted via second messengers (such as cAMP) (Wang *et al.* 2009). The Na+ balance and ENaC status are determined by interplay of the formation and actions of these two types of lipid mediators. PGE_2 also regulates (through G_s-coupled EP_2 and G_q-coupled EP_1) expression of ion carrier Na+/K+-ATPase (Nasrallah *et al.* 2007; Matlhagela and Taub 2006). On the transcriptional level PGE_2 was stimulating expression of β subunit of Na+/K+-ATPase encoded by the ATP1B1 gene.

PGE_2 also stimulates a number of anti-apoptotic signaling cascades in a variety of renal cells. Well established anti-apoptotic effect of Cox-2 is mediated as a general rule by anti-apoptotic signaling by PGE_2. Thus, in the process of autosomal-dominant polycystic kidney disease PGE_2 is released to cyst fluid, binds to EP_2 receptor, causes synthesis of cAMP and protects cystic epithelial cells from apoptosis eventually leading to cyst expansion (Elberg *et al.* 2007). Renal medullary interstitial cells are under significant osmotic/mechanical stress *in vivo* and respond to stress by expression of considerable levels of Cox-2 resulting in PGE_2 production (Carlsen *et al.* 2010). Inhibiting of PGE_2 synthesis in medullary interstitial cells was associated with their death and underlies to NSAID-associated injury in renal medulla (Hao *et al.* 1999). It appears that PGE_2 induces the expression of osmoprotective genes, including Cox-2, in medullary cells and promotes their survival and adaptation to increasing interstitial tonicities (Neuhofer *et al.* 2007). This positive feedback of PGE_2 upon Cox-2 expression during osmotic stress is mediated by binding to EP_2 receptors and resulting activation of cAMP-PKA signaling pathway (Steinert *et al.* 2009).

3.3.2 Contribution of signaling pathways initiated by PGE_2 to the manifestation of the glomerulonephritis

Different types of glomerulonephritis could be classified based on their clinical presentation or histopathology (Khanna 2011). Regardless glomerulonephritis etiology, the deterioration of renal function is often accompanied by a number of pathological processes which all contribute to the progression of renal injury. These prominent features include the progressive accumulation of extracellular matrix components, inflammatory changes, and in several types of glomerulonephritis also proliferation of glomerular mesangial cells and podocytes injury or proliferation (Kurogi 2003; Alchi and Jayne 2010; Couser and Johnson 1994; Gomez-Guerrero *et al.* 2005; Bariety *et al.* 2005). In this and similar sections we will review the potential contribution of particular prostaglandin to the signaling cascades underlying these pathological changes.

PGE_2 had pronounced mitogenic effect upon glomerular mesangial cells (Floege *et al.* 1991a; Floege *et al.* 1991b) and also induced DNA synthesis in glomerular core preparations enriched in mesangial cells (Mahadevan *et al.* 1996). The role of PGE_2 in accumulation of the extracellular matrix and structural components of glomerular basement membrane in glomeruli observed in patients with hypertensive syndromes of pregnancy has been suggested long ago (Foidart *et al.* 1983). Urinary concentrating functions were studied in EP_3 deficient mice and these mice did not loose their ability to concentrate and dilute urine normally in response to physiological stimuli, but urinary osmolarity increased significantly in wild type mice, but not in EP_3 null mice after inhibition of prostaglandin production by

indomethacin (Fleming *et al.* 1998). PGE_2 signaling through EP_4 receptors mediates podocyte injury and affects the glomerular filtration barrier (Stitt-Cavanagh *et al.* 2010).
PGE_2 is synthesized from PGH_2 by terminal PGE synthase mPGES-1. Since deletion or inhibition of mPGES-1 strikingly reduced inflammatory response in mouse models, PGE_2 emerged as an important mediator of inflammation (Ricciotti and Fitzgerald 2011). The progression of glomerulonephritis is accompanied by inflammation and enhanced production of PGE_2, is likely to contribute to inflammatory response, but the majority of studies using mPGES-1 null mice which link PGE_2 to inflammation did not focus on kidney injury (Ricciotti and Fitzgerald 2011). In a recent study mPGES-1 null mice were found to be protected from cisplatin induced nephrotoxicity, but not from acute kidney injury caused by ischemia-reperfusion or endotoxin (Jia *et al.* 2011). Direct evidence of PGE_2 involvement in inflammation will come from an analysis of experimental model of glomerulonephritis induced in mPGES-1 null animals. Due to the signaling via different receptors, PGE_2 is capable of both promoting and opposing the inflammatory response in several disorders (Ricciotti and Fitzgerald 2011; Milatovic *et al.* 2011)

3.4 Renal effect of $PGF_{2\alpha}$

3.4.1 Non-glomerular renal effect of $PGF_{2\alpha}$

$PGF_{2\alpha}$ is generated in different parts of the body, but due to rather quick inactivation by 15-prostaglandin dehydrogenase the half-life of released $PGF_{2\alpha}$ in circulation is less than 1 min. Since $PGF_{2\alpha}$ is sometimes considered as the most likely endothelium-derived contraction factor underlying endothelium-dependent, thromboxane-prostanoid receptor-mediated contractions to acetylcholine in the vasculature (Wong *et al.* 2009), fast inactivation is important for maintenance of normal vascular function. $PGF_{2\alpha}$ activates two spliced isoforms of FP receptor, which are coupled to G_q (Nasrallah *et al.* 2007). In cortical connecting duct $PGF_{2\alpha}$ increases calcium level and through pertussis-toxin sensitive pathway regulates water transport (Hebert *et al.* 2005b) and salt balance (Breyer and Breyer 2001). $PGF_{2\alpha}$ significantly enhanced the ENaC open probability NPo (Wang *et al.* 2009). Latanoprost, agonist of FP receptor, dramatically reduced vasopressin-induced water permeability in microperfused rabbit collecting ducts (Hebert *et al.* 2005a). In summary non-glomerular renal effects of $PGF_{2\alpha}$ are mainly relate to regulation of water and sodium transport.

3.4.2 Contribution of signaling pathways initiated by $PGF_{2\alpha}$ to the manifestation of the glomerulonephritis

Since $PGF_{2\alpha}$ is involved in a number of inflammation and oxidative stress related pathologies (Basu 2010) and could be produced in kidney in substantial amount, it's role in the inflammatory kidney diseases should be considered. Glomerular synthesis of $PGF_{2\alpha}$ (and some other prostaglandins including PGE_2) was stimulated by donors of oxygen radicals, which are likely to stimulate glomerular phospholipases at an early stage of experimental glomerulonephritis (Baud *et al.* 1981). $PGF_{2\alpha}$ is a potent stimulator of glomerular mesangial cell growth and its ability to promote DNA synthesis in quiescent mesangial cells is likely to be mediated by PLC activation as assessed by increased 1,4,5-inositol trisphosphate (IP3) generation and diacylglycerol (DAG) synthesis (Breshnahan *et al.* 1996; Kelefiotis *et al.* 1995). $PGF_{2\alpha}$ also rapidly increases free cytosolic calcium promoting mesangial cell contraction. Through calcium-dependent mechanism $PGF_{2\alpha}$ caused cytosolic acidification of mesangial cells followed by recovery and net alkalinization mediated by enhanced Na(+)-H+ exchange

(Mene *et al.* 1991). Effect of $PGF_{2\alpha}$ on increased glomerular mesangial cells calcium level could modulate glomerular contraction and affect glomerular function in glomerulonephritis.

3.5 Renal effect of PGD_2

3.5.1 Non-glomerular renal effect of PGD_2

There are not many reports about PGD_2 function in kidney. This prostaglandin is among major products of cyclooxygenases in macrophages and in bone marrow and is likely to play role in immunological responses (Padilla *et al.* 2000). It is capable to be converted to prostaglandin 15-deoxy-delta 12,14-PGJ_2 (15d-PGJ_2) that interacts with peroxisome proliferator-activated receptor γ (PPARγ) to promote ROS production and apoptosis in kidney proximal tubule cells (Padilla *et al.* 2000; Nasrallah *et al.* 2007). PGD_2 inhibited TGFβ1-induced epithelial-to-mesanchymal transition in MDCK cells (Zhang *et al.* 2006). In samples of renal papillary tissue PGD_2 modulates phosphatidylcholine biosynthesis through ERK and PLD activation (Fernandez-Tome *et al.* 2004).

3.5.2 Contribution of signaling pathways initiated by PGD_2 to the manifestation of the glomerulonephritis

In cultured mesangial cells 15d-PGJ_2, derivative of PGD_2, inhibited IFNγ-stimulated generation of cytokines presumably by targeting JAK/STAT signaling (Panzer *et al.* 2008). Since synthetic PPARγ ligands failed to produce similar effect, it is likely that in this case 15d-PGJ_2 acted independent of PPARγ interaction. Nevertheless, PPARγ , and correspondingly 15d-PGJ_2, was shown to play protective role in glomerular diseases (Chung *et al.* 2005). PPARγ is known to form heterodimers with 9-cis-retinoic acid receptor (RXRα) and, following ligand activation, to bind to PPARγ-responsive element (PPRE) which are present in the promoters of it's target genes (Kliewer *et al.* 1992). In addition PPARγ is also capable to antagonize the activities of other transcription factors (AP-1, STAT, NF-κB) and thus influence gene expression indirectly (Ricote *et al.* 1998). Although the pathogenesis of glomerulosclerosis is elusive, the imbalance between ECM synthesis and dissolution is the critical determinant of matrix accumulation. This net matrix turnover reflects rapid and specific changes in gene expression controlled by transcription factors that mediate various pathways of cellular injury. PPARγ is such a factor and has recently attracted significant attention for its anti-inflammatory and anti-fibrotic effects against diverse injuries in kidney, liver, lung and heart (Chung *et al.* 2005; Sugawara *et al.* 2010). The most recognized renal effect of agonists of PPARg on diabetic nephropathy is as a rule related to the improved glucose metabolism and insulin resistance. But, there is mounting evidence now that PPARγ also elicits nonmetabolic functions in the progression of glomerular diseases. Thus, PPARγ activation prevented albuminuria and enhanced glomerular ECM gene expression in models of both insulin dependent and independent diabetes and in 5/6 nephrectomized rats (Imano *et al.* 1998; Ma *et al.* 2001; Fujii *et al.* 1997). These effects were observed in the absence of changes in glucose level and systemic blood pressure. In cell culture, PPARγ inhibits ECM gene expression in mesangial cells (Maeda *et al.* 2005; Nicholas *et al.* 2001; Zheng *et al.* 2002). These effects emphasize the anti-fibrotic and anti-inflammatory roles of PPARγ in attenuating the progression of glomerular diseases.

3.6 Non-receptor action of prostaglandins

Even though prostaglandins act as a rule through their specific receptors, some effects of prostaglandins may be non-receptor-mediated. Several studies implied that prostaglandins exerted their diverse effects through post-translational modification of cellular proteins (Kim *et al.* 2007; Takahashi and Breitman 1992; Lecomte *et al.* 1990). Since prostaglandins possess anionic moieties at physiological pH and diffuse poorly through the lipid bilayer (Baroody and Bito 1981; Chan *et al.* 1998), the covalent modification of proteins by prostaglandins should be a carrier-mediated transport process. Several prostaglandins carriers have been cloned and characterized (Schuster 2002). Prostaglandin uptake carrier prostaglandin transporter (PGT) was shown to be expressed in renal collecting ducts and to participate in prostaglandin metabolic inactivation (Nomura *et al.* 2005). Another transporter designated OAT-PG exhibited Na^{+}-independent and saturable transport of PGE_2 and was shown to be present exclusively in the basolateral membrane of the proximal tubules in the kidney (Shiraya *et al.* 2010) (Fig.2). As others prostaglandin transporters, OAT-PG was proposed to be involved in the local PGE_2 clearance and metabolism for the purpose of inactivation of prostaglandin signals in the kidney cortex, but signaling from PGE_2 transported into the cell can't be ruled out. The covalent binding of prostaglandins to proteins has been detected in microsomal cell fractions and in intact platelets (Eling *et al.* 1977; Wilson *et al.* 1979; Anderson *et al.* 1979). It was demonstrated that proteins in HL-60 cells were labeled by PGE_2 (Takahashi and Breitman 1992). PGE_2 possesses a long-chain fatty acid portion that could bind covalently to proteins by an ester bond between its carboxyl group and either a hydroxyl amino acid or a cysteine of a protein. No data, so far, suggest the role of PGE_2-mediated modification of proteins in the progression of renal pathologies. Nevertheless prostaglandin-mediated modification of signaling molecules involved in the progression of glomerulonephritis can't be ruled out and should be kept in mind when renal effects of prostaglandins are observed in cells in the absence of detectable receptors, or in the presence of specific receptor inhibitors/antagonists.

4. Renal regulation of prostaglandin synthesis

4.1 Regulation at the level of availability of arachidonic acid

Liberation of free arachidonic acid from glycerophospholipids is catalyzed by phospholipase A_2 enzymes and presents the initial tightly regulated step in the synthesis of prostaglandins (Shimizu and Wolfe 1990). The diverse phospholipase A_2 enzymes have been classified into eleven groups (Six and Dennis 2000), but cytosolic phospholipase $A_2\alpha$ ($cPLA_2\alpha$), member of Group IV, preferentially hydrolyzes the sn-2 position of glycerophospholipids to produce free arachidonic acid, substrate for cyclooxigenase enzymes (Hirabayashi *et al.* 2004). Mice deficient in $cPLA_2\alpha$ grow normally but are characterized by renal concentration defect and cells derived from these mice produce significantly less amount of prostaglandins (Uozumi and Shimizu 2002). Regulation of $cPLA_2\alpha$ occurs mainly by phosphorylation of regulatory serines, by increasing intracellular Ca^{+2} concentrations and changes in enzyme subcellular localization (Hirabayashi *et al.* 2004). The requirement for extracellular Ca^{+2} and stretch-activated Ca^{+2} channels was shown for cyclic stretching-induced PLA_2 activation and a subsequent release of arachidonic acid in rabbit proximal tubular epithelial cells (Alexander *et al.* 2004). Calcium binding to $cPLA_2\alpha$ promotes its translocation to membrane containing phosphatidylcholine from the cytosol. Binding to membrane anionic phospholipids and phosphorylation of $cPLA_2\alpha$ by either MAPK on Ser505, or by CaMKII on Ser515, or by MAPK-interacting kinase Mnk1 on Ser727 are needed to stabilize $cPLA_2\alpha$ association with the membrane and to increase its intrinsic catalytic activity (Hirabayashi *et al.* 2004).

4.2 Regulation at the level of cyclooxygenases

It is generally accepted that the major mechanism employed by mammalian cells to regulate prostaglandin synthesis is through the control of expression of Cox-2. It is possible however that some alternative mechanisms regulating Cox-2 activity (and ultimately prostaglandin synthesis) exist and are at least partially responsible for the increased production of prostaglandins in glomerular kidney diseases.

4.2.1 Regulation of cyclooxygenases at the level of transcription

Signaling pathways involved in the regulation of Cox-2 expression are relatively well studied (Tsatsanis *et al.* 2006). A rapid and transient expression of Cox-2 was found to be associated with activation of NF kappa B and NF-IL6 transcription factors (Yamamoto *et al.* 1998). The promoter/enhancer region of Cox-2 genes from different mammalian species share a number of modulatory elements, which include cAMP-response element (CRE), nuclear factor (NF)-IL6, NF-κB and activator protein 2 (Kosaka *et al.* 1994). Three of these consensus sequences (CRE, NF-IL6 and NF-κB) have been implicated in agonist-dependent up-regulation of the human Cox-2 (Kosaka *et al.* 1994; Inoue and Tanabe 1997; Inoue and Tanabe 1998); additionally it appears that p53 might negatively regulate Cox-2 expression by binding to the TATA sequence (Subbaramaiah *et al.* 1999). Cox-2 expression is induced by multiple agonists and mitogens including PDGF (Goppelt-Struebe *et al.* 1996), EGF (Saha *et al.* 1999), TGFβ1 (Saha *et al.* 1999) and Endothelin-1 (Kester *et al.* 1994). It is of note that three principal mitogen activated protein kinase (MAPK) pathways ERK, JNK and p38 MAPK are activated by many of the agonists and stimuli capable of stimulating Cox-2 expression (Bokemeyer *et al.* 1996; Widmann *et al.* 1999). Furthermore, a number of MAPK-activated transcription factors are binding to the regions of the promoter of human gene encoding Cox-2 which are involved in the transcriptional activation of the gene (Widmann *et al.* 1999; Kosaka *et al.* 1994). Data obtained with adenovirus mediated gene transfer of constitutively active mutants of members of three principal MAPK signaling cascades provided evidence that enforced stimulation of any of them results in up-regulation of Cox-2 expression (McGinty *et al.* 2000). It looks like MAPK signaling cascades are the convergence point of the many dissimilar stimuli that up-regulate Cox-2.

4.2.2 Regulation of cyclooxygenases at the post-transcriptional pre-translational level

Regulation at the post-transcriptional pre-translational level occurs through regulation of Cox-2 mRNA stability (Tsatsanis *et al.* 2006). It was reported that signaling via p38 MAPK pathway was controlling Cox-2 mRNA stability (Jang *et al.* 2000) and occurred through p38 MAPK-regulated binding of mRNA stabilizing protein human antigen R (HuR) to the AU-rich region of the COX-2 3'-UTR (Subbaramaiah *et al.* 2003). HuR is related to the *Drosophila* embryonic lethal abnormal vision (ELAV) family of proteins, is ubiquitously expressed and was shown to stabilize COX-2 mRNA in human mesangial cells (Doller *et al.* 2007), human tracheal smooth muscle cells (Lin *et al.* 2011) and human keratinocytes exposed to various stimuli (Fernau *et al.* 2010). The involvement of p38 MAPK and HuR in Cox-2 expression was also confirmed by increased level of PGE_2 synthesis (Fernau *et al.* 2010). It is important that increased binding of (HuR) to the mRNAs of Cox-2 was demonstrated not only in cultured cells, but also in the cytoplasmic fractions of renal homogenates from AngII-treated rats (Doller *et al.* 2009).

4.2.3 Regulation of cyclooxygenases at the post- translational level

It seems that the kinetics of prostaglandin synthesis in mammalian cells does not always correlate with the level of cyclooxygenases expression. This suggested that there maybe alternative mechanisms in the cellular regulation of cyclooxygenases activity and ultimately, prostaglandin synthesis. There are not many reports which suggest regulation of catalytic activity of cyclooxygenases at the post-translational level. Until recently only two examples of post-translational regulation of Cox-2 were reported: s-nitrosylation and phosphorylation. iNOS was shown to bind specifically to Cox-2 and S-nitrosylate it, increasing Cox-2 catalytic activity (Kim *et al.* 2005). The same group demonstrated that Cox-2 can be activated by S-nitrosylation after selective binding of nNOS to Cox-2 via nNOS PDZ domain (Tian *et al.* 2008). S-nitrosylation of Cox-2 happened also *in vivo* in atravastatin-treated but not sham-treated rats. Remarkably, Cox-2 was co-immunoprecipitated from myocardial homogenates with iNOS but not with eNOS (Atar *et al.* 2006).

First hint that cyclooxygenase could be regulated by phosphorylation was obtained in cerebral endothelial cells where it was demonstrated that protein tyrosine phosphatase inhibitors rapidly stimulated cyclooxygenase activity resulting in elevated generation of prostaglandins. The protein tyrosine kinase inhibitors genistein and tyrphostins inhibited cyclooxygenase activity (Parfenova *et al.* 1998). It is important that in this study protein synthesis inhibitors were not able to reverse the stimulation of COX activity evoked by PTP inhibitors, suggesting posttranslational modification. The existence of PKC consensus sequences in Cox-2 prompted the investigation whether Cox-2 could be phosphorylated by the serine/threonine protein kinase C (Vezza *et al.* 1996). The obtained data argued against direct Cox-2 phosphorylation by PKC. Thus, even though some indirect evidence suggests that Cox-2 could be regulated by phosphorylation, no specific tyrosine or serine-threonine kinase has been proven to phosphorylate cyclooxygenases and regulate their activity.

We have observed that adenovirus-mediated gene transfer of Cox-2 into renal glomerular mesangial cells resulted in the formation of covalent adducts between Cox-2 and some unknown proteins (detected as high-molecular weight bands recognized by anti-Cox-2 antibodies in western blotting). Formation of these covalent adducts was dependent on Cox-2 enzymatic activity. To identify these proteins which may be involved in regulation of Cox-2 activity, we isolated Cox-2 adducts by affinity purification with Cox-2 antibody and subjected them to tandem mass spectrometry. A following search against mammalian database indicated the presence of a number of proteins, potential candidates for post-translational regulators of Cox-2 activity. It is possible that cross-linking of Cox-2 to some specific proteins spatially co-localized with the enzyme in its natural environment occurs due to spontaneous decomposition of PGH_2 resulting in production of γ-keto aldehydes - levuglandins, which are capable of covalently crosslinking different proteins together through their Lys residues (Iyer *et al.* 1989; Salomon and Miller 1985). One of the proteins cross-linked to Cox-2 was identified as ELMO1 (Engulfment and cell motility 1) (Yang and Sorokin 2011). ELMO1 is a bipartite guanine nucleotide exchange factor (GEF) for the small GTPase Rac 1, which is closely associated with susceptibility to glomerular disease (Shimazaki *et al.* 2005; Leak *et al.* 2009; Pezzolesi *et al.* 2009). ELMO1 was shown to increase fibronectin expression and contribute to the development and progression of chronic glomerular injury (Shimazaki *et al.* 2006). Interaction of endogenous ELMO1 with endogenous Cox-2 was demonstrated in glomerular mesangial cells (Yang and Sorokin 2011). This interaction of ELMO1 with Cox-2 increased Cox-2-mediated fibronectin upregulation, suggesting that ELMO1 serves as a post-translational modulator of Cox-2 activity. Since ELMO1 may participate in ECM accumulation in the pathogenesis of glomerular pathology through modifying Cox-2 activity via protein-protein interaction could play an important role in the development and progression of renal glomerular disease. How exactly interaction with ELMO1 up-regulates Cox-2 activity is not known. One possibility is that interaction with ELMO1 interferes with Cox-2 degradation and preserves Cox-2 for prolonged prostaglandin production. There are two pathways for Cox-2 protein degradation in vivo: Cox-2 can be degraded via the N-glycosylation-dependent endoplasmic reticulum-associated protein degradation pathway or by substrate-dependent degradation which is not inhibited by inhibitors of lysosomal proteases or proteasome inhibitors (Wada *et al.* 2009; Mbonye *et al.* 2008). Future investigation into whether ELMO1 protein interferes with these Cox-2 degradation pathways or contributes to Cox-2 conformational changes which affect its enzymatic activity will help to uncover precise mechanism of ELMO1 action.

4.3 Regulation at the level of prostaglandin synthases

The repertoire of prostaglandin production is determined by the differential expression of terminal prostaglandin synthases in cells located at sites of inflammation (Ricciotti and Fitzgerald 2011). In contrast to cyclooxygenases, there is less known about regulation of PGE-, PGD- and PGF-synthases which convert PGH_2 to PGE_2, PGD_2 and PGF_2 correspondingly. There are three prostaglandin E synthases (PGES): membrane-bound microsomal PGES-1 (mPGES-1), membrane-bound PGES-2 (mPGES-2) and cytosolic PGES (cPGES) (Kudo and Murakami 2005). mPGES-1 is functionally coupled to Cox-2 in preference to Cox-1 and, similar to Cox-2, mPGES-1 expression can be stimulated by proinflammatory stimuli (Kudo and Murakami 2005). Analysis of mPGES-1 promoter revealed that stimulus-inducible mPGES-1 transcription is under control of the transcription factor Egr-1, which binds to the proximal GC box (Naraba *et al.* 2002). Signal transduction pathway comprising phosphatidylcholine-phospholipase C, protein kinase C, NO, cGMP and protein kinas G is important for the induction of mPGES-1 by TNFα (Subbaramaiah *et al.* 2004). mPGES-2 is constitutively expressed, could be coupled either with Cox-1 or Cox-2, and inflammation or tissue damage do not cause increase of mPGES-2 expression (Kudo and Murakami 2005). cPGES is also constitutively expressed but is exclusively coupled with Cox-1. Regulation of cPGES is mediated by phosphorylation by casein kinase 2 (CK2) and Hsp90 acts as an essential scaffold protein to brings cPGES and CK2 in close proximity to allow their efficient functional interaction (Kudo and Murakami 2005). It must be mentioned, that there is some discrepancy in the literature with regard to the role of cPGES and mPGES-2 in PGE synthesis. Analysis of knockout mice deficient in either cPGES or mPGES-2 suggested that cPGES and mPGES-2 do not encode prostaglandin synthases and for that reason mPGES-1-dependent conversion of PGH_2 to PGE_2 may represent the only mechanism by which PGE_2 is produced *in vivo* (Jania *et al.* 2009; Lovgren *et al.* 2007).

5. Effect of glomerulitis on prostaglandin production

5.1 Overexpression of Cox-2 in renal diseases

Overexpression of Cox-2 and increased production of an array of prostaglandins occurs in inflammatory arthritis, several types of cancer, in inflammatory bowel disease (Turini and DuBois 2002) as well as in a number of kidney diseases, namely proliferative glomerulonephritis (Hirose *et al.* 1998; Chanmugam *et al.* 1995), hydronephronic kidney (Seibert *et al.* 1996), hypercalcemia (Mangat *et al.* 1997), hypertension (Khan *et al.* 2001),

diabetic nephropathy (Nasrallah *et al.* 2003; Khan *et al.* 2001) and renal ablation (Schneider and Stahl 1998). In normal kidneys renal Cox-2 expression was shown to localize in the macula densa and associated cortical thick ascending limb and medullary interstitial cells (Harris and Breyer 2001). In patients with active lupus nephritis Cox-2-specific staining was localized mainly in the glomeruli, whereas patients with non-lupus nephropathies had no increase in renal COX-2 expression (Tomasoni *et al.* 1998).
Oxidative stress is significantly higher in patients with proliferative glomerulonephritis, when compared with patients with non-proliferative glomerulonephritis (Markan *et al.* 2008). Oxidative stress is associated with excess of reactive oxygen species (ROS) and signaling pathways triggered by ROS can induce up-regulation of Cox-2 expression and prostaglandin production (Jaimes *et al.* 2008). Isolated glomeruli treated with donor of oxygen radicals increased the synthesis of several prostaglandins including PGE_2 and $PGF_{2\alpha}$ (Baud *et al.* 1981).

5.2 Regulation of prostaglandin synthesis in experimental models of glomerular proliferative diseases

In several in vivo experimental models Cox-2 contributed to progressive kidney injury (Cheng and Harris 2004). Cox-2 inhibition limited progressive injury in 5/6 nephrectomy rats (Fujihara et al. 2003) and also decreased proteinurea and retarded progressive renal injury in rats with renal ablation (Wang et al. 2000). Production of prostaglandins, particularly PGE_2, was shown to contribute to both progression (Hirose *et al.* 1998) and resolution (Hartner *et al.* 2000) of mesangioproliferative glomerulonephritis (GN). Studies with experimental models of glomerular proliferative diseases suggested that regulation of cellular synthesis of prostaglandins *in vivo* occurs at multiple levels. Cox-2 mRNA levels were increased in nephritic mice with MRL-Faslpr lupus nephritis and in mice with anti-glomerular basement membrane (GBM) antibody induced glomerulonephritis (Sun *et al.* 2001). Anti-GBM glomerulonephritis is usually induced by administration of sheep antibody against rat particulate glomerular basement membrane (GBM) and resembles human form of rapidly progressive crescentic nephritis. In the rat model of anti-GBM at the early time points (day 1) infiltration of glomeruli by activated macrophages is a prominent feature while at the late points (days 4, 7 and 14) glomerular cell proliferation and crescent formation are the prominent features (Bokemeyer et al. 1997). In Anti-GBM nephritis there is an increased expression of Cox-2 and enhanced production of prostaglandins in the glomerulus, which may mediate changes in renal hemodynamics (Lianos et al. 1983; Datta et al. 2006). Another experimental model of glomerulonephritis where proliferation of glomerular mesangial cells is a prominent feature is anti-Thy-1.1 model of mesangioproliferative glomerulonephritis. It is a well characterized rat model which closely simulates analogous human diseases with regard to initial mesangiolysis followed by mesangial cell proliferation and accumulation of mesangial matrix (Jefferson and Johnson 1999). Mesangioproliferative lesions start occurring 3–7 days after single injection (Yamamoto and Wilson 1987), and lesions are resolved within several weeks after injecting the antibody. The fact that expression of Cox-2 and $cPLA_2\alpha$ mRNAs was minimal in normal glomerulus and enhanced after induction of this model (Hirose *et al.* 1998) suggested the regulation of prostaglandin production at two levels: liberation of arachidonic acid and transcriptional regulation of Cox-2. Also post-translational regulation of Cox-2 could take place, since expression of the rat *Elmo1* gene was increased in the kidney of unilaterally nephrectomized rats injected with anti-Thy1.1 antibody (Shimazaki *et al.* 2006).

5.3 Mechanisms of renoprotective effect of Cox-2 inhibition

There could be multiple mechanisms by which inhibition of Cox-2 is renoprotective, but the suppression of apoptotic pathways is certainly one of them. It is of note, that glomerular mesangial cell (GMC) apoptosis appears to be the major mechanism for resolution of glomerular hypercellularity in experimental mesangial glomerulonephritis (Badawi 2000). Proliferation of GMC occurs in multiple forms of glomerular immune injury and if continued unopposed, would cause the progression of injury to end stage disease (Lianos 1992). The cell number in glomeruli is controlled by apoptosis, accordingly cell proliferation is counteracted by deletion of extra cells due to apoptotic cell death (Savill 1999). For that reason the failure to undergo apoptosis usually results in unbalanced glomerular cell multiplication; hence, apoptosis has been proposed as an essential mechanism involved in the resolution of a proliferative response. It seems likely that Cox-2 has anti-apoptotic effect, when expressed in renal glomerular cells. Surely, Cox-2 is not the only mediator of the resistance of renal GMC to apoptosis, but Cox-2, acting in concert with other survival factors is expected to contribute to the balance between increase in cell number caused by proliferation and cell elimination by programmed cell death. Both extrinsic (death-receptor initiated) and intrinsic (mitochondria-induced) apoptotic pathways are relevant to renal disease and both of them are likely to be inhibited by Cox-2. Macrophage-derived TNF-α induced apoptosis of mesangial cells in the course of glomerulonephritis and inhibition of NFκB-driven survival pathway promoted TNF-α apoptotic activity (Hirahashi et al. 2000), suggesting the involvement of Cox-2 expression. TNF-α-mediated apoptosis of cultured renal mesangial cells was prevented by Cox-2 expression, either enforced by adenovirus mediated gene transfer or induced by the vasoconstrictor peptide endothelin-1 or the cytokine interleukin-1β (Ishaque *et al.* 2003). Selective Cox-2 inhibition by NS-398 restored TNFα-mediated apoptosis, whereas addition of PGE_2 mimicked Cox-2 effect (Ishaque *et al.* 2003).

Even though it is generally accepted that Cox-2 expression has anti-apoptotic effect, the precise mechanism of Cox-2 anti-apoptotic activity is unknown and remains to be the focus of scientific interest of a number of laboratories. Several mechanisms have been proposed to explain the anti-apoptotic effect of Cox-2 (Cao and Prescott 2002), namely: a) depletion of arachidonic acid, which prevents the activation of neutral sphyngomyelinase and production of ceramide (Cao *et al.* 2000); b) modulation of expression of the anti-apoptotic protein Bcl-2 (Liu *et al.* 1998; Tsujii and DuBois 1995); c) regulation of Akt activation (Hsu *et al.* 2000; Lin *et al.* 2001); d) counteracting NO-mediated apoptotic cell death, either via modulation of expression of prosurvival gene PIN, inhibiting production of NO (Chang *et al.* 2000), or via regulation of cellular susceptibility toward NO (von Knethen and Brune 1997). Among genes activated in mesangial cells by Cox-2 expression and/or addition of prostaglandins is the multi-drug resistance gene (MDR1) which encodes a protein termed P glycoprotein (P-gp). P-gp belongs to the ATP-binding cassette (ABC) family of transporter molecules, which require hydrolysis of ATP to run the transport mechanism. The substrates of P-gp may be endogenous (steroid hormones, cytokines) or xenobiotics (cytostatic drugs). P-gp is known to confer the drug resistance in cancer cells. Only recently has the role of P-gp expressed in normal tissues has been examined. In the kidney P-gp is present in the brush border membrane of the proximal tubule, a site compatible with a role in xenobiotic secretion (Johnstone *et al.* 2000a; Ernest *et al.* 1997). It is also expressed in the mesangium, the thick ascending limb of Henle's loop, and the collecting duct (Ernest *et al.* 1997), locations that are not traditionally associated with drug excretion. P-gp may regulate apoptosis, chloride channel activity, cholesterol methabolism and immune cell function (Ernest *et al.*

1997; Johnstone *et al.* 2000b; Zager 2001). It was shown that Cox-2 regulated P-gp expression in GMC (Patel *et al.* 2002) and rescued GMC from apoptosis induced by adriamycin (Miller *et al.* 2006), suggesting P-gp role in Cox-2-mediated GMC survival (Sorokin 2004). On the contrary, it appears that transgenic mice overexpressing Cox-2 selectively in podocytes were more susceptible to glomerular injury by adriamycin (Cheng *et al.* 2009). It was suggested that basal Cox-2 is important for podocyte survival, but overexpression of podocyte Cox-2 increases susceptibility to podocyte injury (Cheng *et al.* 2009).

5.4 Future directions

Even though inhibitors of cyclooxygenases are capable to induce adverse reactions it is unlikely that efforts would stop to develop drugs affecting prostaglandin production which will be free of this negative aspects. If it would be shown that environmental as well as genetic factors may cause interpatient variability in NSAIDs and COXIBs metabolism and therapeutic effect, it would set the stage for personalized treatment of inflammatory diseases including glomerulonephritis. Only few pharmacogenomics reports have been published to date in nephrology and there is a need to build up efforts in this important research field (Zaza *et al.* 2010). It is reassuring that the susceptibility to crescentic glomerulonephritis was found to be linked to a polymorphism in the promoter region of *Jund*, the gene for the AP-1 transcription factor JunD (Behmoaras *et al.* 2008).
Several studies have established unequivocally that certain widely used inhibitors of cyclooxygenases caused anti-inflammatory and antiproliferative effects independent of cyclooxygenase activity and prostaglandin synthesis inhibition (Tegeder *et al.* 2001). Hence, the possibility to regulate cyclooxygenase activity at the level of protein-protein interactions is of significant interest, because it could set the basis for generation of novel inhibitors of prostaglandin synthesis. A number of signaling proteins, including ELMO1, were identified as candidates for the post-translational regulation of Cox-2 activity. Interaction with ELMO1 increased Cox-2-mediated induction of expression of the extracellular matrix protein fibronectin (Yang and Sorokin 2011). The ability of Cox-2 to induce fibronectin expression depended on the production of PGE_2, implying that an interaction with ELMO1 promoted ability of Cox-2 to synthesize prostaglandins. Thus, the role of ELMO1 could be to increase the synthesis of prostaglandins by Cox-2. One could expect that inhibition of ELMO1/Cox-2 interaction would decrease the biological action of Cox-2 and therefore, represent a novel strategy to attenuate Cox-2 activity in inflammatory renal diseases. It is of note, that exposure to pathological stimuli induced glomerular mesangial cells to produce extracellular matrix proteins (ECM), such as collagens, fibronectin and proteinase inhibitors, resulting in the abnormal accumulation ECM in glomerular mesangium and irreversible glomerular injury (Pezzolesi *et al.* 2009; Wilson *et al.* 1998).

6. Conclusions

Three major levels of cellular control of prostaglandin synthesis are 1) at the level of liberation of free arachidonic acid from glycerophospholipids; 2) at the level of cyclooxygenases, and 3) at the level of terminal prostaglandin synthases. As a rule, prostaglandins exert their actions through specific G-protein coupled receptors even though direct modification of cellular proteins by prostaglandins was also observed. Intra-renal localization of prostaglandins receptors and their coupling to particular G-proteins and, correspondingly, to specific intracellular signaling pathways determine the outcome of renal action of distinct prostaglandins. There is mounting evidence that progression of glomerulitis is accompanied by increased expression of cyclooxygenases (usually inducible isoform Cox-2) and enhanced production of prostaglandins, which have profound effect upon the survival/functioning of glomerular cells and normal performance of glomeruli. Prostaglandins are major mediators of inflammation and continuing treatment with Cox-2 specific inhibitors usually improves functional and structural damage in experimental models associated with changed renal hemodynamics and progressive renal injury. Even though inhibition of renal prostaglandin production is supposed to be renoprotective, prostaglandins also have antiflammatory properties. Currently used inhibitors of cycclooxygenases are not free from adverse effects and their action is not always explained by inhibition of cyclooxygenase activity and prostaglandin synthesis. Therefore, increased understanding of novel mechanisms of regulation of prostaglandin production (such as regulation of cyclooxygenases at the post-translational level) will set the base for the design of new generation of inhibitors of prostaglandin synthesis and will open novel strategies to combat progression of glomerular renal diseases.

7. Acknowledgment

This work was supported by grants to A. Sorokin from National Institutes of Health RO1DK41684 and R21DK088018.

8. References

Alchi B, Jayne D (2010) Membranoproliferative glomerulonephritis. *Pediatr.Nephrol.* 25, 1409-1418.

Alexander LD, Alagarsamy S, Douglas JG (2004) Cyclic stretch-induced cPLA2 mediates ERK 1/2 signaling in rabbit proximal tubule cells. *Kidney Int.* 65, 551-563.

Anderson MW, Crutchley DJ, Chaudhari A, Wilson AG, Eling TE (1979) Studies on the covalent binding of an intermediate(s) in prostaglandin biosynthesis to tissue macromolecules. *Biochim.Biophys.Acta* 573, 40-50.

Arun B, Goss P (2004) The role of COX-2 inhibition in breast cancer treatment and prevention. *Semin.Oncol.* 31, 22-29.

Atar S, Ye Y, Lin Y, Freeberg SY, Nishi SP, Rosanio S, Huang MH, Uretsky BF, Perez-Polo JR, Birnbaum Y (2006) Atorvastatin-induced cardioprotection is mediated by increasing inducible nitric oxide synthase and consequent S-nitrosylation of cyclooxygenase-2. *Am.J.Physiol Heart Circ.Physiol* 290, H1960-H1968.

Audoly LP, Ruan X, Wagner VA, Goulet JL, Tilley SL, Koller BH, Coffman TM, Arendshorst WJ (2001) Role of EP(2) and EP(3) PGE(2) receptors in control of murine renal hemodynamics. *Am.J.Physiol Heart Circ.Physiol* 280, H327-H333.

Badawi AF (2000) The role of prostaglandin synthesis in prostate cancer. *BJU.Int.* 85, 451-462.

Bariety J, Bruneval P, Meyrier A, Mandet C, Hill G, Jacquot C (2005) Podocyte involvement in human immune crescentic glomerulonephritis. *Kidney Int.* 68, 1109-1119.

Baroody RA, Bito LZ (1981) The impermeability of the basic cell membrane to thromboxane-B2' prostacyclin and 6-keto-PGF 1 alpha. *Prostaglandins* 21, 133-142.

Basu S (2010) Bioactive eicosanoids: role of prostaglandin F(2alpha) and F-isoprostanes in inflammation and oxidative stress related pathology. *Mol.Cells* 30, 383-391.

Baud L, Nivez MP, Chansel D, Ardaillou R (1981) Stimulation by oxygen radicals of prostaglandin production by rat renal glomeruli. *Kidney Int.* 20, 332-339.

Behmoaras J, Bhangal G, Smith J, McDonald K, Mutch B, Lai PC, Domin J, Game L, Salama A, Foxwell BM, Pusey CD, Cook HT, Aitman TJ (2008) Jund is a determinant of macrophage activation and is associated with glomerulonephritis susceptibility. *Nat.Genet.* 40, 553-559.

Bek M, Nusing R, Kowark P, Henger A, Mundel P, Pavenstadt H (1999) Characterization of prostanoid receptors in podocytes. *J.Am.Soc.Nephrol.* 10, 2084-2093.

Bell PD, Lapointe JY, Peti-Peterdi J (2003) Macula densa cell signaling. *Annu.Rev.Physiol* 65, 481-500.

Bokemeyer D, Guglielmi KE, McGinty A, Sorokin A, Lianos EA, Dunn MJ (1997) Activation of extracellular signal-regulated kinase in proliferative glomerulonephritis in rats. *J.Clin.Invest* 100, 582-588.

Bokemeyer D, Sorokin A, Dunn MJ (1996) Multiple intracellular MAP kinase signaling cascades. *Kidney Int.* 49, 1187-1198.

Breshnahan BA, Kelefiotis D, Stratidakis I, Lianos EA (1996) PGF2alpha-induced signaling events in glomerular mesangial cells. *Proc.Soc.Exp.Biol.Med.* 212, 165-173.

Breyer MD, Breyer RM (2000) Prostaglandin E receptors and the kidney. *Am.J.Physiol Renal Physiol* 279, F12-F23.

Breyer MD, Breyer RM (2001) G protein-coupled prostanoid receptors and the kidney. *Annu.Rev.Physiol* 63, 579-605.

Buchanan FG, Wang D, Bargiacchi F, DuBois RN (2003) Prostaglandin E2 regulates cell migration via the intracellular activation of the epidermal growth factor receptor. *J.Biol.Chem* 278, 35451-35457.

Cao Y, Pearman AT, Zimmerman GA, McIntyre TM, Prescott SM (2000) Intracellular unesterified arachidonic acid signals apoptosis. *Proc.Natl.Acad.Sci.U.S.A* 97, 11280-11285.

Cao Y, Prescott SM (2002) Many actions of cyclooxygenase-2 in cellular dynamics and in cancer. *J.Cell Physiol* 190, 279-286.

Carlsen I, Donohue KE, Jensen AM, Selzer AL, Chen J, Poppas DP, Felsen D, Frokiaer J, Norregaard R (2010) Increased cyclooxygenase-2 expression and prostaglandin E2 production in pressurized renal medullary interstitial cells. *Am.J.Physiol Regul.Integr.Comp Physiol* 299, R823-R831.

Chan BS, Satriano JA, Pucci M, Schuster VL (1998) Mechanism of prostaglandin E2 transport across the plasma membrane of HeLa cells and Xenopus oocytes expressing the prostaglandin transporter "PGT". *J.Biol.Chem.* 273, 6689-6697.

Chandrasekharan NV, Simmons DL (2004) The cyclooxygenases. *Genome Biol.* 5, 241.

Chang YW, Jakobi R, McGinty A, Foschi M, Dunn MJ, Sorokin A (2000) Cyclooxygenase 2 promotes cell survival by stimulation of dynein light chain expression and inhibition of neuronal nitric oxide synthase activity. *Mol.Cell Biol.* 20, 8571-8579.

Chanmugam P, Feng L, Liou S, Jang BC, Boudreau M, Yu G, Lee JH, Kwon HJ, Beppu T, Yoshida M, . (1995) Radicicol, a protein tyrosine kinase inhibitor, suppresses the expression of mitogen-inducible cyclooxygenase in macrophages stimulated with lipopolysaccharide and in experimental glomerulonephritis. *J.Biol.Chem.* 270, 5418-5426.

Cheng H, Fan X, Guan Y, Moeckel GW, Zent R, Harris RC (2009) Distinct roles for basal and induced COX-2 in podocyte injury. *J.Am.Soc.Nephrol.* 20, 1953-1962.

Cheng HF, Harris RC (2004) Cyclooxygenases, the Kidney, and Hypertension. *Hypertension* 43, 1-6.

Chubb AJ, Fitzgerald DJ, Nolan KB, Moman E (2006) The productive conformation of prostaglandin G2 at the peroxidase site of prostaglandin endoperoxide H synthase: docking, molecular dynamics, and site-directed mutagenesis studies. *Biochemistry* 45, 811-820.

Chung BH, Lim SW, Ahn KO, Sugawara A, Ito S, Choi BS, Kim YS, Bang BK, Yang CW (2005) Protective effect of peroxisome proliferator activated receptor gamma agonists on diabetic and non-diabetic renal diseases. *Nephrology.(Carlton.)* 10 Suppl, S40-S43.

Couser WG, Johnson RJ (1994) Mechanisms of progressive renal disease in glomerulonephritis. *Am.J.Kidney Dis.* 23, 193-198.

Dannenberg AJ, Lippman SM, Mann JR, Subbaramaiah K, DuBois RN (2005) Cyclooxygenase-2 and epidermal growth factor receptor: pharmacologic targets for chemoprevention. *J.Clin.Oncol.* 23, 254-266.

Datta PK, Dhupar S, Lianos EA (2006) Regulatory effects of inducible nitric oxide synthase on cyclooxygenase-2 and heme oxygenase-1 expression in experimental glomerulonephritis. *Nephrol.Dial.Transplant.* 21, 51-57.

Ding YB, Shi RH, Tong JD, Li XY, Zhang GX, Xiao WM, Yang JG, Bao Y, Wu J, Yan ZG, Wang XH (2005) PGE2 up-regulates vascular endothelial growth factor expression in MKN28 gastric cancer cells via epidermal growth factor receptor signaling system. *Exp.Oncol.* 27, 108-113.

Doller A, Gauer S, Sobkowiak E, Geiger H, Pfeilschifter J, Eberhardt W (2009) Angiotensin II induces renal plasminogen activator inhibitor-1 and cyclooxygenase-2 expression post-transcriptionally via activation of the mRNA-stabilizing factor human-antigen R. *Am.J.Pathol.* 174, 1252-1263.

Doller A, Huwiler A, Muller R, Radeke HH, Pfeilschifter J, Eberhardt W (2007) Protein kinase C alpha-dependent phosphorylation of the mRNA-stabilizing factor HuR: implications for posttranscriptional regulation of cyclooxygenase-2. *Mol.Biol.Cell* 18, 2137-2148.

DuBois RN, Abramson SB, Crofford L, Gupta RA, Simon LS, Van De Putte LB, Lipsky PE (1998) Cyclooxygenase in biology and disease. *FASEB J.* 12, 1063-1073.

Elberg G, Elberg D, Lewis TV, Guruswamy S, Chen L, Logan CJ, Chan MD, Turman MA (2007) EP2 receptor mediates PGE2-induced cystogenesis of human renal epithelial cells. *Am.J.Physiol Renal Physiol* 293, F1622-F1632.

Eling TE, Wilson AG, Chaudhari A, Anderson MW (1977) Covalent binding of an intermediate(s) in prostaglandin biosynthesis to guinea pig lung microsomal protein. *Life Sci.* 21, 245-251.

Ernest S, Rajaraman S, Megyesi J, Bello-Reuss EN (1997) Expression of MDR1 (multidrug resistance) gene and its protein in normal human kidney. *Nephron* 77, 284-289.

Fernandez-Tome M, Favale N, Kraemer L, Gabriela MM, Speziale E, Sterin-Speziale N (2004) p44/42(ERK1/2) MAPK and PLD activation by PGD2 preserves papillary phosphatidylcholine homeostasis. *Biochem.Biophys.Res.Commun.* 320, 1055-1062.

Fernau NS, Fugmann D, Leyendecker M, Reimann K, Grether-Beck S, Galban S, Ale-Agha N, Krutmann J, Klotz LO (2010) Role of HuR and p38MAPK in ultraviolet B-induced post-transcriptional regulation of COX-2 expression in the human keratinocyte cell line HaCaT. *J.Biol.Chem.* 285, 3896-3904.

Fitzgerald GA (2004) Coxibs and cardiovascular disease. *N.Engl.J.Med.* 351, 1709-1711.

Fleming EF, Athirakul K, Oliverio MI, Key M, Goulet J, Koller BH, Coffman TM (1998) Urinary concentrating function in mice lacking EP3 receptors for prostaglandin E2. *Am.J.Physiol* 275, F955-F961.

Floege J, Topley N, Resch K (1991a) Regulation of mesangial cell proliferation. *Am.J.Kidney Dis.* 17, 673-676.

Floege J, Topley N, Resch K (1991b) Regulation of mesangial cell proliferation. *Am.J.Kidney Dis.* 17, 673-676.

Foidart JM, Nochy D, Nusgens B, Foidart JB, Mahieu PR, Lapiere CM, Lambotte R, Bariety J (1983) Accumulation of several basement membrane proteins in glomeruli of patients with preeclampsia and other hypertensive syndromes of pregnancy. Possible role of renal prostaglandins and fibronectin. *Lab Invest* 49, 250-259.

Fujihara CK, Antunes GR, Mattar AL, Andreoli N, Malheiros DM, Noronha IL, Zatz R (2003) Cyclooxygenase-2 (COX-2) inhibition limits abnormal COX-2 expression and progressive injury in the remnant kidney. *Kidney Int.* 64, 2172-2181.

Fujii M, Takemura R, Yamaguchi M, Hasegawa G, Shigeta H, Nakano K, Kondo M (1997) Troglitazone (CS-045) ameliorates albuminuria in streptozotocin-induced diabetic rats. *Metabolism* 46, 981-983.

Furberg CD, Psaty BM, Fitzgerald GA (2005) Parecoxib, valdecoxib, and cardiovascular risk. *Circulation* 111, 249.

Gomez-Guerrero C, Hernandez-Vargas P, Lopez-Franco O, Ortiz-Munoz G, Egido J (2005) Mesangial cells and glomerular inflammation: from the pathogenesis to novel therapeutic approaches. *Curr.Drug Targets.Inflamm.Allergy* 4, 341-351.

Goppelt-Struebe M, Stroebel M, Hoppe J (1996) Regulation of platelet-derived growth factor isoform-mediated expression of prostaglandin G/H synthase in mesangial cells. *Kidney Int.* 50, 71-78.

Han C, Michalopoulos GK, Wu T (2006) Prostaglandin E2 receptor EP1 transactivates EGFR/MET receptor tyrosine kinases and enhances invasiveness in human hepatocellular carcinoma cells. *J.Cell Physiol* 207, 261-270.

Hanif R, Pittas A, Feng Y, Koutsos MI, Qiao L, Staiano-Coico L, Shiff SI, Rigas B (1996) Effects of nonsteroidal anti-inflammatory drugs on proliferation and on induction of apoptosis in colon cancer cells by a prostaglandin-independent pathway. *Biochem.Pharmacol.* 52, 237-245.

Hao CM, Komhoff M, Guan Y, Redha R, Breyer MD (1999) Selective targeting of cyclooxygenase-2 reveals its role in renal medullary interstitial cell survival. *Am.J.Physiol* 277, F352-F359.

Harris RC, Breyer MD (2001) Physiological regulation of cyclooxygenase-2 in the kidney. *Am.J.Physiol Renal Physiol* 281, F1-11.

Harris RC, McKanna JA, Akai Y, Jacobson HR, DuBois RN, Breyer MD (1994) Cyclooxygenase-2 is associated with the macula densa of rat kidney and increases with salt restriction. *J.Clin.Invest* 94, 2504-2510.

Hartner A, Pahl A, Brune K, Goppelt-Struebe M (2000) Upregulation of cyclooxygenase-1 and the PGE2 receptor EP2 in rat and human mesangioproliferative glomerulonephritis. *Inflamm.Res.* 49, 345-354.

Hebert RL, Carmosino M, Saito O, Yang G, Jackson CA, Qi Z, Breyer RM, Natarajan C, Hata AN, Zhang Y, Guan Y, Breyer MD (2005a) Characterization of a rabbit kidney prostaglandin F(2{alpha}) receptor exhibiting G(i)-restricted signaling that inhibits water absorption in the collecting duct. *J.Biol.Chem.* 280, 35028-35037.

Hebert RL, Carmosino M, Saito O, Yang G, Jackson CA, Qi Z, Breyer RM, Natarajan C, Hata AN, Zhang Y, Guan Y, Breyer MD (2005b) Characterization of a rabbit kidney prostaglandin F(2{alpha}) receptor exhibiting G(i)-restricted signaling that inhibits water absorption in the collecting duct. *J.Biol.Chem.* 280, 35028-35037.

Helliwell RJ, Adams LF, Mitchell MD (2004) Prostaglandin synthases: recent developments and a novel hypothesis. *Prostaglandins Leukot.Essent.Fatty Acids* 70, 101-113.

Hirabayashi T, Murayama T, Shimizu T (2004) Regulatory mechanism and physiological role of cytosolic phospholipase A2. *Biol.Pharm.Bull.* 27, 1168-1173.

Hirahashi J, Takayanagi A, Hishikawa K, Takase O, Chikaraishi A, Hayashi M, Shimizu N, Saruta T (2000) Overexpression of truncated I kappa B alpha potentiates TNF-alpha-induced apoptosis in mesangial cells. *Kidney Int.* 57, 959-968.

Hirose S, Yamamoto T, Feng L, Yaoita E, Kawasaki K, Goto S, Fujinaka H, Wilson CB, Arakawa M, Kihara I (1998) Expression and localization of cyclooxygenase isoforms and cytosolic phospholipase A2 in anti-Thy-1 glomerulonephritis. *J.Am.Soc.Nephrol.* 9, 408-416.

Hsu AL, Ching TT, Wang DS, song X, Rangnekar VM, Chen CS (2000) The cyclooxygenase-2 inhibitor celecoxib induces apoptosis by blocking Akt activation in human prostate cancer cells independently of Bcl-2. *J.Biol.Chem.* 275, 11397-11403.

Imano E, Kanda T, Nakatani Y, Nishida T, Arai K, Motomura M, Kajimoto Y, Yamasaki Y, Hori M (1998) Effect of troglitazone on microalbuminuria in patients with incipient diabetic nephropathy. *Diabetes Care* 21, 2135-2139.

Imig JD, Breyer MD, Breyer RM (2002) Contribution of prostaglandin EP(2) receptors to renal microvascular reactivity in mice. *Am.J.Physiol Renal Physiol* 283, F415-F422.

Inoue H, Tanabe T (1997) Transcriptional regulation of human prostaglandin-endoperoxide synthase-2 gene in vascular endothelial cells. *Adv.Exp.Med.Biol.* 407, 139-144.

Inoue H, Tanabe T (1998) Transcriptional role of the nuclear factor kappa B site in the induction by lipopolysaccharide and suppression by dexamethasone of cyclooxygenase-2 in U937 cells. *Biochem.Biophys.Res.Commun.* 244, 143-148.

Ishaque A, Dunn MJ, Sorokin A (2003) Cyclooxygenase-2 inhibits tumor necrosis factor alpha-mediated apoptosis in renal glomerular mesangial cells. *J.Biol.Chem.* 278, 10629-10640.

Ishibashi R, Tanaka I, Kotani M, Muro S, Goto M, Sugawara A, Mukoyama M, Sugimoto Y, Ichikawa A, Narumiya S, Nakao K (1999) Roles of prostaglandin E receptors in mesangial cells under high-glucose conditions. *Kidney Int.* 56, 589-600.

Iyer RS, Ghosh S, Salomon RG (1989) Levuglandin E2 crosslinks proteins. *Prostaglandins* 37, 471-480.

Jaimes EA, Zhou MS, Pearse DD, Puzis L, Raij L (2008) Upregulation of cortical COX-2 in salt-sensitive hypertension: role of angiotensin II and reactive oxygen species. *Am.J.Physiol Renal Physiol* 294, F385-F392.

Jang BC, Sanchez T, Schaefers HJ, Trifan OC, Liu CH, Creminon C, Huang CK, Hla T (2000) Serum withdrawal-induced post-transcriptional stabilization of cyclooxygenase-2 mRNA in MDA-MB-231 mammary carcinoma cells requires the activity of the p38 stress-activated protein kinase. *J.Biol.Chem.* 275, 39507-39515.

Jania LA, Chandrasekharan S, Backlund MG, Foley NA, Snouwaert J, Wang IM, Clark P, Audoly LP, Koller BH (2009) Microsomal prostaglandin E synthase-2 is not essential for in vivo prostaglandin E2 biosynthesis. *Prostaglandins Other Lipid Mediat.* 88, 73-81.

Jefferson JA, Johnson RJ (1999) Experimental mesangial proliferative glomerulonephritis (the anti-Thy-1.1 model). *J.Nephrol.* 12, 297-307.

Jendrossek V, Handrick R (2003) Membrane targeted anticancer drugs: potent inducers of apoptosis and putative radiosensitisers. *Curr.Med.Chem.Anti.-Canc.Agents* 3, 343-353.

Jensen BL, Stubbe J, Hansen PB, Andreasen D, Skott O (2001) Localization of prostaglandin E(2) EP2 and EP4 receptors in the rat kidney. *Am.J.Physiol Renal Physiol* 280, F1001-F1009.

Jia Z, Guo X, Zhang H, Wang MH, Dong Z, Yang T (2008) Microsomal prostaglandin synthase-1-derived prostaglandin E2 protects against angiotensin II-induced hypertension via inhibition of oxidative stress. *Hypertension* 52, 952-959.

Jia Z, Wang N, Aoyagi T, Wang H, Liu H, Yang T (2011) Amelioration of cisplatin nephrotoxicity by genetic or pharmacologic blockade of prostaglandin synthesis. *Kidney Int.* 79, 77-88.

Johnstone RW, Ruefli AA, Smyth MJ (2000a) Multiple physiological functions for multidrug transporter P-glycoprotein? *Trends Biochem.Sci.* 25, 1-6.

Johnstone RW, Ruefli AA, Tainton KM, Smyth MJ (2000b) A role for P-glycoprotein in regulating cell death. *Leuk.Lymphoma* 38, 1-11.

Kawanishi S, Hiraku Y (2004) Amplification of anticancer drug-induced DNA damage and apoptosis by DNA-binding compounds. *Curr.Med.Chem.Anti.-Canc.Agents* 4, 415-419.

Kelefiotis D, Bresnahan BA, Stratidakis I, Lianos EA (1995) Eicosanoid-induced growth and signaling events in rat glomerular mesangial cells. *Prostaglandins* 49, 269-283.

Kester M, Coroneos E, Thomas PJ, Dunn MJ (1994) Endothelin stimulates prostaglandin endoperoxide synthase-2 mRNA expression and protein synthesis through a tyrosine kinase-signaling pathway in rat mesangial cells. *J.Biol.Chem.* 269, 22574-22580.

Khan KN, Stanfield KM, Harris RK, Baron DA (2001) Expression of cyclooxygenase-2 in the macula densa of human kidney in hypertension, congestive heart failure, and diabetic nephropathy. *Ren Fail.* 23, 321-330.

Khanna R (2011) Clinical presentation & management of glomerular diseases: hematuria, nephritic & nephrotic syndrome. *Mo.Med.* 108, 33-36.

Kim SF, Huri DA, Snyder SH (2005) Inducible nitric oxide synthase binds, S-nitrosylates, and activates cyclooxygenase-2. *Science* 310, 1966-1970.

Kim WJ, Kim JH, Jang SK (2007) Anti-inflammatory lipid mediator 15d-PGJ2 inhibits translation through inactivation of eIF4A. *EMBO J.* 26, 5020-5032.

Kliewer SA, Umesono K, Noonan DJ, Heyman RA, Evans RM (1992) Convergence of 9-cis retinoic acid and peroxisome proliferator signalling pathways through heterodimer formation of their receptors. *Nature* 358, 771-774.

Kobayashi T, Narumiya S (2002) Function of prostanoid receptors: studies on knockout mice. *Prostaglandins Other Lipid Mediat.* 68-69, 557-573.

Kosaka T, Miyata A, Ihara H, Hara S, Sugimoto T, Takeda O, Takahashi E, Tanabe T (1994) Characterization of the human gene (PTGS2) encoding prostaglandin-endoperoxide synthase 2. *Eur.J.Biochem.* 221, 889-897.

Kudo I, Murakami M (2005) Prostaglandin E synthase, a terminal enzyme for prostaglandin E2 biosynthesis. *J.Biochem.Mol.Biol.* 38, 633-638.

Kurogi Y (2003) Mesangial cell proliferation inhibitors for the treatment of proliferative glomerular disease. *Med.Res.Rev.* 23, 15-31.

Leak TS, Perlegas PS, Smith SG, Keene KL, Hicks PJ, Langefeld CD, Mychaleckyj JC, Rich SS, Kirk JK, Freedman BI, Bowden DW, Sale MM (2009) Variants in intron 13 of the ELMO1 gene are associated with diabetic nephropathy in African Americans. *Ann.Hum.Genet.* 73, 152-159.

Lecomte M, Lecocq R, Dumont JE, Boeynaems JM (1990) Covalent binding of arachidonic acid metabolites to human platelet proteins. Identification of prostaglandin H synthase as one of the modified substrates. *J.Biol.Chem.* 265, 5178-5187.

Lianos EA (1992) Eicosanoids in immune-mediated renal injury. *Semin.Nephrol.* 12, 441-453.

Lianos EA, Andres GA, Dunn MJ (1983) Glomerular prostaglandin and thromboxane synthesis in rat nephrotoxic serum nephritis. Effects on renal hemodynamics. *J.Clin.Invest* 72, 1439-1448.

Lin MT, Lee RC, Yang PC, Ho FM, Kuo ML (2001) Cyclooxygenase-2 inducing Mcl-1-dependent survival mechanism in human lung adenocarcinoma CL1.0 cells. Involvement of phosphatidylinositol 3-kinase/Akt pathway. *J.Biol.Chem.* 276, 48997-49002.

Lin WN, Lin CC, Cheng HY, Yang CM (2011) Regulation of COX-2 and cPLA(2) gene expression by LPS through the RNA-binding protein HuR: involvement of NADPH oxidase, ROS and MAPKs. *Br.J.Pharmacol.*

Liu XH, Yao S, Kirschenbaum A, Levine AC (1998) NS398, a selective cyclooxygenase-2 inhibitor, induces apoptosis and down-regulates bcl-2 expression in LNCaP cells. *Cancer Res.* 58, 4245-4249.

Lovgren AK, Kovarova M, Koller BH (2007) cPGES/p23 is required for glucocorticoid receptor function and embryonic growth but not prostaglandin E2 synthesis. *Mol.Cell Biol.* 27, 4416-4430.

Ma LJ, Marcantoni C, Linton MF, Fazio S, Fogo AB (2001) Peroxisome proliferator-activated receptor-gamma agonist troglitazone protects against nondiabetic glomerulosclerosis in rats. *Kidney Int.* 59, 1899-1910.

Maeda A, Horikoshi S, Gohda T, Tsuge T, Maeda K, Tomino Y (2005) Pioglitazone attenuates TGF-beta(1)-induction of fibronectin synthesis and its splicing variant in human mesangial cells via activation of peroxisome proliferator-activated receptor (PPAR)gamma. *Cell Biol.Int.* 29, 422-428.

Mahadevan P, Larkins RG, Fraser JR, Dunlop ME (1996) Effect of prostaglandin E2 and hyaluronan on mesangial cell proliferation. A potential contribution to glomerular hypercellularity in diabetes. *Diabetes* 45, 44-50.

Mangat H, Peterson LN, Burns KD (1997) Hypercalcemia stimulates expression of intrarenal phospholipase A2 and prostaglandin H synthase-2 in rats. Role of angiotensin II AT1 receptors. *J.Clin.Invest* 100, 1941-1950.

Markan S, Kohli HS, Sud K, Ahuja M, Ahluwalia TS, Sakhuja V, Khullar M (2008) Oxidative stress in primary glomerular diseases: a comparative study. *Mol.Cell Biochem.* 311, 105-110.

Marnett LJ, Rowlinson SW, Goodwin DC, Kalgutkar AS, Lanzo CA (1999) Arachidonic acid oxygenation by COX-1 and COX-2. Mechanisms of catalysis and inhibition. *J.Biol.Chem.* 274, 22903-22906.

Matlhagela K, Taub M (2006) Involvement of EP1 and EP2 receptors in the regulation of the Na,K-ATPase by prostaglandins in MDCK cells. *Prostaglandins Other Lipid Mediat.* 79, 101-113.

Mbonye UR, Yuan C, Harris CE, Sidhu RS, Song I, Arakawa T, Smith WL (2008) Two distinct pathways for cyclooxygenase-2 protein degradation. *J.Biol.Chem.* 283, 8611-8623.

McGinty A, Foschi M, Chang YW, Han J, Dunn MJ, Sorokin A (2000) Induction of prostaglandin endoperoxide synthase 2 by mitogen-activated protein kinase cascades. *Biochem.J.* 352 Pt 2, 419-424.

McGraw DW, Mihlbachler KA, Schwarb MR, Rahman FF, Small KM, Almoosa KF, Liggett SB (2006) Airway smooth muscle prostaglandin-EP1 receptors directly modulate beta2-adrenergic receptors within a unique heterodimeric complex. *J.Clin.Invest* 116, 1400-1409.

Mene P, Dubyak GR, Scarpa A, Dunn MJ (1991) Regulation of cytosolic pH of cultured mesangial cells by prostaglandin F2 alpha and thromboxane A2. *Am.J.Physiol* 260, C159-C166.

Menter DG, Schilsky RL, DuBois RN (2010) Cyclooxygenase-2 and cancer treatment: understanding the risk should be worth the reward. *Clin.Cancer Res.* 16, 1384-1390.

Milatovic D, Montine TJ, Aschner M (2011) Prostanoid signaling: Dual role for prostaglandin E(2) in neurotoxicity. *Neurotoxicology* 32, 312-319.

Miller B, Patel VA, Sorokin A (2006) Cyclooxygenase-2 Rescues Rat Mesangial Cells from Apoptosis Induced by Adriamycin via Upregulation of Multidrug Resistance Protein 1 (P-Glycoprotein). *J.Am.Soc.Nephrol.* 17, 977-985.

Miller SB (2006) Prostaglandins in health and disease: an overview. *Semin.Arthritis Rheum.* 36, 37-49.

Moore BC, Simmons DL (2000) COX-2 inhibition, apoptosis, and chemoprevention by nonsteroidal anti-inflammatory drugs. *Curr.Med.Chem.* 7, 1131-1144.

Morath R, Klein T, Seyberth HW, Nusing RM (1999) Immunolocalization of the four prostaglandin E2 receptor proteins EP1, EP2, EP3, and EP4 in human kidney. *J.Am.Soc.Nephrol.* 10, 1851-1860.

Naraba H, Yokoyama C, Tago N, Murakami M, Kudo I, Fueki M, Oh-Ishi S, Tanabe T (2002) Transcriptional regulation of the membrane-associated prostaglandin E2 synthase gene. Essential role of the transcription factor Egr-1. *J.Biol.Chem.* 277, 28601-28608.

Narumiya S, Sugimoto Y, Ushikubi F (1999) Prostanoid receptors: structures, properties, and functions. *Physiol Rev.* 79, 1193-1226.

Nasrallah R, Clark J, Hebert RL (2007) Prostaglandins in the kidney: developments since Y2K. *Clin.Sci.(Lond)* 113, 297-311.

Nasrallah R, Landry A, Singh S, Sklepowicz M, Hebert RL (2003) Increased expression of cyclooxygenase-1 and -2 in the diabetic rat renal medulla. *Am.J.Physiol Renal Physiol* 285, F1068-F1077.

Neuhofer W, Steinert D, Fraek ML, Beck FX (2007) Prostaglandin E2 stimulates expression of osmoprotective genes in MDCK cells and promotes survival under hypertonic conditions. *J.Physiol* 583, 287-297.

Nicholas SB, Kawano Y, Wakino S, Collins AR, Hsueh WA (2001) Expression and function of peroxisome proliferator-activated receptor-gamma in mesangial cells. *Hypertension* 37, 722-727.

Nomura T, Chang HY, Lu R, Hankin J, Murphy RC, Schuster VL (2005) Prostaglandin signaling in the renal collecting duct: release, reuptake, and oxidation in the same cell. *J.Biol.Chem.* 280, 28424-28429.

Nusing RM, Treude A, Weissenberger C, Jensen B, Bek M, Wagner C, Narumiya S, Seyberth HW (2005) Dominant role of prostaglandin E2 EP4 receptor in furosemide-induced salt-losing tubulopathy: a model for hyperprostaglandin E syndrome/antenatal Bartter syndrome. *J.Am.Soc.Nephrol.* 16, 2354-2362.

Padilla J, Kaur K, Harris SG, Phipps RP (2000) PPAR-gamma-mediated regulation of normal and malignant B lineage cells. *Ann.N.Y.Acad.Sci.* 905, 97-109.

Panzer U, Zahner G, Wienberg U, Steinmetz OM, Peters A, Turner JE, Paust HJ, Wolf G, Stahl RA, Schneider A (2008) 15-deoxy-Delta12,14-prostaglandin J2 inhibits INF-gamma-induced JAK/STAT1 signalling pathway activation and IP-10/CXCL10 expression in mesangial cells. *Nephrol.Dial.Transplant.* 23, 3776-3785.

Parfenova H, Balabanova L, Leffler CW (1998) Posttranslational regulation of cyclooxygenase by tyrosine phosphorylation in cerebral endothelial cells. *Am.J.Physiol* 274, C72-C81.

Patel VA, Dunn MJ, Sorokin A (2002) Regulation of MDR-1 (P-glycoprotein) by cyclooxygenase-2. *J.Biol.Chem.* 277, 38915-38920.

Pezzolesi MG, Katavetin P, Kure M, Poznik GD, Skupien J, Mychaleckyj JC, Rich SS, Warram JH, Krolewski AS (2009) Confirmation of genetic associations at ELMO1 in the GoKinD collection supports its role as a susceptibility gene in diabetic nephropathy. *Diabetes* 58, 2698-2702.

Rahal S, McVeigh LI, Zhang Y, Guan Y, Breyer MD, Kennedy CR (2006) Increased severity of renal impairment in nephritic mice lacking the EP1 receptor. *Can.J.Physiol Pharmacol.* 84, 877-885.

Ricciotti E, Fitzgerald GA (2011) Prostaglandins and inflammation. *Arterioscler.Thromb.Vasc.Biol.* 31, 986-1000.

Ricote M, Li AC, Willson TM, Kelly CJ, Glass CK (1998) The peroxisome proliferator-activated receptor-gamma is a negative regulator of macrophage activation. *Nature* 391, 79-82.

Riedl K, Krysan K, Pold M, Dalwadi H, Heuze-Vourc'h N, Dohadwala M, Liu M, Cui X, Figlin R, Mao JT, Strieter R, Sharma S, Dubinett SM (2004) Multifaceted roles of cyclooxygenase-2 in lung cancer. *Drug Resist.Updat.* 7, 169-184.

Rizzo G, Fiorucci S (2006) PPARs and other nuclear receptors in inflammation. *Curr.Opin.Pharmacol.* 6, 421-427.

Saha D, Datta PK, Sheng H, Morrow JD, Wada M, Moses HL, Beauchamp RD (1999) Synergistic induction of cyclooxygenase-2 by transforming growth factor-beta1 and epidermal growth factor inhibits apoptosis in epithelial cells. *Neoplasia.* 1, 508-517.

Saito O, Guan Y, Qi Z, Davis LS, Komhoff M, Sugimoto Y, Narumiya S, Breyer RM, Breyer MD (2003) Expression of the prostaglandin F receptor (FP) gene along the mouse genitourinary tract. *Am.J.Physiol Renal Physiol* 284, F1164-F1170.

Salomon RG, Miller DB (1985) Levuglandins: isolation, characterization, and total synthesis of new secoprostanoid products from prostaglandin endoperoxides. *Adv.Prostaglandin Thromboxane Leukot.Res.* 15, 323-326.

Satoh T, Moroi R, Aritake K, Urade Y, Kanai Y, Sumi K, Yokozeki H, Hirai H, Nagata K, Hara T, Utsuyama M, Hirokawa K, Sugamura K, Nishioka K, Nakamura M (2006) Prostaglandin D2 plays an essential role in chronic allergic inflammation of the skin via CRTH2 receptor. *J.Immunol.* 177, 2621-2629.

Savill J (1999) Regulation of glomerular cell number by apoptosis. *Kidney Int.* 56, 1216-1222.

Scher JU, Pillinger MH (2005) 15d-PGJ2: the anti-inflammatory prostaglandin? *Clin.Immunol.* 114, 100-109.

Schneider A, Stahl RA (1998) Cyclooxygenase-2 (COX-2) and the kidney: current status and potential perspectives. *Nephrol.Dial.Transplant.* 13, 10-12.

Schuster VL (2002) Prostaglandin transport. *Prostaglandins Other Lipid Mediat.* 68-69, 633-647.

Schweda F, Klar J, Narumiya S, Nusing RM, Kurtz A (2004) Stimulation of renin release by prostaglandin E2 is mediated by EP2 and EP4 receptors in mouse kidneys. *Am.J.Physiol Renal Physiol* 287, F427-F433.

Seibert K, Masferrer JL, Needleman P, Salvemini D (1996) Pharmacological manipulation of cyclo-oxygenase-2 in the inflamed hydronephrotic kidney. *Br.J.Pharmacol.* 117, 1016-1020.

Shimazaki A, Kawamura Y, Kanazawa A, Sekine A, Saito S, Tsunoda T, Koya D, Babazono T, Tanaka Y, Matsuda M, Kawai K, Iiizumi T, Imanishi M, Shinosaki T, Yanagimoto T, Ikeda M, Omachi S, Kashiwagi A, Kaku K, Iwamoto Y, Kawamori R, Kikkawa R, Nakajima M, Nakamura Y, Maeda S (2005) Genetic variations in the gene encoding ELMO1 are associated with susceptibility to diabetic nephropathy. *Diabetes* 54, 1171-1178.

Shimazaki A, Tanaka Y, Shinosaki T, Ikeda M, Watada H, Hirose T, Kawamori R, Maeda S (2006) ELMO1 increases expression of extracellular matrix proteins and inhibits cell adhesion to ECMs. *Kidney Int.* 70, 1769-1776.

Shimizu T, Wolfe LS (1990) Arachidonic acid cascade and signal transduction. *J.Neurochem.* 55, 1-15.

Shiraya K, Hirata T, Hatano R, Nagamori S, Wiriyasermkul P, Jutabha P, Matsubara M, Muto S, Tanaka H, Asano S, Anzai N, Endou H, Yamada A, Sakurai H, Kanai Y (2010) A novel transporter of SLC22 family specifically transports prostaglandins and co-localizes with 15-hydroxyprostaglandin dehydrogenase in renal proximal tubules. *J.Biol.Chem.* 285, 22141-22151.

Silva PJ, Fernandes PA, Ramos MJ (2007) A theoretical study of radical-only and combined radical/carbocationic mechanisms of arachidonic acid cyclooxygenation by prostaglandin H synthase. *Theor Chem Acc* 110, 345-351.

Six DA, Dennis EA (2000) The expanding superfamily of phospholipase A(2) enzymes: classification and characterization. *Biochim.Biophys.Acta* 1488, 1-19.

Smith WL, DeWitt DL, Garavito RM (2000) Cyclooxygenases: structural, cellular, and molecular biology. *Annu.Rev.Biochem.* 69, 145-182.

Sorokin A (2004) Cyclooxygenase-2: potential role in regulation of drug efflux and multidrug resistance phenotype. *Curr.Pharm.Des* 10, 647-657.

Spencer AG, Thuresson E, Otto JC, Song I, Smith T, DeWitt DL, Garavito RM, Smith WL (1999) The membrane binding domains of prostaglandin endoperoxide H synthases 1 and 2. Peptide mapping and mutational analysis. *J.Biol.Chem.* 274, 32936-32942.

Steinert D, Kuper C, Bartels H, Beck FX, Neuhofer W (2009) PGE2 potentiates tonicity-induced COX-2 expression in renal medullary cells in a positive feedback loop involving EP2-cAMP-PKA signaling. *Am.J.Physiol Cell Physiol* 296, C75-C87.

Stitt-Cavanagh EM, Faour WH, Takami K, Carter A, Vanderhyden B, Guan Y, Schneider A, Breyer MD, Kennedy CR (2010) A maladaptive role for EP4 receptors in podocytes. *J.Am.Soc.Nephrol.* 21, 1678-1690.

Stock JL, Shinjo K, Burkhardt J, Roach M, Taniguchi K, Ishikawa T, Kim HS, Flannery PJ, Coffman TM, McNeish JD, Audoly LP (2001) The prostaglandin E2 EP1 receptor mediates pain perception and regulates blood pressure. *J.Clin.Invest* 107, 325-331.

Subbaramaiah K, Altorki N, Chung WJ, Mestre JR, Sampat A, Dannenberg AJ (1999) Inhibition of cyclooxygenase-2 gene expression by p53. *J.Biol.Chem.* 274, 10911-10915.

Subbaramaiah K, Marmo TP, Dixon DA, Dannenberg AJ (2003) Regulation of cyclooxgenase-2 mRNA stability by taxanes: evidence for involvement of p38, MAPKAPK-2, and HuR. *J.Biol.Chem.* 278, 37637-37647.

Subbaramaiah K, Yoshimatsu K, Scherl E, Das KM, Glazier KD, Golijanin D, Soslow RA, Tanabe T, Naraba H, Dannenberg AJ (2004) Microsomal prostaglandin E synthase-1 is overexpressed in inflammatory bowel disease. Evidence for involvement of the transcription factor Egr-1. *J.Biol.Chem.* 279, 12647-12658.

Subbaramaiah K, Zakim D, Weksler BB, Dannenberg AJ (1997) Inhibition of cyclooxygenase: a novel approach to cancer prevention. *Proc.Soc.Exp.Biol.Med.* 216, 201-210.

Sugawara A, Uruno A, Kudo M, Matsuda K, Yang CW, Ito S (2010) Effects of PPARgamma on hypertension, atherosclerosis, and chronic kidney disease. *Endocr.J.* 57, 847-852.

Sugimoto Y, Narumiya S (2007) Prostaglandin E receptors. *J.Biol.Chem.* 282, 11613-11617.

Sun LK, Beck-Schimmer B, Oertli B, Wuthrich RP (2001) Hyaluronan-induced cyclooxygenase-2 expression promotes thromboxane A2 production by renal cells. *Kidney Int.* 59, 190-196.

Takahashi N, Breitman TR (1992) Covalent modification of proteins by ligands of steroid hormone receptors. *Proc.Natl.Acad.Sci.U.S.A* 89, 10807-10811.

Tegeder I, Pfeilschifter J, Geisslinger G (2001) Cyclooxygenase-independent actions of cyclooxygenase inhibitors. *FASEB J.* 15, 2057-2072.

Thun MJ, Henley SJ, Patrono C (2002) Nonsteroidal Anti-inflammatory Drugs as Anticancer Agents: Mechanistic, Pharmacologic, and Clinical Issues. *J.Natl.Cancer Inst.* 94, 252-266.

Thuresson ED, Lakkides KM, Rieke CJ, Sun Y, Wingerd BA, Micielli R, Mulichak AM, Malkowski MG, Garavito RM, Smith WL (2001) Prostaglandin endoperoxide H synthase-1: the functions of cyclooxygenase active site residues in the binding, positioning, and oxygenation of arachidonic acid. *J.Biol.Chem.* 276, 10347-10357.

Tian J, Kim SF, Hester L, Snyder SH (2008) S-nitrosylation/activation of COX-2 mediates NMDA neurotoxicity. *Proc.Natl.Acad.Sci.U.S.A* 105, 10537-10540.

Tomasoni S, Noris M, Zappella S, Gotti E, Casiraghi F, Bonazzola S, Benigni A, Remuzzi G (1998) Upregulation of renal and systemic cyclooxygenase-2 in patients with active lupus nephritis. *J.Am.Soc.Nephrol.* 9, 1202-1212.

Tsatsanis C, Androulidaki A, Venihaki M, Margioris AN (2006) Signalling networks regulating cyclooxygenase-2. *Int.J.Biochem.Cell Biol.* 38, 1654-1661.

Tsujii M, DuBois RN (1995) Alterations in cellular adhesion and apoptosis in epithelial cells overexpressing prostaglandin endoperoxide synthase 2. *Cell* 83, 493-501.

Turini ME, DuBois RN (2002) Cyclooxygenase-2: a therapeutic target. *Annu.Rev.Med.* 53, 35-57.

Uozumi N, Shimizu T (2002) Roles for cytosolic phospholipase A2alpha as revealed by gene-targeted mice. *Prostaglandins Other Lipid Mediat.* 68-69, 59-69.

Vezza R, Habib A, Li H, Lawson JA, Fitzgerald GA (1996) Regulation of cyclooxygenases by protein kinase C. Evidence against the importance of direct enzyme phosphorylation. *J.Biol.Chem.* 271, 30028-30033.

von Euler US (1936) On the specific vaso-dilating and plain muscle stimulating substances from accessory genital glands in man and certain animals (prostaglandin and vesiglandin). *J.Physiol* 88, 213-234.

von Knethen A, Brune B (1997) Cyclooxygenase-2: an essential regulator of NO-mediated apoptosis. *FASEB J.* 11, 887-895.

Wada M, Saunders TL, Morrow J, Milne GL, Walker KP, Dey SK, Brock TG, Opp MR, Aronoff DM, Smith WL (2009) Two pathways for cyclooxygenase-2 protein degradation in vivo. *J.Biol.Chem.* 284, 30742-30753.

Wang JL, Cheng HF, Shappell S, Harris RC (2000) A selective cyclooxygenase-2 inhibitor decreases proteinuria and retards progressive renal injury in rats. *Kidney Int.* 57, 2334-2342.

Wang S, Meng F, Xu J, Gu Y (2009) Effects of lipids on ENaC activity in cultured mouse cortical collecting duct cells. *J.Membr.Biol.* 227, 77-85.

Widmann C, Gibson S, Jarpe MB, Johnson GL (1999) Mitogen-activated protein kinase: conservation of a three-kinase module from yeast to human. *Physiol Rev.* 79, 143-180.

Wilson AG, Kung HC, Anderson MW, Eling TE (1979) Covalent binding of intermediates formed during the metabolism of arachidonic acid by human platelet subcellular fractions. *Prostaglandins* 18, 409-422.

Wilson TW, Alonso-Galicia M, Roman RJ (1998) Effects of lipid-lowering agents in the Dahl salt-sensitive rat. *Hypertension* 31, 225-231.

Wong SL, Leung FP, Lau CW, Au CL, Yung LM, Yao X, Chen ZY, Vanhoutte PM, Gollasch M, Huang Y (2009) Cyclooxygenase-2-derived prostaglandin F2alpha mediates endothelium-dependent contractions in the aortae of hamsters with increased impact during aging. *Circ.Res.* 104, 228-235.

Yamamoto S, Yamamoto K, Kurobe H, Yamashita R, Yamaguchi H, Ueda N (1998) Transcriptional regulation of fatty acid cyclooxygenases-1 and -2. *Int.J.Tissue React.* 20, 17-22.

Yamamoto T, Wilson CB (1987) Quantitative and qualitative studies of antibody-induced mesangial cell damage in the rat. *Kidney Int.* 32, 514-525.

Yang C, Sorokin A (2011) Upregulation of fibronectin expression by COX-2 is mediated by interaction with ELMO1. *Cell Signal.* 23, 99-104.

Yuan C, Rieke CJ, Rimon G, Wingerd BA, Smith WL (2006) Partnering between monomers of cyclooxygenase-2 homodimers. *Proc.Natl.Acad.Sci.U.S.A* 103, 6142-6147.

Zager RA (2001) P glycoprotein-mediated cholesterol cycling determines proximal tubular cell viability. *Kidney Int.* 60, 944-956.

Zaza G, Granata S, Sallustio F, Grandaliano G, Schena FP (2010) Pharmacogenomics: a new paradigm to personalize treatments in nephrology patients. *Clin.Exp.Immunol.* 159, 268-280.

Zhang A, Dong Z, Yang T (2006) Prostaglandin D2 inhibits TGF-beta1-induced epithelial-to-mesenchymal transition in MDCK cells. *Am.J.Physiol Renal Physiol* 291, F1332-F1342.

Zheng F, Fornoni A, Elliot SJ, Guan Y, Breyer MD, Striker LJ, Striker GE (2002) Upregulation of type I collagen by TGF-beta in mesangial cells is blocked by PPARgamma activation. *Am.J.Physiol Renal Physiol* 282, F639-F648.

9

The Role of STAT3 Activation in Glomerulonephritis

Fumio Tsuji, Osamu Katsuta and Hiroyuki Aono
Research and Development Center, Santen Pharmaceutical Co., Ltd.
Japan

1. Introduction

Glomerulonephritis is a renal disease characterized by inflammation of the glomeruli, i.e., small blood vessels, in the kidneys. It may present with isolated hematuria and/or proteinuria or as nephritic syndrome, acute renal failure, or chronic renal failure. Glomerulonephritis has several different pathological patterns that can be broadly grouped into non-proliferative and proliferative types. Non-proliferative types include minimal change glomerulonephritis, focal segmental glomerulosclerosis, and membranous glomerulonephritis. Proliferative types include IgA nephropathy, post-infectious glomerulonephritis, membranoproliferative/mesangiocapillary glomerulonephritis, and rapidly progressive glomerulonephritis (Miller et al., 2010). Of the many factors involved in the inflammatory response, cytokines are the most important factors that bind to their receptors and activate signal transduction pathways. Progress in our understanding of inflammatory signaling pathways has led to the identification of the involvement of nuclear factor-κB (NF-κB), mitogen-activated protein kinases (MAPKs) such as p38, and Janus tyrosine kinase-signal transducer and activator of transcription (JAK-STAT) pathways (O'Neill, 2006). The NF-κB and p38 pathways are activated by the stimulation of interleukin-1 (IL-1) and tumor necrosis factor (TNF). The principal signaling pathways activated by IL-1 and TNF are the NF-κB and stress-activated MAPK pathways, whereas the JAK-STAT pathway is activated by many other cytokines.

2. STAT family

JAK-STAT is an important tyrosine kinase pathway activated by almost all cytokines (Ihle, 2001) that are well known for their role in the progression of renal diseases (Johnson, 1997). The STAT family consists of seven members (Table 1). The STAT proteins are unique transcription factors containing Src homology (SH) 2 and phosphotyrosine-binding domains. The SH2 domain interacts with sites of tyrosine phosphorylation to recruit STATs to receptor complexes. Following tyrosine phosphorylation of STATs, dimerization occurs between the SH2 domains. Tyrosine phosphorylation around amino acid position 700 (STAT1, tyrosine 701; STAT3 tyrosine 705) is essential for dimerization of STATs and the concomitant nuclear translocation of the dimer (Kaptein et al., 1996; Shuai et al., 1993). The basic model of cytokine pathways depends on tyrosine phosphorylation by JAK proteins non-covalently bound to specific receptors. The JAK family consists of four members: JAK1,

JAK2, JAK3, and Tyk2. In addition, the activity of the C-terminal transactivation domain of STATs is at least partially regulated by serine phosphorylation (serine 727 in STAT1 and STAT3) that does not involve the JAK protein (Wen et al., 1995). The kinase responsible for this serine phosphorylation depends on the signaling pathway and cellular context.

Family member	Chromosomal location		Activating cytokines	Phenotype of knockout mice
	Murine	Human		
STAT1	1	2q12–33	IFNs, IL-6	Viable, normal development, IFN functions eliminated, tumors increased, growth control impaired.
STAT2	10	12q13–14.1	IFNs	Viable, normal development, IFN functions affected.
STAT3	11	17q11.2–22	IL-6 family	Embryonic lethal, extraembryonic endoderm defects, cell survival impaired.
STAT4	1	2q12–33	IL-12	Viable, normal development, IL-12 functions eliminated, Th1 differentiation impaired.
STAT5A	11	17q11.2–22	Numerous	Viable, mammary gland deficiency, prolactin responsiveness eliminated.
STAT5B	11	17q11.2–22	Numerous	Viable, partial loss of growth hormone functions.
STAT6	10	12q13–14.1	IL-4, IL-13	Viable, normal development, IL-4 functions eliminated. Th2 differentiation impaired.

Table 1. Properties of STATs.

3. STAT3

STAT3 is a member of the JAK-STAT signaling pathway (Zhong et al., 1995). Cytoplasmic STAT3 in unstimulated cells is activated by recruitment through the SH2 domain to phosphorylated motifs within complexes of cytokine receptors, growth factor receptors, and non-receptor tyrosine kinases. Determination of STAT3 functions based on knockout mice studies have been difficult because mouse embryos die early in embryogenesis, prior to gastrulation (Takeda et al., 1997). STAT3 is essential for the early development of mouse embryos. Recently, some studies have succeeded in isolating STAT3 from individual tissues by the Cre-loxP method (Akira, 2000), which circumvents the problem of embryonic lethality, and revealed the roles of STAT3 in a wide variety of tissues (Table 2). A surprising result from such studies has been the identification of a multitude of and sometimes contradictory roles of STAT3 in biological processes including cell growth, cell growth suppression and apoptosis, and cell motility. The phenotypes resulting from the loss of STAT3 in adult tissues include failure of cell survival, impaired apoptosis, loss of negative feedback regulation, and impaired cell migration and wound healing (Levy & Lee, 2002). Of great current interest is the persistently active STAT3, which occurs in a wide variety of human tumors (Bowman & Jove, 1999). Overexpression and/or elevated protein tyrosine kinase activity of the epidermal growth factor receptor (EGFR), Src, and other protein kinases is associated with the progression of numerous human cancers. As a consequence, growing evidence indicates that abnormal STAT3 signaling in response to hyperactive protein tyrosine kinase activity is frequent in human tumors and is associated with the progression of oncogenesis (Garcia & Jove, 1998). Furthermore, STAT3 can be converted into an oncogene by experimental mutation (Bromberg et al., 1999). A persistently active protein is required because introduction of a dominant-negative form of STAT3 into head and neck cancer cells or multiple myeloma cells causes apoptosis of recipient cancer cells (Bowman et al., 2000). Persistent STAT3 activation in head and neck cancer is associated with mutations in EGFR or mutations that result in the production of excess ligands or normal receptors (Song & Grandis, 2000). In some multiple myelomas, excess production of IL-6 might be the underlying defect (Catlett-Falcone et al., 1999). IL-6-dependent accumulation of long-lived plasma cells occurs due to elevated levels of a key regulatory protein, Bcl-x_L, a member of the Bcl-2 family of proteins that prevent apoptosis. Constitutive activation of STAT3 signaling, an important component of the IL-6 pathway, directly contributes to the induction of Bcl-x_L gene expression. Thus, constitutive activation of STAT3 signaling in response to IL-6 promotes tumor cell survival and malignant progression of multiple myelomas by directly inducing expression of a key apoptosis regulatory protein. All these results suggest that STAT3 may be essential for many cell functions.

Target tissue	Phenotype
Skin	Impaired second hair cycle, wound repair and keratinocyte migration
Thymic epithelium	Age-dependent thymic hypoplasia, hypersensitivity to stress
T lymphocytes	Impaired IL-6-dependent survival and IL-2Rα expression
Monocytes/neutrophils	Enhanced inflammatory responses and Th1 differentiation, chronic colitis
Granulocytes	Enhanced proliferation owing to impaired negative feedback
Mammary epithelium	Defective apoptosis, delayed mammary involution
Liver	Impaired acute phase response
Neurons	Impaired cell survival

Table 2. Tissue-specific roles of STAT3 (Levy & Darnell, 2002).

4. STAT3 in gp130 cytokine signaling

Several cytokines including IL-6, IL-11, leukemia inhibitory factor, oncostatin M, ciliary neurotrophic factor, and cardiotrophin share a gp130 subunit that is required to activate JAKs and STATs (Stahl et al., 1994). These cytokines are competent to activate STAT3 and induce various pleiotrophic responses that include hematopoiesis regulation, immune response, and neuronal differentiation (Snick, 1990). gp130-associated kinases JAK1, JAK2, and Tyk2 become activated on stimulation, and the cytoplasmic tail of gp130 is phosphorylated (Heinrich et al., 1998). STAT3 is recruited to phosphorylated tyrosine residues in the YXXQ motif including the tyrosine residue Y705 of gp130, where it is activated and dimerized. It subsequently enters the nucleus and regulates gene expression (Hirano et al., 2000). STAT3 is essential for gp130-mediated cell survival and G1 to S cell cycle transition signals. Both *c-myc* and *pim* have been identified as target genes of STAT3 and together can compensate for STAT3 in cell survival and cell cycle transition. On the other hand, the SH2 domain-bearing protein tyrosine phosphatase (SHP)-2 is recruited to the phosphorylated tyrosine residue Y759 in gp130, where it becomes activated and forms a complex with adaptor/docking proteins, Gab1 and Gab2, leading to activation of the Ras-MAPK pathway (Hibi & Hirano, 2000). Several *in vitro* experiments have shown that SHP-2- and STAT3-mediated signal transduction pathways initiated through gp130 are involved in growth, differentiation, and gene expression in various cell lines (Fukuda et al., 1996; Hirano et al., 2000; Nakajima et al., 1996). SHP-2-mediated ERK/MAPK activation has been suggested to play a negative role in STAT3-mediated biological responses (Jain et al., 1998; Sengupta et al., 1998). The tyrosine residue Y759 also provides the binding site for the suppressor of cytokine signaling 3 (SOCS3) protein that negatively regulates gp130 signals (Nicholson et al., 2000; Schmitz et al., 2000). To clarify the roles of SHP-2- and STAT3-mediated signal transduction pathways *in vivo*, a series of knock-in mouse lines was generated in which gp130-mediated STAT3 or SHP-2 signals were selectively disrupted. This disruption was achieved by mutating the tyrosine residues in all YXXQ motifs or the tyrosine residue Y759 to phenylalanine ($gp130^{FXXQ/FXXQ}$ and $gp130^{F759/F759}$ mice, respectively) (Ohtani et al., 2000). Analyses of these mice indicated that SHP-2-mediated or Y759-dependent signals negatively regulate the biological responses elicited by STAT3-mediated signals *in vivo* and that the balance of positive and negative signals generated through gp130 is skewed or shifted toward positive STAT3 signaling in $gp130^{F759/F759}$ mice (Fig. 1).

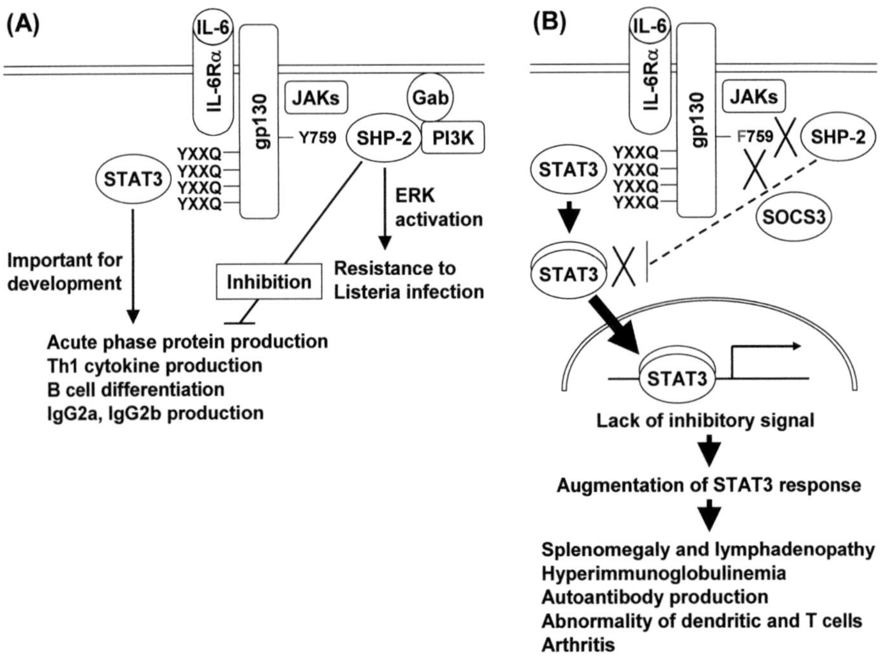

Fig. 1. The role of gp130 signals *in vivo*. A: STAT3/YXXQ and SHP-2/Y759 signals induce responses independent of each other. SHP-2/Y759 signals negatively regulate the biological responses elicited by STAT3-mediated signals. B: The balance of positive and negative signals generated through gp130 is skewed or shifted toward positive STAT3 signaling in $gp130^{F759/F759}$.

The SHP-2 signal-deficient mice ($gp130^{F759/F759}$) were born normally but displayed splenomegaly and lymphadenopathy and an enhanced acute phase reaction. In contrast, the STAT3 signal-deficient mice ($gp130^{FXXQ/FXXQ}$) died perinatally, similar to the gp130-deficient mice. The $gp130^{F759/F759}$ mice showed prolonged gp130-induced STAT3 activation. Importantly, these mice in a mixed background with 129 and C57BL/6 spontaneously develop a rheumatoid arthritis-like autoimmune disease in old age (Atsumi et al., 2002). The mice show severe immunological abnormalities, including autoantibody production, increased memory/activated T cells, impaired thymic negative selection, and peripheral clonal deletion. Development of a rheumatoid arthritis-like disease is entirely dependent on mature lymphocytes, but abnormally enhanced homeostatic proliferation of CD4 T cells is caused by augmented production of IL-7 by non-hematopoietic stromal cells through a STAT3-dependent process (Sawa et al., 2006). In mice showing hyperactivation of STAT1/STAT3, T cell recruitment and CCL5/RANTES expression is enhanced (McLoughlin et al., 2005). A recent study described an IL-17A-triggered positive-feedback loop of IL-6 signaling that involved activation of the transcription factors NF-κB and STAT3 in fibroblasts (Ogura et al., 2008). Although the underlying mechanisms by which STAT3 regulates tissue fibrosis are not fully understood, its activation is required for upregulation of transforming growth factor (TGF)-β signaling, activation/proliferation of myofibroblasts, and deposition of extracellular matrix proteins (Ma & Zhuang, 2011). All these results suggest that STAT3 plays an important role in the function of multiple cells.

5. STAT3 activation in renal cells

Various factors show STAT3 activation in glomerular mesangial and proximal tubule cells. High glucose activates the growth-promoting enzyme JAK2 and its latent STAT transcription factors (STAT1, STAT3, and STAT5) and increases TGF-β and fibronectin synthesis in mesangial cells (Wang et al., 2002). High glucose-induced tyrosine phosphorylation of JAK2, STAT1, and STAT3 as well as TGF-β and fibronectin synthesis are abolished by a specific JAK2 inhibitor, AG-490. However, antisense oligonucleotide studies have shown that STAT1 activation is more important than STAT3 activation for TGF-β and fibronectin synthesis. Angiotensin II induces phosphorylation of JAK2, STAT1, STAT3, STAT5A/STAT5B and SHP-2, and angiotensin II-induced phosphorylation is enhanced by high glucose levels (Amiri et al., 2002). Angiotensin II-induced growth and collagen IV synthesis are also increased under high glucose conditions. Transfection of glomerular mesangial cells with JAK2 antisense oligonucleotides blocks angiotensin II-induced growth and collagen IV synthesis under both normal and high glucose conditions.

In renal proximal tubule cells, IL-6 increases phosphorylation of STAT3, phosphoinositide-3 kinase (PI3K)/Akt, MAPKs, and NF-κB (Lee et al., 2007). IL-6 also stimulates α-methyl-D-[^{14}C]glucopyranoside uptake, which is indicative of active transport in renal proximal tubule cells. The increased uptake can be blocked by pretreatment with a STAT3 inhibitor, a PI3K inhibitor, an Akt inhibitor, MAPK inhibitors, and NF-κB inhibitors. High glucose also induces activation of Raf-1, p42/p44 MAPK, JAK2, STAT1, and STAT3 (but not STAT5) in renal tubular epithelial cells (Huang et al., 2007). Moreover, severe oxidative stress leads to tyrosine phosphorylation of STAT3 at Y705 (Arany et al., 2006). This event depends on the activation of EGFR and JAK2 and is directly linked to cell death because inhibition of STAT3 function enables cells to survive severe oxidative stress.

6. STAT3 activation in an animal model of glomerulonephritis

In an animal model of mesangial proliferative glomerulonephritis induced by the injection of anti-Thy1.1 antibody, STAT3 is phosphorylated in mesangial cells (Yanagita et al., 2001a). STAT3 phosphorylation peaks 8 days after the anti-Thy1.1 injection. Inhibition of growth arrest-specific gene 6 by the extracellular domain of its receptor Axl or warfarin abolishes STAT3 phosphorylation (Yanagita et al., 2001a) and inhibits mesangial cell proliferation (Yanagita et al., 2001b) *in vivo*. STAT3 can be expressed and activated in the kidneys of rats with immune complex glomerulonephritis using BSA as an antigen (Zhang et al., 2005). These rats also have increased macrophage infiltration (detected by a surface marker for monocytes/macrophages, ED-1), with some cells showing simultaneous expression of p-STAT3 and ED-1; this may contribute to inflammatory proliferation in the glomeruli and accumulation of extracellular matrix proteins. Inhibition of angiotensin-converting enzyme (ACE) with fosinopril downregulates STAT3 activation and ED-1 influx, and these effects may attenuate renal damage in this model. Hyperglycemia induces activation of JAK2 and STATs, including STAT3, *in vivo* (Banes et al., 2004). Phosphorylation of JAK2, STAT1, STAT3, and STAT5 in the glomeruli by streptozotocin (STZ) injection is reduced in rats treated with the ACE inhibitor captopril, angiotensin II type 1 receptor antagonist candesartan, or AG-490. Furthermore, both candesartan and AG-490 inhibit STZ-induced increases in urinary protein excretion. Knockdown of STAT3 activity *in vivo* prevents diabetic glomerulopathy (Lu et al., 2009). While the number of glomeruli does not differ between diabetic STAT3 knockdown and reference mice, the diabetic STAT3 knockdown mice exhibit significantly less proteinuria, mesangial expansion, glomerular cell proliferation, and macrophage infiltration than the diabetic reference mice. Reduction in STAT3 activity abrogates the stimulation of inflammatory markers, including IL-6, intercellular adhesion molecule-1, and monocyte chemotactic protein (MCP)-1, and blocks nuclear translocation of NF-κB. JAK2-STAT3 proteins may be involved in the early kidney damage associated with diabetes. AG490 also ameliorates adriamycin-induced nephritic syndrome in mice (Li et al., 2007). JAK-STAT signaling is activated in adriamycin nephropathy. Phosphorylation of JAK2, STAT1, and STAT3 is significantly inhibited by AG490. Proteinuria, glomerulosclerosis, tubulointerstitial lesions, and renal α-smooth muscle actin expression are significantly suppressed by AG490 treatment. In addition, AG490 inhibits MCP-1 mRNA expression accompanied by reduced interstitial infiltration of macrophages and T cells. Activation of JAK-STAT signaling is involved in the progression of glomerular diseases with proteinuria. While AG490 inhibits phosphorylation of STAT1 and STAT3, a novel selective inhibitor of STAT3, S3I-201, has been synthesized. S3I-201 preferentially inhibits STAT3 DNA-binding activity and diminishes tyrosine phosphorylation of STAT3 (Siddiquee et al., 2007). In a mouse model of renal interstitial fibrosis induced by unilateral ureteral obstruction, STAT3 was activated and administration of S3I-201 attenuated both STAT3 activation and extracellular matrix protein deposition following injury (Pang et al., 2010). S3I-201 reduced infiltration of the injured kidney by inflammatory cells and suppressed injury-induced expression of fibronectin, α-smooth muscle actin, and collagen type 1 proteins, as well as expression of multiple cytokines. Furthermore, S3I-201 inhibited proliferation and preferentially induced apoptosis in renal interstitial fibroblasts of the obstructed kidney. Inhibition of STAT3 signaling may hold therapeutic potential for fibrotic kidney diseases. IL-6 expression is increased in S-(1,2 dichlorovinyl)-L-cysteine-induced acute renal tubule necrosis (Vaidya et al., 2003) and renal ischemia-reperfusion injury (Lemay et al., 2000) in mice. IL-6-deficient mice are resistant to

$HgCl_2$-induced acute kidney injury compared with wild-type mice (Nechemia-Arbely et al., 2008). IL-6 expression and STAT3 activation in renal tubular epithelial cells is significantly increased during the development of injury, suggesting active IL-6 signaling. Activation of the JAK-STAT pathway in renal and non-renal cells in kidney diseases is shown in Fig. 2.

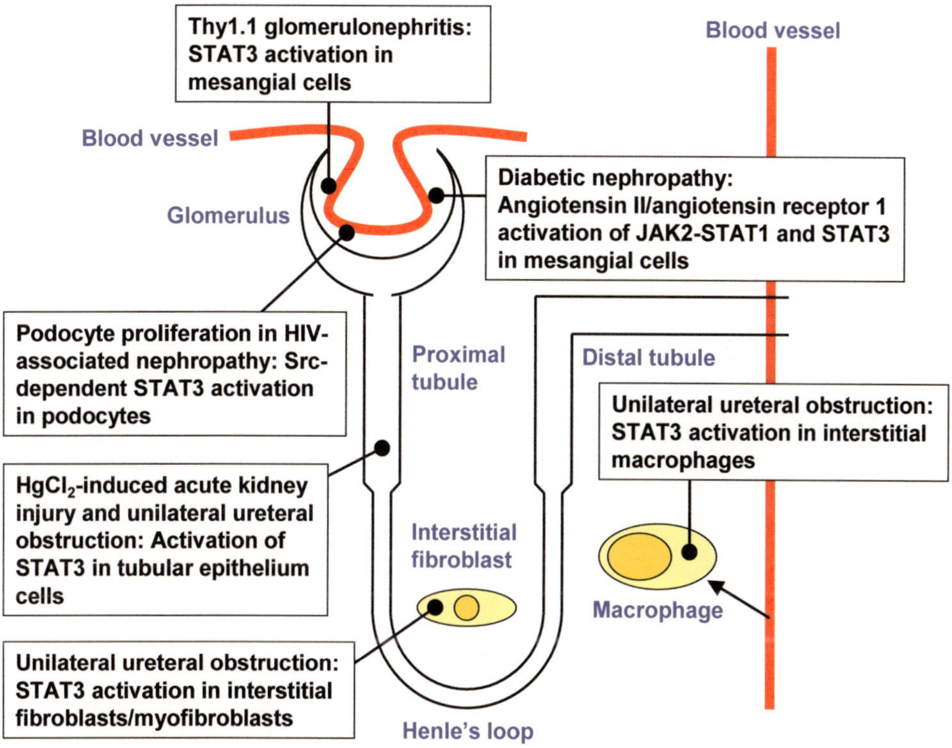

Fig. 2. Activation of the JAK-STAT pathway in renal and non-renal cells in kidney diseases (Chuang & He, 2010).

We have generated a series of knock-in mouse lines with several genetic backgrounds in which gp130-mediated STAT3 or SHP-2 signals are selectively disrupted. gp130 is a shared receptor of the IL-6 cytokine family (Ohtani et al., 2000). We found that characteristic abnormalities in C57BL/6 background $gp130^{F759/F759}$ mice included not only spontaneous polyarthritis but also glomerulonephritis (Fig. 3, only in females) (Tsuji et al., 2009). However, spontaneous glomerulonephritis did not develop in DBA/1J background mice, indicating that genetic background may affect the development of disease.

7. STAT3 activation in human glomerulonephritis

In vitro and animal studies have shown that an increase in STAT3 activity may play a critical role in the development of glomerulonephritis. Few studies have investigated the role of STAT3 activation in human renal diseases, but one study has identified STAT3 activation in the normal human kidney and a marked increase in this activation in many forms of glomerulonephritis (Arakawa et al., 2008). The correlation of STAT3 activation with clinical and histological parameters suggests that this pathway plays an important role in the pathogenesis of kidney diseases. In addition, mesangial expansion and podocyte loss in the glomeruli are important early features of diabetic nephropathy. JAK1, JAK2, and JAK3 as well as STAT1 and STAT3 are expressed at higher levels in patients with diabetic nephropathy than in control subjects (Berthier et al., 2009). Immunohistochemistry showed strong JAK2 staining in glomerular and tubulointerstitial compartments of patients with diabetic nephropathy compared with control subjects. These data suggest a direct relationship between tubulointerstitial JAK-STAT expression and the progression of kidney failure in patients with type 2 diabetic nephropathy and can be used to distinguish progressive human diabetic nephropathy. Further studies are needed to clarify the role of STAT3 activation in human glomerulonephritis.

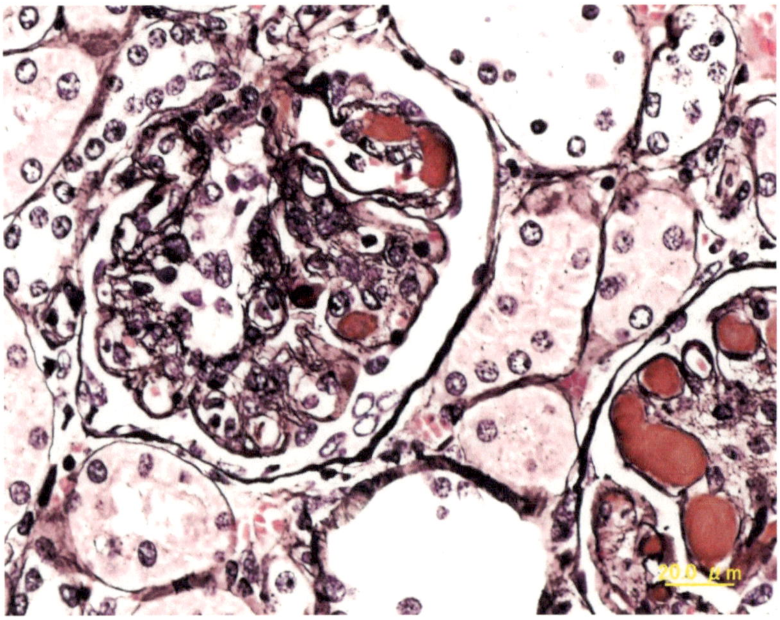

Fig. 3. Glomerulonephritis in a gp130$^{F759/F759}$ mouse (female, 12 months). Deposition of hyaline droplets in the subendothelial zone is shown.

8. Conclusions

The JAK-STAT pathway is a pleiotropic cascade essential to cytokine and growth hormone receptor signaling. Signaling through the JAK-STAT pathway is important for the kidney's response to injury in disease. STAT3 activation is observed in an animal model of glomerulonephritis and human glomerulonephritis, and the STAT3 pathway inhibition ameliorates the renal conditions in some animal models. Further studies are needed to clarify the role of STAT3 activation in human glomerulonephritis, but the STAT3 pathway inhibition may be one of the potential therapeutic approaches for renal diseases.

9. References

Akira, S. (2000). Roles of STAT3 defined by tissue-specific gene targeting. *Oncogene*, Vol.19, No.21, pp. 2607-2611, ISSN 0950-9232

Amiri, F.; Shaw, S.; Wang, X.; Tang, J.; Waller, J.L.; Eaton, D.C. & Marrero, M.B. (2002). Angiotensin II activation of the JAK/STAT pathway in mesangial cells is altered by high glucose. *Kidney International*, Vol.61, No.5, pp. 1605-1616, ISSN 0085-2538

Arakawa, T.; Masaki, T.; Hirai, T.; Doi, S.; Kuratsune, M.; Arihiro, K.; Kohno, N. & Yorioka, N. (2008). Activation of signal transducer and activator of transcription 3 correlates with cell proliferation and renal injury in human glomerulonephritis. *Nephrology Dialysis Transplantation*, Vol.23, No.11, pp. 3418-3426, ISSN 0931-0509

Arany, I.; Megyesi, J.K.; Nelkin, B.D. & Safirstein, R.L. (2006). STAT3 attenuates EGFR-mediated ERK activation and cell survival during oxidant stress in mouse proximal tubular cells. *Kidney International*, Vol.70, No.4, pp. 669-674, ISSN 0085-2538

Atsumi, T.; Ishihara, K.; Kamimura, D.; Ikushima, H.; Ohtani, T.; Hirota, S.; Kobayashi, H.; Park, S.; Saeki, Y.; Kitamura, Y. & Hirano, T. (2002). A point mutation of Tyr-759 in interleukin 6 family cytokine receptor subunit gp130 causes autoimmune arthritis. *The Journal of Experimental Medicine*, Vol.196, No.7, pp. 979-990, ISSN 0022-1007

Banes, A.K.; Shaw, S.; Jenkins, J.; Redd, H.; Amiri, F.; Pollock, D.M. & Marrero, M.B. (2004). Angiotensin II blockade prevents hyperglycemia-induced activation of JAK and STAT proteins in diabetic rat kidney glomeruli. *American Journal of Physiology Renal Physiology*, Vol.286, No.4, pp. F653-F659, ISSN 0363-6127

Berthier, C.C.; Zhang, H.; Schin, M.; Henger, A.; Nelson, R.G.; Yee, B.; Boucherot, A.; Neusser, M.A.; Cohen, C.D.; Carter-Su, C.; Argetsinger, L.S.; Rastaldi, M.P.; Brosius, F.C. & Kretzler, M. (2009). Enhanced expression of janus kinase-signal transducer and activator of transcription pathway members in human diabetic nephropathy. *Diabetes*, Vol.58, No.2, 469-477, ISSN 0012-1797

Bowman, T. & Jove, R. (1999). STAT proteins and cancer. *Cancer Control*, Vol.6, No.6, pp. 615-619, ISSN 1073-2748

Bowman, T.; Garcia, R.; Turkson, J. & Jove, R. (2000). STATs in oncogenesis. *Oncogene*, Vol.19, No.21, pp. 2474-2488, ISSN 0950-9232

Bromberg, J.F.; Wrzeszczynska, M.H.; Devgan, G.; Zhao, Y.; Pestell, R.G.; Albanese, C. & Darnell, J.E., Jr. (1999). Stat3 as an oncogene. *Cell*, Vol.98, No., pp. 295-303, ISSN 0092-8674

Catlett-Falcone, R.; Landowski, T.H.; Oshiro, M.M.; Turkson, J.; Levitzki, a.; Savino, R.; Ciliberto, G.; Moscinski, L.; Fernández-Luna, J.L.; Nuñez, G.; Dalton, W.S. & Jove, R. (1999). Constitutive activation of Stat3 signaling confers resistance to apoptosis in human U266 myeloma cells. *Immunity*, Vol.10, No.1, pp. 105-115, ISSN 1074-7613

Chuang, P.Y. & He, J.C. (2010). JAK/STAT signaling in renal diseases. *Kidney International*, Vol.78, No.3, pp. 231-234, ISSN 0085-2538

Fukada, T.; Hibi, M.; Yamanaka, Y.; Takahashi-Tezuka, M.; Fujitani, Y.; Yamaguchi, T.; Nakajima, K. & Hirano, T. (1996). Two signals are necessary for cell proliferation induced by a cytokine receptor gp130: involvement of STAT3 in anti-apoptosis. *Immunity*, Vol.5, No.5, pp. 449-460, ISSN 1074-7613

Garcia, R. & Jove, R. (1998). Activation of STAT transcription factors in oncogenic tyrosine kinase signaling. *Journal of Biomedical Science*, Vol.5, No.2, pp. 79-85, ISSN 1423-0127

Heinrich, P.C.; Behrmann, I.; Müller-Newen, G.; Schaper, F. & Graeve, L. (1998). Interleukin-6-type cytokine signalling through the gp130/Jak/STAT pathway. *Biochemical Journal*, Vol.334, No.2, pp. 297-314, ISSN 0264-6021

Hibi, M. & Hirano, T. (2000). Gab-family adapter molecules in signal transduction of cytokine and growth factor receptors, and T and B cell antigen receptors. *Leukemia & Lymphoma*, Vol.37, No.3-4, pp. 299-307, ISSN 1042-8194

Hirano, T.; Ishihara, K. & Hibi, M. (2000). Roles of STAT3 in mediating the cell growth, differentiation and survival signals relayed through the IL-6 family of cytokine receptors. *Oncogene*, Vol.19, No.21, pp. 2548-2556, ISSN 0950-9232

Huang, J.S.; Chuang, L.Y.; Guh, J.Y.; Huang, Y.J. & Hsu, M.S. (2007). Antioxidants attenuate high glucose-induced hypertrophic growth in renal tubular epithelial cells. *American Journal of Physiology Renal Physiology*, Vol.293, No.4, pp. F1072-F1082, ISSN 0363-6127

Ihle, J.N. (2001). The Stat family in cytokine signaling. *Current Opinion in Cell Biology*, Vol.13, No.2, pp. 211-217, ISSN 0955-0674

Jain, N. ; Zhang, T.; Fong, S.L.; Lim, C.P. & Cao, X. (1998). Repression of Stat3 activity by activation of mitogen-activated protein kinase (MAPK). *Oncogene*, Vol.17, No.24, pp. 3157-3167, ISSN 0950-9232

Johnson, R.J. (1997). Cytokines, growth factors and renal injury: where do we go now? *Kidney International*, Vol.52, Suppl.63, pp. S2-S6, ISSN 0085-2538

Kaptein, A.; Paillard, V. & Saunders, M. (1996). Dominant negative Stat3 mutant inhibits interleukin-6-induced Jak-STAT signal transduction. *The Journal of Biological Chemistry*, Vol.271, No.11, pp. 5961-5964, ISSN 0021-9258

Lee, Y.J.; Heo, J.S.; Suh, H.N.; Lee, M.Y. & Han, H.J. (2007). Interleukin-6 stimulates α-MG uptake in renal proximal tubule cells: involvement of STAT3, Pi3K/Akt, MAPKs, and NF-kB. *American Journal of Physiology Renal Physiology*, Vol.293, No.4, pp. F1036-F1046, ISSN 0363-6127

Lemay, S.; Rabb, H.; Postler, G. & Singh, A.K. (2000). Prominent and sustained up-regulation of gp130-signaling cytokines and of the chemokine MIP-2 in murine renal ischemia-reperfusion injury. *Transplantation*, Vol.69, No.5, pp. 959-963, ISSN 0041-1337

Levy, D.E. & Darnell, J.E. (2002). STATs: Transcriptional control and biological impact. *Nature Reviews Molecular Cell Biology*, Vol.3, No.9, pp. 651-662, ISSN 1471-0072

Levy, D.E. & Lee, C. (2002). What does STAT3 do? *The Journal of Clinical Investigation*, Vol.109, No.9, pp. 1143-1148, ISSN 0021-9738

Li, R.; Yang, N.; Zhang, L.; Huang, Y.; Zhang, R.; Wang, F.; Luo, M.; Liang, Y. & Yu, X. (2007). Inhibition of JAK/STAT signaling ameliorates mice experimental nephritic syndrome. *American Journal of Nephrology*, Vol.27, No.6, pp. 580-589, ISSN 0250-8095

Lu, T.C.; Wang, Z.H.; Feng, X.; Chuang, P.Y.; Fang, W.; Shen, Y.; Levy, D.E.; Xiong, H.; Chen, N. & He, J.C. (2009). Knockdown of Stat3 activity in vivo prevents diabetic glomerulopathy. *Kidney International*, Vol.76, No.1, pp. 63-71, ISSN 0085-2538

Ma, L. & Zhuang, S. (2011). The role of STAT3 in tissue fibrosis. *Current Chemical Biology*, Vol.5, No.1, pp. 44-51, ISSN 1872-3136

McLoughlin, R.M.; Jenkins, B.J.; Grail, D.; Williams, A.S.; Fielding, C.A.; Parker, C.R.; Ernst, M.; Topley, N. & Jones, S.A. (2005). IL-6 trans-signaling via STAT3 directs T cell infiltration in acute inflammation. *Proceedings of the National Academy of Sciences of the United States of America*, Vol.102, No.27, pp. 9589-9594, ISSN 0027-8424

Miller, F.P.; Vandome, A.F. & McBrewster J. (2010). *Glomerulonephritis*, Alphascript Publishing, ISBN 978-613-1-76981-8, USA

Nakajima, K.; Yamanaka, Y.; Nakae, K.; Kojima, H.; Ichiba, M.; Kiuchi, N.; Kitaoka, T.; Fukada, T.; Hibi, M. & Hirano, T. (1996). A central role for Stat3 in IL-6-induced regulation of growth and differentiation in M1 leukemia cells. *The EMBO Journal*, Vol.15, No.14, pp. 3651-3658, ISSN 0261-4189

Nechemia-Arbely, Y.; Barkan, D.; Pizov, G.; Shriki, A.; Rose-John, S.; Galun, E. & Axelrod, J.H. (2008). IL-6/IL-6R axis plays a critical role in acute kidney injury. *Journal of the American Society of Nephrology*, Vol.19, No.6, pp. 1106-1115, ISSN 1046-6673

Nicholson, S.E.; De Souza, D.; Fabri, L.J.; Corbin, J.; Willson, T.A.; Zhang, J.; Silva, A.; Asimakis, M.; Farley, A.; Nash, A.D.; Metcalf, D.; Hilton, D.J.; Nicola, N.A. & Baca, M. (2000). Suppressor of cytokine signaling-3 preferentially binds to the SHP-2-binding site on the shared cytokine receptor subunit gp130. *Proceedings of the National Academy of Sciences of the United States of America*, Vol.97, No.12, pp. 6493-6498, ISSN 0027-8424

Ogura, H.; Murakami, M.; Okuyama, Y.; Tsuruoka, M.; Kitabayashi, C.; Kanamoto, M.; Nishimura, M.; Iwakura, Y. & Hirano, T. (2008). Interleukin-17 promotes autoimmunity by triggering a positive-feedback loop via interleukin-6 induction. *Immunity*, Vol.29, No.4, pp. 628-636, ISSN 1074-7613

Ohtani, T.; Ishihara, K.; Atsumi, T.; Nishida, K.; Kaneko, Y.; Miyata, T.; Itoh, S.; Narimatsu, M.; Maeda, H.; Fukada, H.; Itoh, M.; Okano, H.; Hibi, M. & Hirano, T. (2000). Dissection of signaling cascades through gp130 in vivo: Reciprocal roles for STAT3- and SHP2-mediated signals in immune responses. *Immunity*, Vol.12, No.1, pp. 95-105, ISSN 1074-7613

O'Neill, L.A.J. (2006). Targeting signal transduction as a strategy to treat inflammatory diseases. *Nature Reviews Drug Discovery*, Vol.5, No.7, pp. 549-563, ISSN 1474-1776

Pang, M.; Ma, L.; Gong, R.; Tolbert, E.; Mao, H.; Ponnusamy, M.; Chin, Y.E.; Yan, H.; Dworkin, L.D. & Zhuang, S. (2010). A novel STAT3 inhibitor, S3I-201, attenuates renal interstitial fibroblast activation and interstitial fibrosis in obstructive nephropathy. *Kidney International*, Vol.78, No.3, pp. 257-268, ISSN 0085-2538

Sawa, S.; Kamimura, D.; Jin, G.H.; Morikawa, H.; Kamon, H.; Nishihata, M.; Ishihara, K.; Murakami, M. & Hirano, T. (2006). Autoimmune arthritis associated with mutated interleukin (IL)-6 receptor gp130 is driven by STAT3/IL-7-dependent homeostatic proliferation of CD4+ T cells. *The Journal of Experimental Medicine*, Vol.203, No.6, pp. 1459-1470, ISSN 0022-1007

Schmitz, J.; Weissenbach, S.; Haan, S.; Heinrich, P.C. & Schaper, F. (2000). SOCS3 exerts its inhibitory function on interleukin-6 signal transduction through the SHP2 recruitment site of gp130. *The Journal of Biological Chemistry*, Vol.275, No.17, pp. 12848-12856, ISSN 0021-9258

Sengupta, T.K.; Talbot, E.S.; Scherle, P.A. & Ivashkiv, L.B. (1998). Rapid inhibition of interleukin-6 signaling and Stat3 activation mediated by mitogen-activated protein kinases. *Proceedings of the National Academy of Sciences of the United States of America*, Vol.95, No.19, pp. 11107-11112, ISSN 0027-8424

Shuai, K.; Stark, G.R.; Kerr, I.M. & Darnell, J.E., Jr. (1993). A single phosphotyrosine residue of Stat91 required for gene activation by interferon-gamma. *Science*, Vol.261, No.5129, pp. 1744-1746, ISSN 0036-8075

Siddiquee, K.; Zhang, S.; Guida, W.C.; Blaskovich, M.A.; Greedy, B.; Lawrence, H.R.; Yip, M.L.R.; Jove, R.; McLaughlin, M.M.; Lawrence, N.J.; Sebti, S.M. & Turkson, J. (2007).

Selective chemical probe inhibitor of Stat3, identified through structure-based virtual screening, induces antitumor activity. *Proceedings of the National Academy of Sciences of the United States of America*, Vol.104, No.18, pp. 7391-7396, ISSN 0027-8424

Snick, J.V. (1990). Interleukin-6: An overview. *Annual Review of Immunology*, Vo.8, pp. 253-278, ISSN 0732-0582

Song, J.I. & Grandis, J.R. (2000). STAT signaling in head and neck cancer. *Oncogene*, Vol.19, No.21, pp. 2489-2495, ISSN 0950-9232

Stahl, N.; Boulton, T.G.; Farruggella, T.; Ip, N.Y.; Davis, S.; Witthuhn, B.A.; Quelle, F.W.; Silvennoien, O.; Barbieri, G.; Pellegrini, S.; Ihle, J.N. & Yancopoulos, G.D. (1994). Association and activation of Jak-Tyk kinases by CNTF-LIF-OSM-IL-6 beta receptor components. *Science*, Vol.263, No.5143, pp. 92-95, ISSN 0036-8075

Takeda, K.; Noguchi, K.; Shi, W.; Tanaka, T.; Matsumoto, M.; Yoshida, N.; Kishimoto, T. & Akira, S. (1997). Targeted disruption of the mouse Stat3 gene leads to early embryonic lethality. *Proceedings of the National Academy of Sciences of the United States of America*, Vol.94, No.8, pp. 3801-3804, ISSN 0027-8424

Tsuji, F.; Yoshimi, M.; Katsuta, O.; Takai, M.; Ishihara, K. & Aono, H. (2009). Point mutation of tyrosine 759 of the IL-6 family cytokine receptor, gp130, augments collagen-induced arthritis in DBA/1J mice. *BMC Musculoskeletal Disorders*, Vol.10, No.23, ISSN 1471-2474

Vaidya, V.S.; Shankar, K.; Lock, E.A.; Dixon, D. & Mehendale, H. (2003). Molecular mechanisms of renal tissue repair in survival from acute renal tubule necrosis: role of ERK1/2 pathway. *Toxicologic Pathology*, Vol.31, No.6, pp. 604-618, ISSN 0192-6233

Wang, X.; Shaw, S.; Amiri, F.; Eaton, D.C. & Marrero, M.B. (2002). Inhibition of the JAK/STAT signaling pathway prevents the high glucose-induced increase in TGF-β and fibronectin synthesis in mesangial cells. *Diabetes*, Vol.51, No.12, pp. 3505-3509, ISSN 0012-1797

Wen, Z.; Zhong, Z. & Darnell, J.E., Jr. (1995). Maximal activation of transcription by Stat1 and Stat3 requires both tyrosine and serine phosphorylation. *Cell*, Vol.82, No.2, pp. 241-250, ISSN 0092-8674

Yanagita, M.; Arai, H.; Nakano, T.; Ohashi, K.; Mizuno, K.; Fukatsu, A.; Doi, T. & Kita, T. (2001a). Gas6 induces mesangial cell proliferation via latent transcription factor STAT3. *The Journal of Biological Chemistry*, Vol.276, No.45, pp. 42364-42369, ISSN 0021-9258

Yanagita, M.; Arai, H.; Ishii, K.; Nakano, T.; Ohashi, K.; Mizuno, K.; Vernum, B.; Fukatsu, A.; Doi, T. & Kita, T. (2001b). Gas6 regulates mesangial cell proliferation through Axl in experimental glomerulonephritis. *The American Journal of Pathology*, Vol.158, No.4, pp. 1423-1432, ISSN 0002-9440

Zhang, W.; Chen, X.; Shi, S.; Wei, R.; Wang, J.; Yamanaka, N. & Hong, Q. (2005). Expression and activation of STAT3 in chronic proliferative immune complex glomerulonephritis and the effect of fosinopril. *Nephrology Dialysis Transplantation*, Vol.20, No.5, pp. 892-901, ISSN 0931-0509

Zhong, Z.; Wen, Z. & Darnell, J.E., Jr. (1994). Stat3: a STAT family member activated by tyrosine phosphorylation in response to epidermal growth factor and interleukin-6. *Science*, Vol.264, No.5155, pp. 95-98, ISSN 0036-8075

10

Role of the Mammalian Target of Rapamycin (mTOR) Signalling Pathway in Podocytes in Glomerular Disease

Lena Succar, David CH Harris and Gopala K Rangan
Centre for Transplant and Renal Research,
Westmead Millennium Institute, The University of Sydney
Australia

1. Introduction

The key intrinsic cell of the glomerulus is the podocyte, which is described as the "organiser and caretaker" of glomerular structure and function (Leeuwis et al., 2010). Podocytes (also known as visceral epithelial cells) are terminally differentiated pericyte-like epithelial cells that form the outer exocapillary layer of the glomerular filtration barrier. They have a critical function in maintaining normal glomerular capillary permeability and functional integrity (Marshall and Shankland, 2007). The aim of this chapter is to summarize the current research on the contribution of podocytes to the disease process in glomerulonephritis in connection to the mTOR signaling pathway.

During glomerular development, the podocyte has a central role in integrating signals from the other glomerular resident cells to form the proper basic structure of the glomerular filtration unit (Eremina and Quaggin, 2004). Podocytes line the outer aspect of the glomerular basement membrane (GBM) and physiologically have a unique and complex cytostructure consisting of three morphologically and functionally distinct segments: a cell body, foot processes and the slit diaphragm (Mundel and Kriz, 1995). Major processes arise from the cell body and split into foot processes. The foot processes contain an actin-based cytoskeleton that is linked to the glomerular basement membrane at focal contacts (Faul et al., 2007). Podocyte foot processes form a highly branched interdigitating network which enwrap the glomerular capillaries, and are connected by the slit diaphragm. Three distinct membrane compartments form the foot processes: the basal side, the apical side, and the slit filtration diaphragm. The basal side connects the podocyte to the GBM with several types of integrins and dystroglycans (Pavenstadt et al., 2003). It also plays a role in endocytosis of albumin and IgG trapped in the GBM, offering possibilities for drug delivery (Eyre J, 2007) (Akilesh S, 2008). The apical side contains negatively charged proteins such as podocalyxin, a sialoglycoprotein, and podoplanin which form a glycocalyx layer and thereby contribute to charge-selectivity of the glomerular filtrate (Koop et al., 2008) (Orlando RA, 2001) (Kerjaschki D, 1984).

The slit diaphragm is the most complex layer of the glomerular filtration barrier, with a constant width of 40 nm (Tryggvason et al., 2006, Benzing, 2004). The main function of the slit diaphragm is to form a size-selective barrier for proteins and since many of the slit diaphragm proteins are phosphorylated, this contributes to the charge-selective element (Tryggvason K,

2001). Podocyte-specific multiprotein complexes, similar to adherens junctions, extend between the filtration slits, closely interact with the actin cytoskeleton, influencing signaling pathways and motility of the podocyte (Lee et al., 2009) (Burt et al., 2007) and thereby establishing the final barrier to urinary protein loss (Somlo and Mundel, 2000).

The proteins which make up the slit diaphragm system are nephrin, Neph1, Neph2, podocin, fatty acid transporter tumor suppressor homolog-1 (FAT1) and FAT2, and the calcium channel transient receptor potential cation 6 (TRPC6) and cadherins (Harita Y, 2008) (Yaoita et al., 2005) (Liu G, 2003) (Dryer SE, 2010) . Linker proteins such as CD2-associated protein (CD2AP), and Nck connect the slit diaphragm to the actin skeleton (Coward et al., 2005) (Jones et al., 2009). Also, proteins that are directly part of the slit diaphragm but are involved in regulating the actin cyskeleton include synaptopodin, the GTPase dynamin and cytoplasmic Cathepsin L (CatL) (Sever S, 2007). Nephrin, a member of the immunoglobulin family, is regarded as the critical structural component of the slit diaphragm of podocytes as it is composed of an extracellular and intracellular domain capable of transducing signals between neighboring podocytes, and is the protein that bridges the distance between interdigitating foot processes (Zhu et al., 2008). Encoded by the NPHSI gene, both humans and experimental mice models lacking nephrin or a mutation in the NPHSI gene are born without typical slit diaphragms and exhibit severe podocyte abnormalities and massive proteinuria in utero and at birth (Kuusniemi et al., 2006). The Src family kinase Fyn, controls the phosphorylation of nephrin and when phosphorylated together with CD2AP and podocin, phosphoinositide-3-OH kinase (PI3K)-dependent Akt activation is induced, which is thought to inhibit podocyte apoptosis (Huber et al., 2003). Phosphorylation of nephrin also promotes Nck-dependent actin rearrangements, indicating an important role for nephrin in preventing foot process effacement (Verma et al. 2006). The transmembrane proteins Neph1 and Neph2 are structurally related to nephrin, containing extracellular IgG-like motifs, and interact with nephrin during intracellular signaling. FAT1 and FAT2, like Neph1 and Neph2, are part of the slit diaphragm but contain cadherin-like repeats (Tryggvason et al., 2006). Podocin is a membrane-associated intracellular protein, and is involved in the organization of the slit diaphragm complex, interacting with both nephrin and CD2AP (Schwarz et al., 2001). CD2AP is linked to nephrin, podocin and the actin cytoskeleton, transducing signals to the actin cytoskeleton. Recently, attention has focused on TRPC6, a calcium channel present in the slit diaphragm complex interacting with both nephrin and podocin, and involved in podocyte mechanosensation and regulation of gene transcription (Moller et al., 2009). Synaptopodin, an actin-binding protein, is present in the foot process and involved in actin elongation through α-actinin-4 by modulating RhoA signaling (Asanuma et al., 2005) (Asanuma et al., 2006). The GTPase dynamin is also involved in actin modulation, and both GTP-bound dynamin and unphosphorylated synaptopodin are direct targets of the proteolytic activity of the cysteine protease Cathepsin L (Reiser et al., 2004). Undoubtedly, an intricate alignment of the slit diaphragm proteins is pivotal for proper filtration and renal function and disruption to the expression or function of these proteins alters the intercellular junctions and cytoskeletal structures of the foot processes and the cell takes on an effaced phenotype, pathologically known as effacement. Thus, foot processes effacement is identified as the hallmark in the development of proteinuric kidney disease (Kwoh et al., 2006) (Perysinaki GS, 2011).

As well as having the role of maintaining glomerular structural and functional integrity, podocytes also play a key role in autocrine signalling. Podocytes are essential suppliers of

vascular endothelial growth factor A (VEGF-A) to the glomerular capillary endothelium and with glomerular endothelial cells, they are among the few cell types where VEGF-A is expressed throughout life (Tufro et al., 1999) (Simon et al., 1995). In addition, injured podocytes have been reported to upregulate expression of the transmembrane protein B7-1 (or CD80) on their surface, normally expressed on B cells and other antigen-presenting cells (Reiser J, 2004). To illustrate, in response to B7-1 activation due to binding of LPS to toll-like receptor-4 (TLR4), the podocyte slit diaphragm is rearranged leading to proteinuria, a response not seen in B7-1 knockout mice (Reiser J, 2004), suggesting that the podocyte is part of the innate immune system and has a role in danger signaling (Reiser J, 2004) (D'Agati, 2008).
Clearly, the podocyte is a highly complex cell involved in maintaining normal capillary health, other glomerular cells and structures as well as being a gateway for the perm-selectivity of the glomerular filtrate. Given the terminally differentiated nature of podocytes, loss of these cells cannot be compensated by regenerative proliferation. Thus an intricate alignment of the slit diaphragm proteins is pivotal for proper filtration and renal function. Hence, podocytes are key contributors to glomerular disease and understanding the cellular mechanisms governing their response to injury is imperative to the development of therapeutic strategies to directly protect podocytes in disease situations from advancing to kidney sclerosis.

2. Role of podocytes in glomerular disease

Glomerular diseases (including diabetic kidney disease) are the most common cause of end-stage kidney failure throughout the world. They comprise a variety of heterogenous disorders that are due to acute or chronic injury of the renal glomeruli. Whether they are a primary disease process or a secondary manifestation of a systemic disease process, the working paradigm is that they all converge onto few pathways of disease progression.
Over the last decade, immense knowledge has emerged implicating podocytes as key players in a broad range of glomerular diseases. Injury to the podocytes is the initiating cause of many renal diseases, leading to proteinuria with possible progression to end-stage renal disease (Leeuwis et al., 2010). Human podocytopathies include focal and segmental glomerular sclerosis (FSGS), minimal change disease, membranous nephropathy, collapsing glomerulopathy and diabetic nephropathy and more recently podocytes have also been in implicated in proliferative forms of GN such as crescentic glomerulonephritis (Thorner et al., 2008) (Moeller et al., 2004) . The filtration barrier is the major pathogenic site in almost all glomerular diseases and its study is therefore of clinical significance. When podocytes are injured, as in many forms of glomerulonephritides, the podocytes respond by retracting their foot processes into their cell bodies to form flattened dense epithelium, morphologically designated foot process effacement (Harita et al., 2006) (Mundel and Shankland, 2002). These podocytic changes lead to precipitous protein leakage into the urine, which over a chronic period of time culiminates in the development of glomerulosclerosis and end-stage kidney failure (Smoyer and Mundel, 1998). Thus, the intrinsic defect in the cytoskeletal proteins renders podocytes non-functional as the actin cytoskeletal organisation changes from parallel contractile bundles into a dense network, culminating in foot processes effacement, subsequent proteinuria and sclerosis.
Podocyte contribution is essential to the formation of glomerular crescent as they populate cellular crescents in human and experimental models of CGN (Thorner et al., 2008) (Bariety et al., 2005) (Moeller et al., 2004) (Le Hir et al., 2001). So far, the earliest documentation of

podocyte response to injury in a model of crescentic glomerulonephritis is from the ultrastructural studies conducted by Le Hir et al., 2001, whereby podocytes formed bridges glomerular tuft area and Bowman's capsule in mice ten days injection with rabbit anti-GBM serum (Le Hir et al., 2001). These findings were the first to provide a link between the initial inflammatory injury processes occurring within the endocapillary compartment of the glomerular tuft and the formation of a multilayered cellular crescent in bowman's space (Le Hir et al., 2001). What causes these presumably terminally differentiated visceral cells to acquire a phenotype favourable for cytoskeletal reorganisation leading to contact with the parietal basement membrane of Bowman's capsule, culminating in the formation of podocyte bridges is yet to be explored.

3. The mammalian target of rapamycin complex signal transduction pathway

The coordinated control of cell growth to produce a genetically predetermined cell size, shape, survival and proliferation is greatly influenced by a ubiquitously expressed serine/threonine kinase known as the mammalian target of rapamycin (mTOR). mTOR functions to regulate a variety of cellular activites that are sensitive to environmental stress (Foster, 2007) (Sabatini, 2006). Our current understanding of mTOR dates back to the initial discoverers of its inhibitor, Rapamycin, about three decades ago on the Southern Pacific Ocean island named Easter Island, known as "Rapa Nui" by the language of its native Polynesian inhabitants (Yang and Guan, 2007). The bacterial strain, Streptomyces hygroscopicus, which was first isolated from this island secrete a potent anti-fungal macrolide that was named rapamycin after the location of its discovery (Yang and Guan, 2007). Rapamycin was initially developed as an anti-fungal agent (Loewith, 2011). However, its major application quickly developed after rapamycin was proven to have immunosuppressive and anti-proliferative properties (Yang and Guan 2007). To date, rapamycin (or sirolimus) has become routinely used clinically for immunosuppression in organ transplantation, prevention of restenosis post-angioplasty, and chemotherapy in a variety of cancers (Dobashi et al., 2009) (Yang and Guan, 2007).
mTORC1 Signaling pathway: mTOR is the downstream effector protein belonging to the phosphatidylinositol (PIKK)-related kinase family with a predicted molecular weight of 290kDa, and is part of the PI-3 Kinase pathway which is part of the tyrosine kinase activation cascade (Vogt, 2001). The physiological importance of the primordial mTOR is undoubtedly demonstrated by the fact that the knockout of mTOR in mice is embryonically lethal (Gangloff et al., 2004) (Murakami M, 2004). In mammalian cells, mTOR signaling consist of two distinct multiprotein complexes named mTOR Complex-1 (TOR-raptor-GβL) and mTOR Complex-2 (TOR-rictor-GβL), and each complex is evolutionarily conserved from yeast to mammalian eukaryotes with distinct and essential roles in maintenance of cell function and structure (Loewith R, 2002). It is now well established that the raptor-containing mTOR complex (mTORC1) is rapamycin-sensitive (Sabatini et al., 1994), whereas the rictor-containing mTOR complex (mTORC2) is rapamycin-insensitive (Sarbassov et al., 2006). In contrast to mTORC1, mTORC2 regulates growth factor signalling, cell survival (AKT) and cytoskeletal reorganization (Facchinetti et al., 2008) (Bhaskar PT, 2007) (Jacinto et al., 2004). However, as much of our current understanding of mTOR is limited to mTORC1, because of the availability and wide use of rapamycin. The factors promoting mTORC2 activation are not well defined and may be controlled by the activation states of multiple mTORC1 effector proteins (Gossage L, 2010).

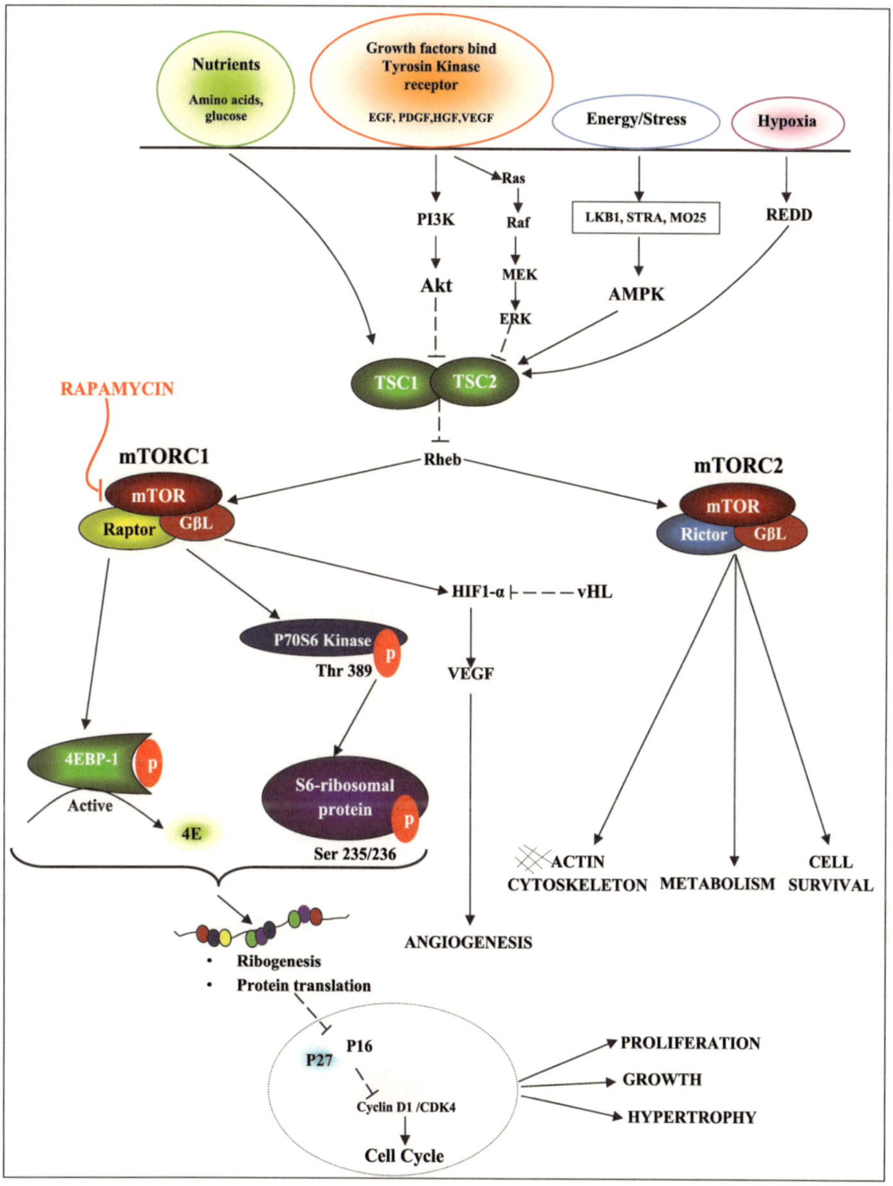

Fig. 1. **Mammalian target of rapamycin (mTOR) signaling pathway.** mTOR incorporates growth factor activation from the tyrosine receptor kinase to control several catabolic and anabolic processes that collectively determine cell growth and metabolism. mTOR is an atypical serine/threonine kinases. In response to growth factors, Akt phosphorylates and inactivates TSC1-TSC2, allowing Rheb to activate mTOR. Low energy (cellular energy status) inhibits mTORC by activating AMPK, which phosphorylates and activates TSC1-TSC2. mTOR controls protein synthesis by phosphorylating and inactivating the translational inhibitor 4EBP-1 and by phosphorylating and activating P70S6 kinase. mTORC2 promotes cell survival through direct phosphorylation of serine 473 in the hydrophobic motif of AKT. The immunosuppressant rapamycin in complex with FKBP inhibits mTOR when bound to raptor.

Activities of mTORC1: The mTORC1 arm of mTOR signaling pathway promotes cell cycle progression through G_1-phase and proliferation through multiple molecular mechanisms. mTORC1 signaling functions via the two earliest recognized and best-characterised downstream effector proteins namely, SK1 (p70 ribosomal protein S6 kinase 1) and eukaryotic initiation factor (eIF) 4E-binding protein 1 (4EBP1) that are involved in the regulated control of protein synthesis/ribosome biogenesis and cap-dependent translation initiation (Yang and Guan 2007). The pathway is activated as follows: Firstly, mTOR incorporates growth factor activation from the tyrosine kinase receptor to activate AKT via phosphorylation at the threonine-308 residue site, which results in phosphorylation and subsequent inactivation of the endogenous mTOR complexes inhibitors, the tuberous sclerosis complexes-1 and 2 (TSC1-TSC2). Upon phosphorylation of TSC1-TSC2 heterodimer, Rheb is released which positively regulates mTORC1 for activation via phosphorylation at the serine 2448 site (Yang and Guan 2007). The activation of mTORC1 results in increased protein synthesis by phosphorylating and inactivating the translational inhibitor 4E-BP and by phosphorylating and activating S6 kinase (S6K). S6K, in addition to phosphorylating various translational targets. It also phosphorylates and inhibits insulin receptor substrate 1 (IRS-1) as part of a negative feedback loop that attenuates insulin signaling. mTORC2 promotes cell survival through direct phosphorylation of serine 473 in the hydrophobic motif of AKT. The immunosuppressant rapamycin in complex with FKBP binds and inhibits mTOR when bound to raptor. Activation of the protein kinase p70 S6 kinase ($p70^{S6k}$) and subsequent phosphorylation of 40S subunit of the S6 ribosomal protein regulates the translation of ribosome proteins and components of the translational machinery. mTORC1 also phosphorylates 4E-BP1, which releases it from the translation factor, eIF-4E, and allows the latter to initiate translation of messenger RNAs. TORC1 also regulates proliferation through modulation of cell cycle regulatory proteins, involving the cyclin D1/E-cyclin-dependent kinase (Cdk)-2/4-retinoblastoma pathway (Berthet and Kaldis, 2007). In particular, eIF4E regulates the translation of the Cyclin D1 and D3 genes, which leads to reduced formation of cyclinD3-cdk4 kinase (Hleb M, 2004). TORC1 activation is correlated with the protein expression of cdk2 (Chen et al., 2009) and also increases the expression of $p27^{kip1}$ (the endogenous inhibitor of cdks 2 and 4), through undefined mechanisms (Sun et al., 2008) (Wang et al., 2001). mTORC1 is also a negative regulator of autophagy (one of the major systems which regulate cellular protein degradation) (Meijer and Codogno, 2004).

The earliest recognized and best-studied mTORC1 downstream effector proteins are SK1 (p70 ribosomal protein S6 kinase 1) and eukaryotic initiation factor (eIF) 4E-binding protein 1 (4EBP1). Under basal conditions, S6KI and 4EBP1 are bound to eIF3 and remain inactive (Holz MK, 2005) mTOR-dependent phosphorylation of 4EBP1 releases eIF4E, initiating cap-dependent de novo translation of various species of mRNA (Brunn et al., 1997 and Gingras et al., 2004). Another set of downstream effectors of mTOR are the serine/threonine protein kinases, S6 kinase 1 (S6K1) and S6 kinase 2 (S6K2), both of which are responsible for phosphorylation of the 40S ribosomal protein S6 (rpS6) (Murakami et al., 2004, Sarbassov et al., 2004 and Shima et al., 1998). mTOR activation of S6K results in phosphorylation of S6 ribosomal protein, leading to recruitment of the 40S ribosome subunit and translation of 5'-terminal oligopyrimidine tract (5'TOP) mRNA (Jefferies et al., 1997). These 5'TOP mRNA encode primarily ribosomal proteins and other components of the translational apparatus (Meyuhas et al., 2000). Thus, by controlling S6K activity, mTOR also regulates the abundance of translational machinery. Under favorable growth conditions, mTOR is activated and S6K and 4E-BP1 are phosphorylated, leading to new RNA and protein synthesis. Proliferation of intrinsic glomerular cells, characterized by increased RNA and protein synthesis with DNA replication and cell division is fundamental in crescent formation in crescentic glomerulonephritis. It may well be that mTOR plays a critical role in this disease process. Thus, the judicious attenuation of proliferation with mTOR inhibitors may potentially provide an option to limiting the progression of renal injury from progressing to crescentic glomerulonephritis.

4. Implication of mTOR signaling in renal disease

The availability of the mTOR inhibitor ($mTOR_i$) rapamycin, which is used clinically as an immunosuppressant drug to prevent rejection in organ transplantation, has helped to identify a large signaling network around mTOR signaling leading to extensive studies for its effect on cell proliferation and apoptosis not just in cancer but in both human and experimental in vivo and in vitro models of glomerular disease. Nevertheless, whilst some studies suggest mTOR inhibition by rapamycin might halt or reverse glomerulopathies (Mori H, 2009) (Inoki, 2008) (Lloberas et al., 2006) (Sakaguchi et al., 2006) (Rangan and Coombes, 2007) other studies documented an increase in proteinuria and glomerulosclerosis in patients and in animal models following rapamycin treatment (Torras J, 2009) (Amer and Cosio, 2009) (Munivenkatappa et al., 2010) (Letavernier et al., 2007), suggesting a significance for mTORC1 signaling in endogenous and compensatory regenerative repair of renal cells in glomerulopathies. To add, most studies regarding the role of mTOR signaling in renal disease are based on pharmacological intervention with rapamycin (and as mTORC1 is expressed in resident as well as infiltrating cells) this approach does not allow for distinguishing the specific role of blocking mTORC1 in intrinsic renal cells. Furthermore, off-target effects have been described with long-standing application of rapamycin, most notably the inhibition of mTORC2 (Sarbassov et al., 2006). Therefore, tissue-specific analysis of mTOR signaling is required for an in-depth understanding of the functional and cell autonomous role of mTOR in diabetic nephropathy and other glomerular diseases.

5. Role of TORC1 in normal podocyte biology

The mTOR signalling pathway has emerged as having an important role in maintaining podocyte survival and cytoskeletal structure. Recently, elegant studies by Godel et al. and Inoki et al., conducted in conditional knockout mice, have comprehensively verified the critical role that TORC1 plays in maintaining normal podocyte function and glomerular architecture. Godel et al. showed that podocyte-specific deletion of TORC1 ($Raptor^{flox/flox}$) in conditional knockout mice caused heavy proteinuria at 8 weeks of age, associated with development of segmental glomerulsclerosis (particulary in juxtamedullary glomeruli), reduced expression of slit diaphragm proteins (nephrin, podocin and Par3), foot process effacement and increased mortality after 8 months of age. The dependence of normal podocyte biology on TORC1 was also determined by genetic background (with conditional TORC1 deletion in ICR mice being more prone to proteinuria than those from a C57BL/6 background) as well as age (suppression of TORC1 was more resistant in causing proteinuria in adult mice). Godel and co-authors also demonstrated that the combined inactivation of TORC1 and TORC2 (using $Raptor/Rictor^{podocyte}$ conditional mice) caused a rapid onset of nephrotic syndrome, FSGS, renal failure and death by 8 weeks of age.

Using an alternative approach, Inoki et al. examined the effects of over-activation of TORC1 in podocytes using podocyte-specific deletion of TSC1 (a negative regulator of TORC1 activation). These studies showed that high TORC1 activation led to mesangial expansion and glomerulosclerosis, proteinuria, podocyte body enlargement and foot process effacement and a reduction in podocyte number (partly due to reduced podocyte attachment) and death due to renal failure by 14 weeks. The molecular and cellular changes underlying these morphological changes included mislocalization of nephrin, cellular dedifferentiation and conversion to a fibroblastic phenotype (as determined by increased expression of desmin and redistribution of zonula occluden-1) and promoted endoplasmic reticulum stress. These effects were rapamycin-sensitive and reversible if attenuated at an early stage, but not after prolonged over-activation. Taken together, the studies by Godel et al. and Inoki et al. highlight that glomerular TORC1 activity in podocytes must kept under low finely regulated levels, with both complete suppression as well as over-expression of TORC1 having deleterious effects on podocyte structure and function.

The molecular mechanisms by which TORC1 regulates normal podocyte function is not yet fully understood. Previous in vitro studies investigating the effects of TORC1 inhibition with sirolimus in cultured podocytes have shown that the TORC1 regulates at least three physiological functions which are essential for normal podocyte surivial as well as functioning of the glomerular filtration barrier: (i) podocytes produce VEGF (an important angiogenic peptide that maintains the normal integrity of the glomerular-endothelial barrier (Eremina, Baelde, & Quaggin, 2007), in a TORC1 dependent manner; (ii) TORC1 may regulate pro-survival pathways in podocytes. At present, there is only indirect evidence to support this hypothesis. Nephrin and CD2-associated protein (CD2AP) constitutively regulate PI3K and Akt, both of which are upstream of TORC1 (Huber et al., 2003). Nephrin is a transmembrane protein expressed in podocytes and is linked to the cytoskeleton by CD2AP (Pavenstadt, Kriz, & Kretzler, 2003). Both are critical factors that maintain the normal function of the slit diaphragm of the podocytes and the glomerular filtration barrier (Pavenstadt et al., 2003). Given that mutations in the genes encoding nephrin or CD2AP lead to FSGS, these studies raise the possibility that their downstream pathways involve TORC1 (Kwoh, Shannon, Miner, & Shaw, 2006). This postulate has recently been confirmed in two studies showing that sirolimus reduced Akt phosphorylation in cultured podocytes (Letavernier et al., 2008; Vollenbroeker et al., 2008). Akt is a cytoplasmic serine/threonine kinase that regulates programmed cell death by phosphorylating substrates that regulate apoptosis (such as caspase-9, XIAP, MM2); (iii) Lastly, sirolimus altered the cytoskeletal structure of podocytes in vitro. The latter may be due to inhibitory effects on Akt, TORC2 and Wt1(Letavernier et al., 2008; Vollenbroeker et al., 2008). In vitro, podocytes exposed to sirolimus (20 ng/ml) for 48 hours developed a more roundshaped morphology with reorganization of cytoskeleton and redistribution of actin filaments and focal adhesion proteins (viniculin) to the periphery of the cell (Letavernier et al., 2008; Vollenbroeker et al., 2008). These effects may lead to reduced cell adhesion and migration (Vollenbroeker et al., 2008).

6. Role of TORC1 in podocytes in human and animal models of glomerular disease

Glomerular diseases can be classified according to changes in podocyte number and differentiation, as proposed by Shankland and colleagues (Griffin et al. 2003)(Figure 2). Podocyte number is normal or decreased in minimal change disease, focal segmental glomerulosclerosis and diabetic kidney disease, whereas it is increased with an dedifferentiated phenotype in HIV nephropathy, collapsing variant of focal segmental glomerulosclerosis and crescentic glomerulonephritis. Loss of Podocytes (due to cell death and detachment from the glomerular basement membrane) is a key determinant of progression to kidney failure, regardless of the cause. Our knowledge about the role of TORC1 in podocytes in glomerular disease is incomplete and is summarised and discussed below.

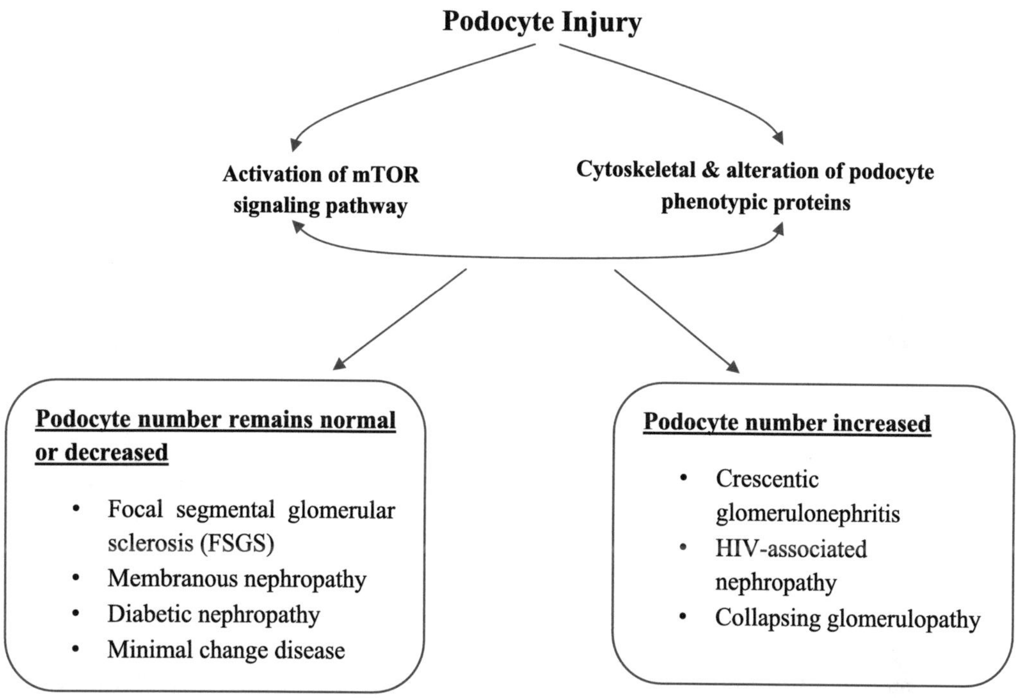

Fig. 2. Classification of glomerular diseases according to changes in podocyte number and differentiation, as proposed by Shankland and colleagues (Griffin et al. 2006).

6.1 Glomerular diseases in which podocyte number decreased or normal

Minimal change disease/focal segmental glomerulosclerosis. Several studies have examined the effects of sirolimus in animal models of glomerular diseases associated with heavy proteinuria and reduced or normal podocyte number. These models resemble the human counterparts of FSGS and minimal change disease. Both everolimus and sirolimus were renoprotective when administered during the early stages of non-immune FSGS induced by either puromycin (Daniel et al., 2000) or adriamycin (Rangan and Coombes, 2007) in rats. In adriamycin nephropathy, commencement of sirolimus during the established, but early phase of disease (day 14 to 49), attenuated the increase in kidney weight, glomerular capillary tuft enlargement, glomerulosclerosis and tubulointerstitial fibrosis as well as renal cortical TGF-β (Rangan and Coombes, 2007), whereas interstitial inflammation and peritubular myofibroblast accumulation were unaffected. Interestingly, the examination of sirolimus on proteinuria and subsequent podocyte damage in two contrasting renal disease models, with clearly different pathophysiological mechanisms (a glomerular toxicoimmunological model induced by puromycin aminonucleoside, and a chronic hyperfiltration and inflammatory model by mass reduction), both treated with a fixed high sirolimus dose revealed, significant increases in proteinuria, together with a significant fall in podocin immunofluorescence, as well as clear additional damage to podocyte foot processes (Torras et al., 2009). Conversely, after mass reduction, rapamycin produced lower levels of proteinuria and amelioration of inflammatory and pro-fibrotic damage. In contrast to the puromycin model, higher glomerular podocin and nephrin expression and amelioration of glomerular ultrastructural damage were found (Torras et al., 2009). Thus these studies suggest sirolimus has dual opposing effects, with proteinuria and podocyte damage aggravation in the glomerular model and a nephro-protective effect in the chronic inflammatory tubulointerstitial model. To add, sirolimus has also been reported to damage podocytes in rats with protein overload nephropathy (Cia et al., 2011). Collectively these findings indicate that sirolimus produces slight alterations in podocyte structure when acting on healthy podocytes, but it clearly worsens those podocytes damaged by other concomitant injury.

In humans with FSGS, the role of TORC1 in podocytes in disease pathogenesis has not been directly evaluated. Clinical trial evidence however suggests that TORC1 has a dichotomous role (congruent with data from TORC1-conditional knockout mice) indicating that its role in disease is finely balanced. (Pollak, 2008, Fervenza et al., 2004, Tumlin et al., 2006, Cho et al., 2007, Aymanns et al., 2006). In a prospective open label trial, conducted by Tumlin and colleagues (Tumlin et al., 2006), sirolimus induced complete remission (defined as <300mg protein/24h after 6 months) in 4 of the 21 patients, and partial remission (defined as a 50% reduction of baseline proteinuria) in 8 of the 21 patients tested within the 6 month period. Twelve of the responsive patients, along with 2 others who saw a 30% reduction in proteinuria continued sirolimus therapy for another 6 months. In these patients, baseline proteinuria fell significantly within the first 6 months, however this decline in proteinuria became statistically insignificant from the period of 6 months to 12 months. Overall, the study found that sirolimus was able to stabilize the renal function of patients with FSGS, by not only reducing proteinuria, but also glomerular pore size and increasing glomerular ultrafiltration coefficient (Fervenza et al., 2004). On the other hand, Patel and colleagues (Patel et al., 2005) reported that a combination of tacrolimus with sirolimus was beneficial in reducing proteinuria and inducing remission in a patient with a long history of refractory minimal change nephropathy. In contrast, other smaller pilot studies in humans highlighted the possible nephrotoxic effects of sirolimus in patients with FSGS (Tumlin et al., 2006, Cho et al., 2007). A common observation amongst all the studies was that a longer duration of disease was associated with resistance to sirolimus therapy and a risk for renal dysfunction. Therefore, genetic factors, stage of disease and level of TORC1 inhibition may be factors underlying these variable results in humans.

Membranous nephropathy. The effects of sirolimus have been examined in both the passive and active Heymann nephritis model of membranous nephropathy (Cavallo, 1994), but the specific effects on podocytes has not been assessed. In a nephrectomized model of passive Heyman nephritis, sirolimus reduced the expression of pro-inflammatory and pro-fibrotic genes, tubulointerstitial inflammation and fibrosis as well as compensatory renal hypertrophy (Bonegio et al., 2005). In the active model, sirolimus exhibited protective effects during both the induction as well as the chronic phases (Naumovic et al., 2007). The efficacy of sirolimus in human membranous nephropathy is currently being evaluated in an NIH-sponsored clinical trial.

Diabetic kidney disease. Sirolimus is known to prevent the development of diabetes in non-obese diabetic mouse, which is an autoimmune model of insulin-dependent diabetes, presumably due to immunomodulatory effects (Baeder et al., 1992). In the kidney, the expression of mTORC1 is upregulated in animals with diabetes, possibly through an AMPK-dependent manner (Lee et al., 2007). In addition, several groups have investigated the role of sirolimus and mTORC1 in mediating renal injury associated with diabetes. These studies showed that sirolimus reduced renal hypertrophy associated with hyperglycaemia and that it also has some anti-inflammatory and anti-fibrotic effects (Yang et al., 2007, Sataranatarajan et al., 2007, Lee et al., 2007, Sakaguchi et al., 2006, Lloberas et al., 2006, Nagai et al., 2005). For example, the treatment of rats with streptozotocin (STZ)-induced diabetes with sirolimus from week 16 to 20 reduced albuminuria, phosphorylated Akt and mTORC1 expression and growth factor expression of TGF-β1 (Lloberas et al., 2006). These effects were comparable to diabetic animals treated with insulin (Lloberas et al., 2006). Sirolimus had similar effects in db/db mice with diabetes (Sataranatarajan et al., 2007). The effects of sirolimus in human diabetic nephropathy have not been directly evaluated. However, Senior and colleagues reported in a retrospective case series, 3 out 62 clinical islet transplant recipients developed proteinuria when converted from CNI-based regimen to a CNI-free/sirolimus-based treatment (Senior et al., 2005). At least two of the three patients had underlying established diabetic nephropathy, which progressed following islet transplantation. Another five patients developed microalbuminuria. The proteinuria improved with increased doses of CNI, suggesting that the mechanisms of proteinuria may be similar to that described for patients with chronic allograft nephropathy (CAN) (i.e. partly due to CNI withdrawal) (Senior et al., 2005).

Chronic kidney disease. In the remnant kidney model in rats and mice, 5/6th of the kidneys are removed either by nephrectomy or infarction through the selective ligation of the renal arteries. This model recapitulates some of the features associated with chronic kidney progression in humans. In this model, divergent effects of mTOR inhibitors have been observed, but this may depend on the timing of their administration, similar to what was observed in the glomerular disease models described earlier (Diekmann et al., 2007, Vogelbacher et al., 2007). For example, Vogelbacher and co-workers found that starting everolimus three days after induction of the model, suppressed glomerular endothelial and mesangial cell proliferation, and worsened structural renal injury and proteinuria (Vogelbacher et al., 2007). In contrast, when sirolimus was started at week 6, it improved proteinuria, fibrosis and inflammation (Diekmann et al., 2007). Sirolimus attenuated glomerular VEGF production in both studies and paradoxically increased serum levels of VEGF (Diekmann et al., 2007).

6.2 Glomerular diseases in which podocyte number increased

Crescentic glomerulonephritis. mTORC1 may mediate both the immunopathogenesis as well as the local glomerular cell proliferation that occurs in crescentic glomerulonephritis. For example, in mice the overexpression of HIF-1α (Ding et al., 2006). Two recent studies have evaluated the effects of sirolimus in murine models of crescentic glomerulonephritis. In mice, prophylactic treatment with sirolimus, 5 days prior to disease induction, decreased the proliferation of inflammatory cells and autologous antibody production, but did not alter the lymph node expression of CD4+CD25-FoxP3 regulatory cells was detected (Hochegger et al., 2008). In contrast, when sirolimus was commenced on day 14 of established disease, deleterious effects occurred, including an increase in proteinuria and worsening of inflammatory cell infiltration (Hochegger et al., 2008). In rats with crescentic glomerulonephritis induced by nephrotoxic serum, treatment with sirolimus during the early stage (1 day after immunization) reduced glomerular cell proliferation, tubulointerstitial damage and fibrinoid necrosis, as well as increasing urine volume and preventing the decline in renal function (Succar et al., 2007). Of note, the degree of histopathological protection following sirolimus treatment was much greater in the tubulointerstitial compartment than in the glomerulus, and was associated with reductions in both the glomerular and tubulointerstitial phosphorylation of the S6 ribosomal protein (Succar et al., 2007).

HIV-nephropathy. The most common, or "classical", type of HIV-associated nephropathy (HIVAN) is a collapsing FSGS, though other forms of kidney disease may also occur with HIV (Medapalli, 2011) (Kimmel et al., 2003). Both glomerular and tubular lesions are characterized by a proliferative phenotype in HIVAN, and mTORC1 pathway was been implicated to contribute to the development of the HIVAN phenotype, as demonstrated in Kumar et al., 2010, whereby, renal tissues of transgenic mice showed enhanced phosphorylation of p70S6 kinase, 4EBP1 and eIF4B, HIF1-α, VEGF and an associated diminished phosphorylation of eEF2 (Kumar D, 2010). Here transgenic mice receiving rapamycin not only showed inhibition of the mTOR-associated downstream signaling but also displayed attenuated renal lesions suggesting that the mTOR pathway contributes to the HIVAN phenotype and that inhibition of the mTOR pathway can be used as a therapeutic strategy to alter the course of HIVAN (Kumar D, 2010).

7. Therapeutic implications of targeting TORC1 in podocytes in therapy of human glomerular diseases

The foregoing data clearly support that the TORC pathway has an important role in the pathogenesis of glomerular disease. However, our knowledge in human disease is in its infancy and there remain several significant challenges in translating the known role of TORC in podocytes to the therapy of human glomerular disease. Firstly, further studies are needed to confirm the expression and functional role of TORC in human disease. Biopsy studies of the localization of TORC pathway in glomerular disease are essential. Furthermore, serial assessment of biomarkers indication TORC activity will allow the level of expression to be determined according to stage of disease. Such assessment may include the expression of TORC in podocytes of the urine. Second, further refinements in the way in which TORC is modulated in vivo are required. This may require evaluation of low-dose sirolimus in conjunction with assessment of biomarkers that modulate the bioactivity of TORC; the development of more specific drug-inhibitors that target the TORC pathway as well as more specific methods of drug-delivery that target the podocyte. In essence, further data in humans is currently lacking and currently essential for furthering the role of TORC modulation in podocytes.

8. Summary and conclusions

Podocytes form the final barrier to protein loss, which explains why podocyte injury is typically associated with marked proteinuria. Indeed, all forms of glomerular disease are characterized by some degree of podocyte abnormality. Recent advancement in the understanding of the role of mTOR signalling pathway have emphasized the important role this key cell signalling transduction pathway plays in podocyte function both in normal and disease conditions. However, much more work is still needed to understand how mTOR signalling in podocytes can be modulated to allow the effective therapy of human glomerular disease.

9. References

Akilesh S, H. T., Wu H, Wang G, Hartleben B, Kopp JB, Miner JH, Roopenian DC, Unanue ER, Shaw AS 2008. Podocytes use FcRn to clear IgG from the glomerular basement membrane. *Proc Natl Acad Sci USA,* 105, 967-972.

Amer, H. & Cosio, F. G. 2009. Significance and management of proteinuria in kidney transplant recipients. *J Am Soc Nephrol,* 20, 2490-2.

Asanuma, K., Kim, K., Oh, J., Giardino, L., Chabanis, S., Faul, C., Reiser, J. & Mundel, P. 2005. Synaptopodin regulates the actin-bundling activity of alpha-actinin in an isoform-specific manner. *J Clin Invest,* 115, 1188-98.

Asanuma, K., Yanagida-Asanuma, E., Faul, C., Tomino, Y., Kim, K. & Mundel, P. 2006. Synaptopodin orchestrates actin organization and cell motility via regulation of RhoA signalling. *Nat Cell Biol,* 8, 485-91.

Aymanns, C., Voehringer, M., Rasche, F. M. & Keller, F. 2006. Effects of sirolimus on proteinuria and renal function in focal segmental glomerulonephritis. *Int J Clin Pharmacol Ther,* 44, 675-6.

Baeder, W. L., Sredy, J., Sehgal, S. N., Chang, J. Y. & Adams, L. M. 1992. Rapamycin prevents the onset of insulin-dependent diabetes mellitus (IDDM) in NOD mice. *Clin Exp Immunol,* 89, 174-8.

Bariety, J., Bruneval, P., Meyrier, A., Mandet, C., Hill, G. & Jacquot, C. 2005. Podocyte involvement in human immune crescentic glomerulonephritis. *Kidney Int,* 68, 1109-19.

Benzing, T. 2004. Signaling at the slit diaphragm. *J Am Soc Nephrol,* 15, 1382-1391.

Berthet, C. & Kaldis, P. 2007. Cell-specific responses to loss of cyclin-dependent kinases. *Oncogene,* 26, 4469-77.

Bhaskar PT, H. N. 2007. The two TORCs and Akt. *Dev Cell,* 12, 487-502.

Bonegio, R. G., Fuhro, R., Wang, Z., Valeri, C. R., Andry, C., Salant, D. J. & Lieberthal, W. 2005. Rapamycin ameliorates proteinuria-associated tubulointerstitial inflammation and fibrosis in experimental membranous nephropathy. *J Am Soc Nephrol,* 16, 2063-72.

Burt, D., Salvidio, G., Tarabra, E., Barutta, F., Pinach, S., Dentelli, P., Camussi, G., Perin, P. C. & Gruden, G. 2007. The monocyte chemoattractant protein-1/cognate CC chemokine receptor 2 system affects cell motility in cultured human podocytes. *Am J Pathol,* 171, 1789-99.

Cavallo, T. 1994. Membranous nephropathy. Insights from Heymann nephritis. *Am J Pathol,* 144, 651-8.

Chen, S. J., Nakahara, T., Takahara, M., Kido, M., Dugu, L., Uchi, H., Takeuchi, S., Tu, Y. T., Moroi, Y. & Furue, M. 2009. Activation of the mammalian target of rapamycin signalling pathway in epidermal tumours and its correlation with cyclin-dependent kinase 2. *Br J Dermatol,* 160, 442-5.

Cho, M. E., Hurley, J. K. & Kopp, J. B. 2007. Sirolimus therapy of focal segmental glomerulosclerosis is associated with nephrotoxicity. *Am J Kidney Dis,* 49, 310-7.

Coward, R. J., Foster, R. R., Patton, D., Ni, L., Lennon, R., Bates, D. O., Harper, S. J., Mathieson, P. W. & Saleem, M. A. 2005. Nephrotic plasma alters slit diaphragm-dependent signaling and translocates nephrin, Podocin, and CD2 associated protein in cultured human podocytes. *J Am Soc Nephrol,* 16, 629-37.

D'agati, V. D. 2008. Podocyte injury in focal segmental glomerulosclerosis: Lessons from animal models (a play in five acts). *Kidney Int,* 73, 399-406.

Daniel, C., Ziswiler, R., Frey, B., Pfister, M. & Marti, H. P. 2000. Proinflammatory effects in experimental mesangial proliferative glomerulonephritis of the immunosuppressive agent SDZ RAD, a rapamycin derivative. *Exp Nephrol,* 8, 52-62.

Diekmann, F., Rovira, J., Carreras, J., Arellano, E. M., Banon-Maneus, E., Ramirez-Bajo, M. J., Gutierrez-Dalmau, A., Brunet, M. & Campistol, J. M. 2007. Mammalian target of rapamycin inhibition halts the progression of proteinuria in a rat model of reduced renal mass. *J Am Soc Nephrol,* 18, 2653-60.

Ding, M., Cui, S., Li, C., Jothy, S., Haase, V., Steer, B. M., Marsden, P. A., Pippin, J., Shankland, S., Rastaldi, M. P., Cohen, C. D., Kretzler, M. & Quaggin, S. E. 2006. Loss of the tumor suppressor Vhlh leads to upregulation of Cxcr4 and rapidly progressive glomerulonephritis in mice. *Nat Med,* 12, 1081-7.

Dobashi, Y., Suzuki, S., Sato, E., Hamada, Y., Yanagawa, T. & Ooi, A. 2009. EGFR-dependent and independent activation of Akt/mTOR cascade in bone and soft tissue tumors. *Mod Pathol,* 22, 1328-40.

Dryer SE, R. J. 2010. TRPC6 channels and their binding partners in podocytes: role in glomerular filtration and pathophysiology. Review. *Am J Physiol Renal Physiol* 299, 689-701

Eremina, V. & Quaggin, S. E. 2004. The role of VEGF-A in glomerular development and function. *Curr Opin Nephrol Hypertens,* 13, 9-15.

Eyre J, I. K., Grubb BD, Saleem MA, Mathieson PW, Brunskill NJ, Christensen EI, Topham PS 2007. Statin-sensitive endocytosis of albumin by glomerular podocytes. *Am J Physiol Renal Physiol,* 292, 674-681

Facchinetti, V., Ouyang, W., Wei, H., Soto, N., Lazorchak, A., Gould, C., Lowry, C., Newton, A. C., Mao, Y., Miao, R. Q., Sessa, W. C., Qin, J., Zhang, P., SU, B. & Jacinto, E. 2008. The mammalian target of rapamycin complex 2 controls folding and stability of Akt and protein kinase C. *Embo J,* 27, 1932-43.

Faul, C., Asanuma, K., Yanagida-Asanuma, E., Kim, K. & Mundel, P. 2007. Actin up: regulation of podocyte structure and function by components of the actin cytoskeleton. *Trends Cell Biol,* 17, 428-37.

Fervenza, F. C., Fitzpatrick, P. M., Mertz, J., Erickson, S. B., Liggett, S., Popham, S., Wochos, D. N., Synhavsky, A., Hippler, S., Larson, T. S., Bagniewski, S. M. & Velosa, J. A. 2004. Acute rapamycin nephrotoxicity in native kidneys of patients with chronic glomerulopathies. *Nephrol Dial Transplant,* 19, 1288-92.

Foster, D. A. 2007. Regulation of mTOR by phosphatidic acid? *Cancer Res,* 67, 1-4.

Gangloff, Y. G., Mueller, M., Dann, S. G., Svoboda, P., Sticker, M., Spetz, J. F., Um, S. H., Brown, E. J., Cereghini, S., Thomas, G. & Kozma, S. C. 2004. Disruption of the mouse mTOR gene leads to early postimplantation lethality and prohibits embryonic stem cell development. *Mol Cell Biol,* 24, 9508-16.

Gossage L, E. T. 2010. Targeting multiple kinase pathways: a change in paradigm. *Clin Cancer Res,* 16, 1973-1978.

Griffin, S. V., Petermann, A. T., Durvasula, R. V. & Shankland, S. J. 2003. Podocyte proliferation and differentiation in glomerular disease: role of cell-cycle regulatory proteins. *Nephrol Dial Transplant,* 18 Suppl 6, vi8-13.

Guan, F., Villegas, G., Teichman, J., Mundel, P. & Tufro, A. 2006. Autocrine VEGF-A system in podocytes regulates podocin and its interaction with CD2AP. *Am J Physiol Renal Physiol,* 291, F422-8.

Harita Y, K. H., Kosako H, Tezuka T, Sekine T, Igarashi T, Hattori S 2008. Neph1, a component of the kidney slit diaphragm, is tyrosine-phosphorylated by the Src family tyrosine kinase and modulates intracellular signaling by binding to Grb2. *J Biol Chem* 283, 9177-9186.

Harita, Y., Miyauchi, N., Karasawa, T., Suzuki, K., Han, G. D., Koike, H., Igarashi, T., Shimizu, F. & Kawachi, H. 2006. Altered expression of junctional adhesion molecule 4 in injured podocytes. *Am J Physiol Renal Physiol,* 290, F335-44.

Hleb M, M. S., Wagner EF, Hanna NN, Sharma N, Park J, Li XC, Strom TB, Padbury JF, Tseng YT, Sharma S 2004. Evidence for cyclin D3 as a novel target of rapamycin in human T lymphocytes. *J Biol Chem,* 279, 31948-31955.

Hochegger, K., Jansky, G. L., Soleiman, A., Wolf, A. M., Tagwerker, A., Seger, C., Griesmacher, A., Mayer, G. & Rosenkranz, A. R. 2008. Differential effects of rapamycin in anti-GBM glomerulonephritis. *J Am Soc Nephrol,* 19, 1520-9.

Holz MK, B. B., Gygi SP, Blenis J 2005. mTOR and S6K1 mediate assembly of the translation preinitiation complex through dynamic protein interchange and ordered phosphorylation events. *Cell,* 123, 569-580.

Huber, T. B., Hartleben, B., Kim, J., Schmidts, M., Schermer, B., Keil, A., Egger, L., Lecha, R. L., Borner, C., Pavenstadt, H., Shaw, A. S., Walz, G. & Benzing, T. 2003. Nephrin and CD2AP associate with phosphoinositide 3-OH kinase and stimulate AKT-dependent signaling. *Mol Cell Biol,* 23, 4917-28.

Inoki, K. 2008. Role of TSC-mTOR pathway in diabetic nephropathy. *Diabetes Res Clin Pract,* 82 Suppl 1, S59-62.

Jacinto, E., Loewith, R., Schmidt, A., Lin, S., Ruegg, M. A., Hall, A. & Hall, M. N. 2004. Mammalian TOR complex 2 controls the actin cytoskeleton and is rapamycin insensitive. *Nat Cell Biol,* 6, 1122-8.

Jones, N., New, L. A., Fortino, M. A., Eremina, V., Ruston, J., Blasutig, I. M., Aoudjit, L., Zou, Y., Liu, X., Yu, G. L., Takano, T., Quaggin, S. E. & Pawson, T. 2009. Nck proteins maintain the adult glomerular filtration barrier. *J Am Soc Nephrol,* 20, 1533-43.

Kerjaschki D, S. D., Farquhar MG 1984. Identification and characterization of podocalyxin--the major sialoprotein of the renal glomerular epithelial cell. *J Cell Biol,* 98, 1591-1596.

Kimmel, P. L., Barisoni, L. & Kopp, J. B. 2003. Pathogenesis and treatment of HIV-associated renal diseases: lessons from clinical and animal studies, molecular pathologic correlations, and genetic investigations. *Ann Intern Med,* 139, 214-26.

Koop, K., Eikmans, M., Wehland, M., Baelde, H., Ijpelaar, D., Kreutz, R., Kawachi, H., Kerjaschki, D., De Heer, E. & Bruijn, J. A. 2008. Selective loss of podoplanin protein expression accompanies proteinuria and precedes alterations in podocyte morphology in a spontaneous proteinuric rat model. *Am J Pathol,* 173, 315-26.

Kumar D, K. S., Yadav A, Sataranatarajan K, Kasinath BS, Chander PN, Singhal PC 2010. HIV-associated nephropathy: role of mammalian target of rapamycin pathway. *Am J Pathol,* 177, 813-821.

Kuusniemi, A. M., Merenmies, J., Lahdenkari, A. T., Holmberg, C., Salmela, K., Karikoski, R., Rapola, J. & Jalanko, H. 2006. Glomerular sclerosis in kidneys with congenital nephrotic syndrome (NPHS1). *Kidney Int,* 70, 1423-31.

Kwoh, C., Shannon, M. B., Miner, J. H. & Shaw, A. 2006. Pathogenesis of nonimmune glomerulopathies. *Annu Rev Pathol,* 1, 349-74.

Le Hir, M., Keller, C., Eschmann, V., Hahnel, B., Hosser, H. & Kriz, W. 2001. Podocyte bridges between the tuft and Bowman's capsule: an early event in experimental crescentic glomerulonephritis. *J Am Soc Nephrol,* 12, 2060-71.

Lee, E. Y., Chung, C. H., Khoury, C. C., Yeo, T. K., Pyagay, P. E., Wang, A. & Chen, S. 2009. The monocyte chemoattractant protein-1/CCR2 loop, inducible by TGF-beta, increases podocyte motility and albumin permeability. *Am J Physiol Renal Physiol,* 297, F85-94.

Lee, M. J., Feliers, D., Mariappan, M. M., Sataranatarajan, K., Mahimainathan, L., Musi, N., Foretz, M., Viollet, B., Weinberg, J. M., Choudhury, G. G. & Kasinath, B. S. 2007. A role for AMP-activated protein kinase in diabetes-induced renal hypertrophy. *Am J Physiol Renal Physiol,* 292, F617-27.

Leeuwis, J. W., Nguyen, T. Q., Dendooven, A., Kok, R. J. & Goldschmeding, R. 2010. Targeting podocyte-associated diseases. *Adv Drug Deliv Rev,* 62, 1325-36.

Letavernier, E., Bruneval, P., Mandet, C., Van Huyen, J.-P. D., Pã©Raldi, M.-N. L., Helal, I., Noã«L, L.-H. L. N. & Legendre, C. 2007. High Sirolimus Levels May Induce Focal Segmental Glomerulosclerosis De Novo. *Clinical Journal of the American Society of Nephrology,* 2, 326-333.

Liu G, K. B., Kurfis J, Rahmanuddin S, Kanwar YS, Chugh SS 2003. Neph1 and nephrin interaction in the slit diaphragm is an important determinant of glomerular permeability. *J Clin Invest,* 112, 209-221.

Lloberas, N., Cruzado, J. M., Franquesa, M., Herrero-Fresneda, I., Torras, J., Alperovich, G., Rama, I., Vidal, A. & Grinyo, J. M. 2006. Mammalian target of rapamycin pathway blockade slows progression of diabetic kidney disease in rats. *J Am Soc Nephrol,* 17, 1395-404.

Loewith, R. 2011. A brief history of TOR. *Biochem Soc Trans,* 39, 437-42.

Loewith R, J. E., Wullschleger S, Lorberg A, Crespo JL, Bonenfant D, Oppliger W, Jenoe P, Hall MN 2002. Two TOR complexes, only one of which is rapamycin sensitive, have distinct roles in cell growth control. *Molecular Cell,* 10, 457-468.

Marshall, C. B. & Shankland, S. J. 2007. Cell cycle regulatory proteins in podocyte health and disease. *Nephron Exp Nephrol,* 106, e51-9.

Medapalli, R. K., He, J. C, Klotman, P. E. 2011. HIV-associated nephropathy: pathogenesis. *Curr Opin Nephrol Hypertens,* 20, 306-11.

Meijer, A. J. & Codogno, P. 2004. Regulation and role of autophagy in mammalian cells. *Int J Biochem Cell Biol,* 36, 2445-62.

Moeller, M. J., Soofi, A., Hartmann, I., Le Hir, M., Wiggins, R., Kriz, W. & Holzman, L. B. 2004. Podocytes populate cellular crescents in a murine model of inflammatory glomerulonephritis. *J Am Soc Nephrol,* 15, 61-7.

Moller, C. C., Flesche, J. & Reiser, J. 2009. Sensitizing the Slit Diaphragm with TRPC6 ion channels. *J Am Soc Nephrol,* 20, 950-3.

Mori H, I. K., Masutani K, Wakabayashi Y, Komai K, Nakagawa R, Guan KL, Yoshimura A 2009. The mTOR pathway is highly activated in diabetic nephropathy and rapamycin has a strong therapeutic potential. *Biochem Biophys Res Commun,* 384, 471-475.

Mundel, P. & Kriz, W. 1995. Structure and function of podocytes: an update. *Anat Embryol (Berl),* 192, 385-97.

Mundel, P. & Shankland, S. J. 2002. Podocyte biology and response to injury. *J Am Soc Nephrol,* 13, 3005-15.

Munivenkatappa, R., Haririan, A., Papadimitriou, J. C., Drachenberg, C. B., Dinits-Pensy, M. & Klassen, D. K. 2010. Tubular epithelial cell and podocyte apoptosis with de novo sirolimus based immunosuppression in renal allograft recipients with DGF. *Histol Histopathol,* 25, 189-96.

Murakami M, I. T., Maeda M, Oshiro N, Hara K, Edenhofer F, Kiyama H, Yonezawa K, Yamanaka S 2004. mTOR is essential for growth and proliferation in early mouse embryos and embryonic stem cells. *Mol Cell Biol,* 24, 6710-6718.

Nagai, K., Matsubara, T., Mima, A., Sumi, E., Kanamori, H., Iehara, N., Fukatsu, A., Yanagita, M., Nakano, T., Ishimoto, Y., Kita, T., Doi, T. & Arai, H. 2005. Gas6 induces Akt/mTOR-mediated mesangial hypertrophy in diabetic nephropathy. *Kidney Int,* 68, 552-61.

Naumovic, R., Jovovic, D., Basta-Jovanovic, G., Miloradovic, Z., Mihailovic-Stanojevic, N., Aleksic, T. & Jovanovic, D. 2007. Effects of rapamycin on active Heymann nephritis. *Am J Nephrol,* 27, 379-89.

Orlando Ra, T. T., Zak B, Schmieder S, Benoit VM, Mcquistan T, Furthmayr H, Farquhar MG 2001. The glomerular epithelial cell anti-adhesin podocalyxin associates with the actin cytoskeleton through interactions with ezrin. *J Am Soc Nephrol,* 12, 1589-1598.

Patel, P., Pal, S., Ashley, C., Sweny, P. & Burns, A. 2005. Combination therapy with sirolimus (rapamycin) and tacrolimus (FK-506) in treatment of refractory minimal change nephropathy, a clinical case report. *Nephrol Dial Transplant,* 20, 985-7.

Pavenstadt, H., Kriz, W. & Kretzler, M. 2003. Cell biology of the glomerular podocyte. *Physiol Rev,* 83, 253-307.

Perysinaki GS, M. D., Bertsias G, Giannopoulou I, Kyriakou K, Nakopoulou L, Boumpas DT, Daphnis E 2011. Podocyte main slit diaphragm proteins, nephrin and podocin, are affected at early stages of lupus nephritis and correlate with disease histology. *Lupus.*

Pollak, M. R. 2008. Focal segmental glomerulosclerosis: recent advances. *Curr Opin Nephrol Hypertens,* 17, 138-142.

Rangan, G. K. & Coombes, J. D. 2007. Renoprotective effects of sirolimus in non-immune initiated focal segmental glomerulosclerosis. *Nephrol Dial Transplant,* 22, 2175-82.

Reiser, J., Oh, J., Shirato, I., Asanuma, K., Hug, A., Mundel, T. M., Honey, K., Ishidoh, K., Kominami, E., Kreidberg, J. A., Tomino, Y. & Mundel, P. 2004. Podocyte migration during nephrotic syndrome requires a coordinated interplay between cathepsin L and alpha3 integrin. *J Biol Chem,* 279, 34827-32.

Reiser J, O. J., Shirato I, Asanuma K, Hug A, Mundel TM, Honey K, Ishidoh K, Kominami E, Kreidberg JA, Tomino Y, Mundel P 2004. Podocyte migration during nephrotic syndrome requires a coordinated interplay between cathepsin L and alpha3 integrin. *J Biol Chem,* 279, 34827-34832.

Sabatini, D. M. 2006. mTOR and cancer: insights into a complex relationship. *Nat Rev Cancer,* 6, 729-34.

Sabatini, D. M., Erdjument-Bromage, H., Lui, M., Tempst, P. & Snyder, S. H. 1994. RAFT1: a mammalian protein that binds to FKBP12 in a rapamycin-dependent fashion and is homologous to yeast TORs. *Cell,* 78, 35-43.

Sakaguchi, M., Isono, M., Isshiki, K., Sugimoto, T., Koya, D. & Kashiwagi, A. 2006. Inhibition of mTOR signaling with rapamycin attenuates renal hypertrophy in the early diabetic mice. *Biochem Biophys Res Commun,* 340, 296-301.

Sarbassov, D. D., Ali, S. M., Sengupta, S., Sheen, J. H., Hsu, P. P., Bagley, A. F., Markhard, A. L. & Sabatini, D. M. 2006. Prolonged rapamycin treatment inhibits mTORC2 assembly and Akt/PKB. *Mol Cell,* 22, 159-68.

Sataranatarajan, K., Mariappan, M. M., Lee, M. J., Feliers, D., Choudhury, G. G., Barnes, J. L. & Kasinath, B. S. 2007. Regulation of elongation phase of mRNA translation in diabetic nephropathy: amelioration by rapamycin. *Am J Pathol,* 171, 1733-42.

Schwarz, K., Simons, M., Reiser, J., Saleem, M. A., Faul, C., Kriz, W., Shaw, A. S., Holzman, L. B. & Mundel, P. 2001. Podocin, a raft-associated component of the glomerular slit diaphragm, interacts with CD2AP and nephrin. *J Clin Invest,* 108, 1621-9.

Senior, P. A., Paty, B. W., Cockfield, S. M., Ryan, E. A. & Shapiro, A. M. 2005. Proteinuria developing after clinical islet transplantation resolves with sirolimus withdrawal and increased tacrolimus dosing. *Am J Transplant,* 5, 2318-23.

Sever S, A. M., Nankoe SR, Möller CC, Ko D, Wei C, Henderson J, Del Re EC, Hsing L, Erickson A, Cohen CD, Kretzler M, Kerjaschki D, Rudensky A, Nikolic B, Reiser J

2007. Proteolytic processing of dynamin by cytoplasmic cathepsin L is a mechanism for proteinuric kidney disease. *J Clin Invest,* 117, 2095-2104.

Simon, M., Grone, H. J., Johren, O., Kullmer, J., Plate, K. H., Risau, W. & Fuchs, E. 1995. Expression of vascular endothelial growth factor and its receptors in human renal ontogenesis and in adult kidney. *Am J Physiol,* 268, F240-50.

Smoyer, W. E. & Mundel, P. 1998. Regulation of podocyte structure during the development of nephrotic syndrome. *J Mol Med,* 76, 172-83.

Somlo, S. & Mundel, P. 2000. Getting a foothold in nephrotic syndrome. *Nat Genet,* 24, 333-5.

Succar L, Lai-Kwon J, Nikolic-Paterson D. & Rangan, G.K. 2007. Inhibition of mTOR reduces crescent formation and improves renal function in experimental crescentic glomerulonephritis (abstract). *J Am Soc Nephrol* 18, 399A

Sun, D., Toan, X., Zhang, Y., Chen, Y., Lu, R., Wang, X. & Fang, J. 2008. Mammalian target of rapamycin pathway inhibition enhances the effects of 5-aza-dC on suppressing cell proliferation in human gastric cancer cell lines. *Sci China C Life Sci,* 51, 640-7.

Thorner, P. S., Ho, M., Eremina, V., Sado, Y. & Quaggin, S. 2008. Podocytes contribute to the formation of glomerular crescents. *J Am Soc Nephrol,* 19, 495-502.

Torras J, H.-F. I., Gulias O, Flaquer M, Vidal A, Cruzado JM, Lloberas N, Franquesa M, Grinyó JM 2009. Rapamycin has dual opposing effects on proteinuric experimental nephropathies: is it a matter of podocyte damage? *Nephrol Dial Transplant,* 24, 3632-3640.

Tryggvason, K., Patrakka, J. & Wartiovaara, J. 2006. Hereditary proteinuria syndromes and mechanisms of proteinuria. *N Engl J Med,* 354, 1387-401.

Tryggvason K, W. J. 2001. Molecular basis of glomerular permselectivity. *Curr Opin Nephrol Hypertens,* 10, 543-549.

Tufro, A., Norwood, V. F., Carey, R. M. & Gomez, R. A. 1999. Vascular endothelial growth factor induces nephrogenesis and vasculogenesis. *J Am Soc Nephrol,* 10, 2125-34.

Tumlin, J. A., Miller, D., Near, M., Selvaraj, S., Hennigar, R. & Guasch, A. 2006. A prospective, open-label trial of sirolimus in the treatment of focal segmental glomerulosclerosis. *Clin J Am Soc Nephrol,* 1, 109-16.

Verma, R., Kovari, I., Soofi, A., Nihalani, D., Patrie, K. & Holzman, L. B. 2006. Nephrin ectodomain engagement results in Src kinase activation, nephrin phosphorylation, Nck recruitment, and actin polymerization. *J Clin Invest,* 116, 1346-59.

Vogelbacher, R., Wittmann, S., Braun, A., Daniel, C. & Hugo, C. 2007. The mTOR inhibitor everolimus induces proteinuria and renal deterioration in the remnant kidney model in the rat. *Transplantation,* 84, 1492-9.

Vogt, P. K. 2001. PI 3-kinase, mTOR, protein synthesis and cancer. *Trends Mol Med,* 7, 482-4.

Wang, W., Chan, Y. H., Lee, W. & Chan, L. 2001. Effect of rapamycin and FK506 on mesangial cell proliferation. *Transplant Proc,* 33, 1036-7.

Yang, Q. & Guan, K. L. 2007. Expanding mTOR signaling. *Cell Res,* 17, 666-81.

Yang, Y., Wang, J., Qin, L., Shou, Z., Zhao, J., Wang, H., Chen, Y. & Chen, J. 2007. Rapamycin prevents early steps of the development of diabetic nephropathy in rats. *Am J Nephrol,* 27, 495-502.

Yaoita, E., Kurihara, H., Yoshida, Y., Inoue, T., Matsuki, A., Sakai, T. & Yamamoto, T. 2005. Role of Fat1 in cell-cell contact formation of podocytes in puromycin aminonucleoside nephrosis and neonatal kidney. *Kidney Int,* 68, 542-51.

Zhu, J., Sun, N., Aoudjit, L., Li, H., Kawachi, H., Lemay, S. & Takano, T. 2008. Nephrin mediates actin reorganization via phosphoinositide 3-kinase in podocytes. *Kidney Int,* 73, 556-66.

11

Renin-Angiotensin System Activation and Extracellular Signal-Regulated Kinases in Glomerulonephritis

Maki Urushihara and Yukiko Kinoshita
Department of Pediatrics, Institute of Health Biosciences, The University of Tokushima Graduate School Tokushima, Japan

1. Introduction

Abnormal extracellular matrix (ECM) remodeling is a prominent biological feature of progressive glomerulonephritis (GN), and leads to glomerular dysfunction and sclerosis (Kagami et al., 2001; Prols et al., 1999). This condition is pathologically manifested in all the three major cells types of the glomerulus, and is characterized by the accumulation of fibronectin, laminin, and collagen in the diseased glomeruli (Kagami et al., 2004; Schnaper et al., 2003). Published genetic data (Boute et al., 2000; Kaplan et al., 2000; Patrakka et al., 2000) and the finding of podocyte abnormalities in transgenic mouse models of glomerulosclerosis (Shih et al., 1999) and patients with focal segmental glomerulosclerosis (Srivastava et al., 2001) suggest that the visceral epithelial cell plays a significant role. This assertion is supported by earlier data implicating potential epithelial cell stressors, such as glomerular hypertension, hyperfiltration, or hypertrophy in sclerosis (Brenner, 1985). Some models implicate the endothelial cells in the sclerotic process (Akaoka et al., 1995; Lee et al., 1995b). Still others suggest a role for the mesangial cells (MC) (Habib, 1973). As seen in human GN and experimental rat GN models, activated MCs acquire increased mitogenicity and migratory activity, and exhibit de novo synthesis of α-smooth muscle actin (α-SMA) and interstitial collagen (Hugo et al., 1996; Johnson, 1994). In addition, filtered macromolecules may be trapped in the mesangium, initiating an inflammatory response that could play a role in stimulating ECM synthesis. A unifying hypothesis that includes participation of all the cellular elements of the glomerulus can be constructed. Glomerular capillary hypertension, or a genetic or acquired abnormality in podocyte adhesion or structure, permits hyperfiltration of macromolecules. Paracrine signals from the injured podocyte stimulate endothelial cell expression of leukocyte adhesion molecules and impair endothelial cell fibrinolytic activity. Signals from epithelial or endothelial cells to the mesangium, or direct delivery of proinflammatory substances through the glomerular filtrate, initiates a process that culminates in the accumulation of ECM (Schnaper and Kopp, 2003). Mesangial expansion infringes on the capillary spaces, decreasing filtration surface area in the glomerular tuft. A major concept emerging from molecular cell biological studies is that pathological mesangial remodeling in progressive kidney disease is caused by uncontrolled interactions between MCs, ECM, and growth factors (Rupprecht et al., 1996). Recent efforts have been directed towards modeling the cellular events regulating glomerular ECM turnover. Clarifying the molecular and cellular mechanisms responsible for pathological ECM remodeling may help to elucidate the pathogenesis of progressive glomerular sclerosis (Gruden et al., 2000; Krepinsky et al., 2003). A variety of physiological, pharmacological, and molecular approaches have been used to study how various mediators initiate or modify intracellular signaling pathways to cause mesangial cell matrix accumulation. These factors include transforming growth factor (TGF)-β (Border and Noble, 1997), basic fibroblast growth factor (bFGF) (Haseley et al., 1999), platelet-derived growth factor (PDGF) (Haseley et al., 1999), angiotensin II (Ang II) (Mezzano et al., 2001), connective tissue growth factor (CTGF) (Gupta et al., 2000), and various eicosanoids (Ledbetter et al., 1990).

2. The renin-angiotensin system (RAS) in GN

The RAS plays an important role in fluid and electrolyte homeostasis, the development of hypertension, and the progression of renal disease (Anderson et al., 1986; Navar et al., 1999). Recently, the focus of interest on the RAS has shifted towards the role of the local RAS in specific tissues (Dzau and Re, 1994). The local RAS in the kidney has several pathophysiological functions not only in regulating blood pressure, but also in renal cell growth and production of glomerulosclerosis, which is induced during the development of renal fibrosis (Kagami et al., 1994; Ruiz-Ortega and Egido, 1997). Indeed, previous studies have shown that RAS blockades have beneficial effects in rats and humans with various renal diseases, and these effects are often considerably more significant than their suppressive effects on blood pressure (Horita et al., 2004; Ravid et al., 1998). Chronic GN, which results in substantial renal damage, is frequently characterized by relentless progression to end-stage renal disease. Renal Ang II, whose production is enhanced in chronic GN, can elevate the intraglomerular pressure, increase glomerular cell hypertrophy, and augment ECM accumulation (Brunner, 1992; Kohan, 1998). Ang II antagonists or synthesis inhibitors markedly decelerate, and can even prevent, renal deterioration in renal disease (Anderson et al., 1986; Brunner, 1992; Giatras et al., 1997; Lafayette et al., 1992). This may be a reflection of the relatively short-term nature and small sample size of these studies, but may also be an indication that factors other than Ang II play an important role in the progression of GN.

3. Mitogen-activated protein kinase (MAPK)

The MAPK signaling pathway is a highly conserved module involved in various cellular functions, including cell proliferation, survival, differentiation, and migration (Fig. 1). Extracellular stimuli, such as growth factors and environmental stress, induce sequential activation of the MAPK cascade. At least four members of the MAPK family have been identified: extracellular signal-regulated kinase 1/2 (ERK1/2), p38, c-Jun N-terminal kinase (JNK), and ERK5 (Nishimoto and Nishida, 2006). The cascade allows for signal amplification, modulation, and specificity in response to different stimuli (Ferrell, 1996; Rose et al., 2010). As with many signaling pathways, complex regulatory mechanisms are utilized to direct the functional outcome mediated by MAPKs. The prototypic ERK1/2 pathway is found to be mainly responsive to stimulation by growth factors (Ramos, 2008), while p38 and JNK are collectively called stress-activated MAPKs (SAPKs) due to their induction by physical, chemical, and physiological stressors (Kyriakis and Avruch, 2001). In addition, the ERK5 pathway is implicated in both growth and stress signaling (Hayashi et al., 2004). The specificity and efficiency of MAPK signaling pathways are often dictated by specific docking and bindings partners (Jacobs et al., 1999; Raman et al., 2007; Remenyi et al., 2005). These include positive and negative modulators and scaffolding proteins that help to bring upstream and downstream signaling components together (Dhanasekaran et al., 2007; Morrison and Davis, 2003; Pearson et al., 2001). Thus, MAPKs form complex signaling networks that can be induced by a large array of external stimuli, and can achieve highly specific cellular effects through multitudes of regulatory mechanisms (Rose et al., 2010).

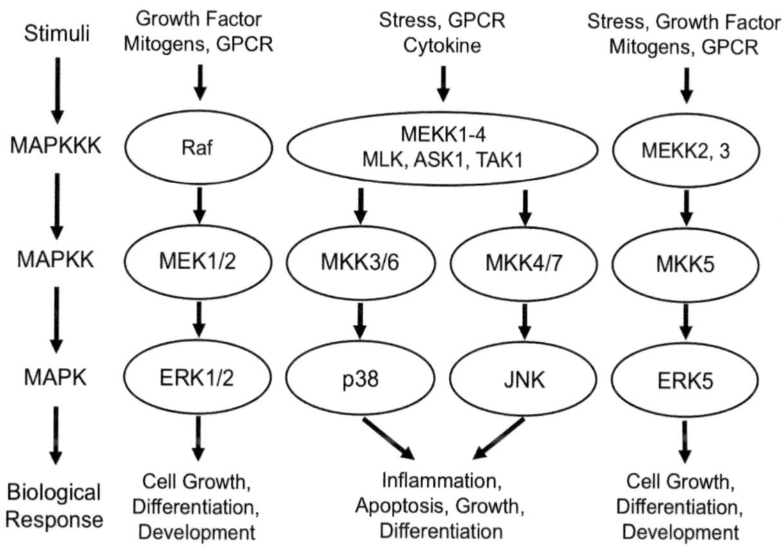

Fig. 1. Mitogen-activated protein kinase (MAPK) signaling. GPCR, G protein-coupled receptor; MLK, Mixed lineage kinase; TAK, TGF-β activated kinase; ASK, Apoptosis signal-regulating kinase.

3.1 ERK1/2

ERK1 and ERK2 are isoforms of the classical MAPK. Both ERK1 and ERK2 are activated by MAP/ERK kinase 1 (MEK1) and MEK2, which are members of the MAPKK family (Nishimoto and Nishida, 2006). After stimulation by a variety of mitogens, including peptide growth factors, MEK1/2 is activated by MAPKKK-mediated phosphorylation. These MAPKKKs include Raf and Mos. MEK1/2 then phosphorylates threonine and tyrosine residues in the Thr-Glu-Tyr (TEY) sequence of ERK1/2, thereby activating it. Activated ERK1/2 phosphorylates many substrates, including transcription factors, such as Elk1 and c-Myc, and protein kinases, such as ribosomal S6 kinase (RSK). Subsequently, immediate early genes, such as c-Fos, are induced. At the cellular level, ERK1/2 regulates cell cycle progression, proliferation, cytokinesis, transcription, differentiation, senescence, cell death, migration, GAP junction formation, actin and microtubule networks, and cell adhesion (Ramos, 2008). Owing to its role in cellular biology, ERK1/2 is a prominent player in physiological settings, influencing the immune system and heart development and participating in the cellular response to many hormones, growth factors, and insulin. The ERK1/2 pathway is activated not only by growth factors, serum, and phorbol esters, but also by G protein-coupled receptors (GPCR), cytokines, microtubule disorganization, and other stimuli (Goldsmith and Dhanasekaran, 2007; McKay and Morrison, 2007; Raman et al., 2007). Prototypically, binding of growth factors (such as FGF) to their respective receptor tyrosine kinases (RTK) activates Ras, which recruits and activates Raf (MAP3K) at the plasma membrane. Once activated, Raf phosphorylates and activates MEK1/2. MEK1/2, in turn, activates ERK1/2 by phosphorylation of the Thr and Tyr residues in the conserved TEY motif within its regulatory loop. Activated ERK1/2 can phosphorylate downstream proteins, including many transcription factors, in the cytoplasm or nucleus.

3.2 ERK5

ERK5, also known as big MAP kinase 1 (BMK1), is twice the size of the other MAPKs (Lee et al., 1995a; Zhou et al., 1995). Since it is activated by oxidative stress and hyperosmolarity, ERK5 was initially documented as a MAPK family member activated by stress stimuli (Abe et al., 1996). Subsequently, ERK5 was also shown to be activated in response to serum, one of the well-known activators of ERK1/2 (Kato et al., 1997). Once activated, ERK5 exerts its kinase activity on a number of other protein kinases and transcription factors in both the cytosol and the nucleus. Furthermore, unlike other MAPKs, ERK5 has been shown to function directly as a transcriptional activator (Akaike et al., 2004; Kasler et al., 2000). Diverse biological roles of ERK5, including cell survival, differentiation, proliferation, and growth, have also been identified. ERK5 is reported to play a physiological role in neuronal survival, endothelial cell response to sheer stress, prostate and breast cancer, cardiac hypertrophy, and atherosclerosis (Hayashi and Lee, 2004; Nishimoto and Nishida, 2006; Wang and Tournier, 2006). Nerve growth factor, Ang II, high glucose, and other stimulators of ERK1/2 can also increase ERK5 activity (Kamakura et al., 1999). Similar to the ERK1/2 pathway, the MEK-ERK5 pathway is blocked by MEK inhibitors (Kamakura et al., 1999). Thus, there are similarities between the activation modes and functions of the ERK5 and ERK1/2 pathways. However, recent studies have also identified some distinctive features of the ERK5 and ERK1/2 pathway (Mulloy et al., 2003; Squires et al., 2002).

4. MAPKs in GN

A number of former studies have reported that the MAPK pathway plays a crucial role in the development of renal diseases. Bokemeyer et al. reported that ERK1/2 activation occurs in the rat Thy-1 model of mesangioproliferative nephritis, and that inhibition of the ERK1/2 pathway results in a significant reduction in mesangial cell proliferation in this model (Bokemeyer et al., 2000; Bokemeyer et al., 2002). The glomerular ERK1/2 was maximally activated on day 6 and represents a putative mediator of the proliferative response in mesangioproliferative GN. In addition, ERK1/2 activation in human glomerulopathies is associated with cell proliferation, histological lesions, and renal dysfunction (Masaki et al., 2004). Thus, these studies showing ERK activation in damaged glomeruli raise the possibility that ERK1/2 is an important signal molecule for acute inflammation-induced cellular proliferation in GN.

ERK5 was originally shown to be activated by stress stimuli or serum (Kamakura et al., 1999; Kato et al., 1997). Other stimuli, such as oxidative stress, Ang II, and high glucose, can also activate ERK5 in various cell types (Kato et al., 2000). Previous reports have demonstrated that ERK5 is activated in the glomeruli of diabetic nephropathy rat models, but not in normal control rats. High glucose also induces ERK5 activation in cultured MCs in vitro (Suzaki et al., 2004). It was suggested that ERK5 might be involved in glomerular injury during the pathogenesis of diabetic nephropathy.

4.1 Animal experiments

We have established a progressive model of mesangioproliferative GN, as previously described (Nakamura et al., 1999). Briefly, rats (n = 36) were uninephrectomized, and, 1 week later, administered with a single intravenous injection of 2 mg of nephritogenic anti-Thy-1 monoclonal antibody 1-22-3. This monoclonal antibody recognizes a critical epitope of the Thy-1.1 molecule on the mesangial cell surface. Upon binding to its epitope, the antibody induces severe complement-dependent mesangial cell injury. The injection of monoclonal antibody 1-22-3 into uninephrectomized rats induced chronic progressive glomerulosclerosis with marked proteinuria. Control rats (n = 6) only received a vehicle. Six rats were sacrificed at each time point (days 3, 7, 14, 28, and 56 after the monoclonal antibody injection). In addition, 6 rats were sacrificed as baseline controls (0 h) prior to the injection of monoclonal antibody 1-22-3, and 5 rats (Nx group) were injected with PBS one week post-uninephrectomy and sacrificed on day 56 after the injection.

The right kidney of each rat was removed, immediately fixed in 10% buffered-formalin, embedded in paraffin, cut into 4-μm sections, and stained with periodic acid-Schiff (PAS) reagent. The mean glomerular cell number, which was based on the total glomerular cell count per glomerular cross section after PAS staining, was calculated for 30 glomeruli/kidney. A pathologist, who was blinded to the other findings, semi-quantitatively analyzed the glomerulosclerosis score. The percentage of each glomerulus occupied by the mesangial matrix was estimated and assigned a code, according to the following system: 0, 0%; 0.5, 1-5%; 1, 5-25%; 2, 25-50%; 3, 50-75%; and 4, >75%. Frozen sections (3 μm) were fixed in acetone, incubated with a rabbit anti-phospho-ERK5 antibody at 4°C overnight, and then incubated with a FITC-conjugated donkey anti-rabbit IgG antibody. To evaluate the level of glomerular staining with each antibody, we performed a semi-quantitative analysis, according to the following scoring system: 0, diffuse, very weak or no mesangial staining; 1+, 1-25% of glomerular tufts exhibit focal increases in mesangial staining; 2+, 25-50% of glomerular tufts exhibit strong mesangial staining; 3+, 50-75% of glomerular tufts exhibit strong mesangial staining; and 4+, >75% of glomerular tufts exhibit strong mesangial staining. For each kidney section, 30 glomeruli were selected at random and evaluated in a blinded fashion by the same pathologist. The mean value per section was then calculated. Formalin-fixed tissue sections (3 μm) were deparaffinized with xylene and rehydrated through a graded series of ethanol. Endogenous peroxidase was blocked by incubation with hydrogen peroxide, and the samples were heated at 121°C for 15 minutes in 0.01 mol/L citrate buffer (pH 6.0) for antigen retrieval. Next, the sections were incubated at 4°C for 24 hours with an anti-phospho-ERK1/2 antibody diluted in PBS containing 1% BSA. After washing with PBS, the sections were incubated with a biotinylated secondary antibody and avidin-biotin-peroxidase complex (ABC Elite; Vector Laboratories, Burlingame, CA), and developed with 3,3′-diaminobenzidine. Each section was counterstained with Mayer's hematoxylin, dehydrated, and coverslipped. The phospho-ERK1/2-positive cells in 30 full-size glomeruli were counted, and the mean value was calculated.

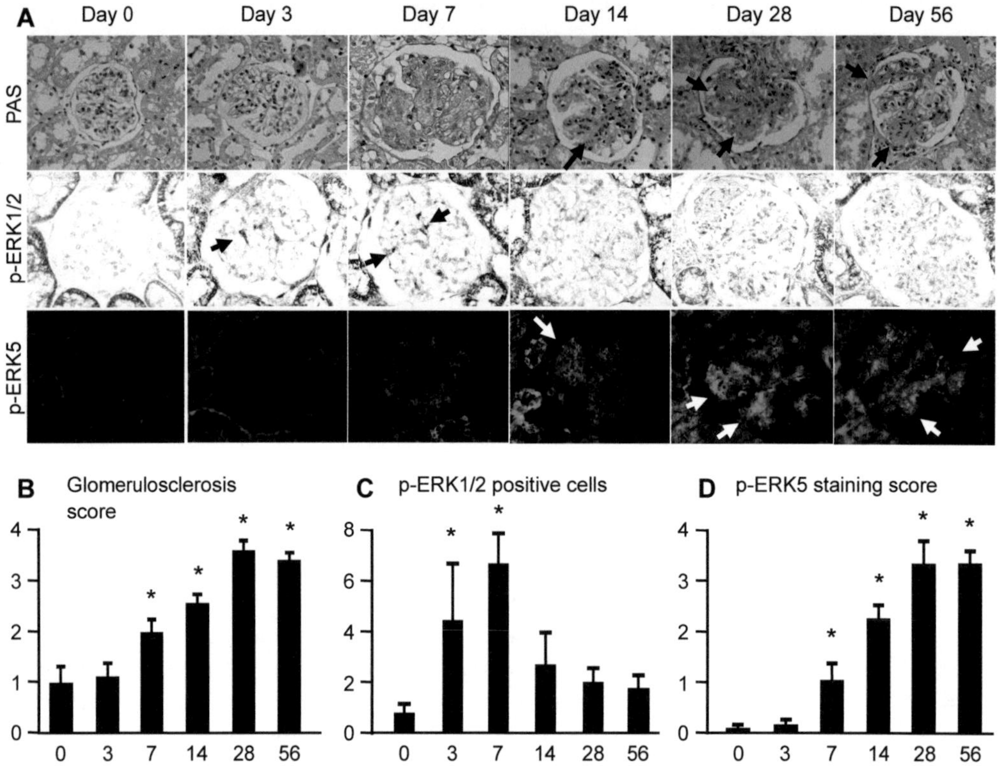

Fig. 2. Time course studies in glomerular histology and expression of phospho-ERK1/2 (p-ERK1/2) and phospho-ERK5 (p-ERK5) in normal and glomerulonephritis (GN) rats. A: analysis of glomerular histology on periodic acid-Schiff (PAS)-stained sections and sections immunostained with anti-p-ERK1/2 or anti-p-ERK5 antibody. Magnification, ×200. B: semi-quantitative assessment of glomerular ECM accumulation in normal and GN rats. C: semi-quantitative assessment of glomerular p-ERK1/2 expression. D: semi-quantitative assessment of glomerular p-ERK5 expression. Values are mean +/- SD. *P < 0.05 vs rats at day 0.

4.2 ERK1/2 and ERK5 expression in rat models of progressive GN

Early induction of ERK1/2 phosphorylation was detected on days 3 and 7 of GN. A significant increase in phosphorylated ERK1/2 was not seen in the late phase of GN. In contrast to the time course of glomerular ERK1/2 phosphorylation, glomerular phospho-ERK5 expression was very weak on day 3. However, the level of this expression increased in the expanded mesangial area by day 7, and dramatically increased in a typical mesangial pattern by days 28 and 56 (Fig. 2). The level of glomerular phospho-ERK5 expression closely paralleled the glomerulosclerosis score during the course of chronic anti-Thy-1-induced GN ($P < 0.05$). Treatment of GN rats with an Ang II type 1 receptor blocker (ARB) resulted in a significant decrease in phospho-ERK5 expression, accompanied by remarkable histological improvement. We have also previously reported that increased ERK5 phosphorylation is associated with MC proliferation and ECM accumulation in the glomeruli of 52-week-old OLETE rats, a model of type 2 diabetic mellitus (DM) (Suzaki et al., 2004). Bokemeyer et al. demonstrated that glomerular ERK1/2 is maximally activated on day 6 and that blocking the ERK1/2 pathway using a specific inhibitor results in a significant reduction in mesangial cell proliferation in mesangioproliferative GN (Bokemeyer et al., 2000; Bokemeyer et al., 2002). Thus, these studies demonstrating ERK activation in damaged glomeruli suggest the possibility that ERK1/2 is an important signal molecule for acute inflammation-induced cellular proliferation, and that ERK5 may participate in the development of chronic glomerular lesions in GN.

5. MAPK in glomerular cells

Ang II stimulates ERK1/2 activation via NADPH oxidase-dependent reactive oxygen species (ROS) production in cultured rat MCs (Gorin et al., 2004). Therefore, we examined whether oxidative stress mediates the effects of Ang II on ERK5 phosphorylation in MCs. Cultured rat MCs were established from intact glomeruli of Sprague-Dawley rats. MCs were pretreated with ARB or diphenylene iodonium (DPI) before stimulation with Ang II or H_2O_2. MCs were serum-starved for 48 hours in serum-free RPMI 1640 medium, prior to stimulation with H_2O_2 and/or Ang II in the presence or absence of reagents. Ang II-induced ERK5 phosphorylation in MCs was blocked by the pretreatment with ARB but not DPI, indicating that Ang II-induced ERK5 phosphorylation was mediated by the Ang II type 1 receptor and not by the Ang II-induced NAD(P)H oxidase-dependent ROS production (Urushihara et al., 2010). Furthermore, the costimulation of MCs with Ang II and H_2O_2 resulted in a synergistic increase in ERK5 phosphorylation, compared to the stimulation of MCs with either Ang II or H_2O_2 (Urushihara et al., 2010). These findings suggest that Ang II directly induces ERK5 phosphorylation via NADPH in an oxidase-independent manner, and that ROS and Ang II could each induce ERK5 phosphorylation in MCs through different signaling pathways.

5.1 ERK5-specific knockdown in cultured rat mesangial cells (MC)

To examine the endogenous function of ERK5 in MCs, we used the small interfering (si) RNA technique for ERK5 gene silencing. MCs were transiently transfected with a mixture of three ERK5-specific siRNAs, using the lipofection method. After incubation in a low-serum-containing medium (5% FBS) for 18 hours, the serum concentration was adjusted to that of complete medium and the cells were cultured further. A non-silencing siRNA that did not target any known mammalian genes was used as a negative control. The transfection efficiency, determined under the same experimental conditions by counting the number of fluorescently labeled siRNA-transfected cells using a fluorescence microscope, was ~80%. Inhibition of ERK5 expression was verified by quantitative real-time PCR and western blot analysis. Further, we evaluated the viability of siRNA-transfected cells cultured for 24 hours in serum-free medium using the WST-1 assay for determining cell survival rate. The WST-1 assay was performed using a cell counting kit, according to the manufacturer's protocol. Briefly, siRNA-transfected cells grown in 96-well plates were washed with PBS, and 10 μL of the WST-1 reagent was added to 100 μL of cell culture medium in each well. After incubation for 8 hours, the absorbance of the samples was measured at 450 nm (test) and 690 nm (reference) with a microplate reader. Additionally, we measured the soluble collagen levels in culture supernatants after 24 hours of incubation in serum-free medium using a Sircol collagen assay. This assay measures the total collagen secreted from cultured cells. Briefly, cells were cultured for 24 hours with or without treatment, and supernatants were collected. One milliliter of Sirius red, an anionic dye that specifically reacts with basic side chain groups of collagens, was added to 200 μL of the supernatant and incubated with gentle rotation for 30 minutes at room temperature. After centrifugation, the collagen-bound dye was resolublized in 1 mL of 0.5 M NaOH, and the absorbance at 540 nm was measured.

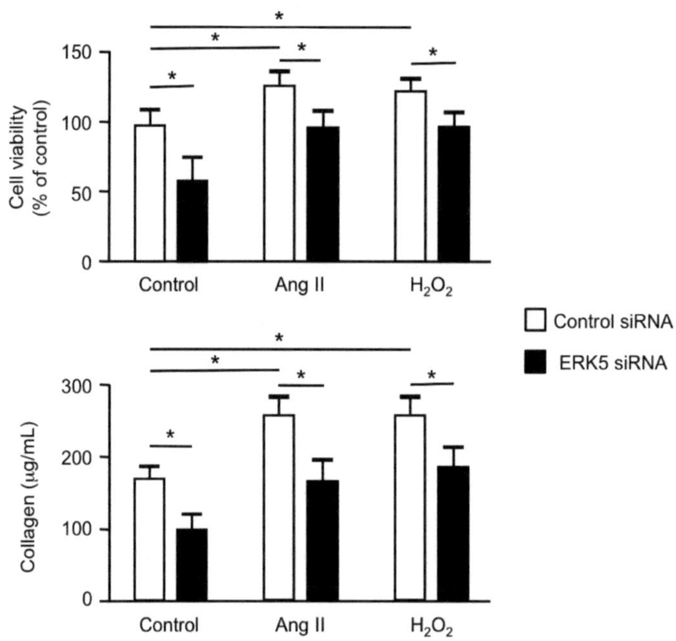

Fig. 3. Effects of Angiotensin II (Ang II) or H_2O_2 on cell viability and collagen secretion in ERK5 siRNA-transfected MCs. MCs were transfected with non-silencing siRNA (control siRNA) or ERK5-specific siRNA (ERK5 siRNA) and stimulated with Ang II (100 nM) or H_2O_2 (50 µM) after incubation in serum-free medium for 24 hours. Cell viability was evaluated using the WST-1 assay (8 hours; top), and collagen secretion in culture supernatants was evaluated by the Sircol assay (24 hours; bottom). Values are mean +/- SD. *$P < 0.05$ between groups as indicated.

5.2 Cell viability and collagen secretion

Using the WST-1 and Sircol assays, significant concentration-dependent decreases in both cell viability and soluble collagen secretion were observed in ERK5 siRNA-transfected, but not control siRNA-transfected MCs. Next, the effect of oxidative stress and Ang II on ECM accumulation and cell viability, and the involvement of ERK5 in these processes were examined. As seen in Fig. 3, Ang II and H_2O_2 significantly increased both cell viability and soluble collagen secretion in control siRNA-transfected MCs ($P < 0.05$). Transfection of ERK5 siRNA significantly reduced Ang II- or H_2O_2-induced increases in MC viability and collagen secretion compared to control siRNA transfection ($P < 0.05$).

Many studies have demonstrated that the ERK5 pathway controls cellular processes, such as proliferation, survival, differentiation, and ECM metabolism in pathophysiological conditions (Chang and Karin, 2001; Kyriakis and Avruch, 2001; Nishimoto and Nishida, 2006). We investigated the involvement of MC ERK5 expression in chronic progressive GN using in vitro and in vivo studies. We found that both cell viability and soluble collagen secretion were induced by Ang II or H_2O_2 in control MCs. These changes were significantly inhibited in ERK5 siRNA-transfected MCs, suggesting a possible role for ERK5 expression in the sustained MC proliferation and pathological ECM accumulation observed in progressive GN. Furthermore, the data obtained from the treatment of GN rats with ARB indicate that Ang II is an inducer of MC ERK5 phosphorylation in vivo, and support the involvement of Ang II-induced ERK5 phosphorylation in progressive glomerular lesions. In general, the repair of proliferative GN-induced damage requires the regression of the proliferated glomerular cells by apoptosis and the appropriate removal of the accumulated pathological ECM (Shimizu et al., 1995). Based on our results, the activation of an ERK5 signal may not only induce prolonged MC survival, but also enhance the secretion of pathological collagen I within damaged glomeruli, thereby contributing to the development of progressive GN.

6. Conclusion

The present study has revealed that phospho-ERK1/2 and phospho-ERK5 expression in the glomeruli are markedly increased in an experimental model of progressive GN. Glomerular ERK1/2 activation seems to play an important role in acute inflammation-induced cellular proliferation in the development of GN. Furthermore, the enhancement of ERK5 phosphorylation by Ang II appears to be linked to the increased MC viability and pathological ECM accumulation in the chronic glomerular lesions in GN (Fig. 4). We, therefore, propose that the controlled regulation of glomerular ERK1/2 and ERK5 activation could provide the basis for an effective therapeutic strategy for preventing the progression of GN.

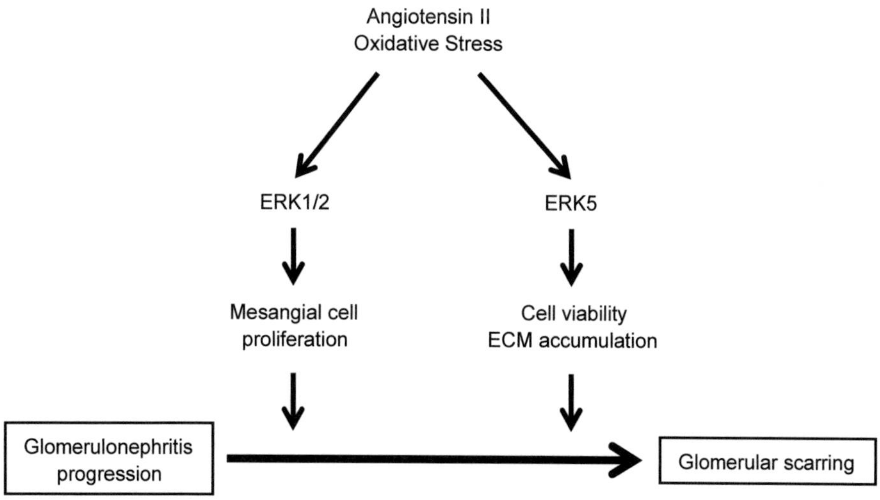

Fig. 4. ERK1/2 and ERK5 signaling during the course of progressive GN.

7. References

Abe, J.; Kusuhara, M.; Ulevitch, R.J.; Berk, B.C. & Lee, J.D. (1996). Big mitogen-activated protein kinase 1 (BMK1) is a redox-sensitive kinase. *J Biol Chem* 271, pp. 16586-16590.

Akaike, M.; Che, W.; Marmarosh, N.L.; Ohta, S.; Osawa, M.; Ding, B.; Berk, B.C.; Yan, C. & Abe, J. (2004). The hinge-helix 1 region of peroxisome proliferator-activated receptor gamma1 (PPARgamma1) mediates interaction with extracellular signal-regulated kinase 5 and PPARgamma1 transcriptional activation: involvement in flow-induced PPARgamma activation in endothelial cells. *Mol Cell Biol* 24, pp. 8691-8704.

Akaoka, K.; White, R.H. & Raafat, F. (1995). Glomerular morphometry in childhood reflux nephropathy, emphasizing the capillary changes. *Kidney Int* 47, pp. 1108-1114.

Anderson, S.; Rennke, H.G. & Brenner, B.M. (1986). Therapeutic advantage of converting enzyme inhibitors in arresting progressive renal disease associated with systemic hypertension in the rat. *J Clin Invest* 77, pp. 1993-2000.

Bokemeyer, D.; Ostendorf, T.; Kunter, U.; Lindemann, M.; Kramer, H.J. & Floege, J. (2000). Differential activation of mitogen-activated protein kinases in experimental mesangioproliferative glomerulonephritis. *J Am Soc Nephrol* 11, pp. 232-240.

Bokemeyer, D.; Panek, D.; Kramer, H.J.; Lindemann, M.; Kitahara, M.; Boor, P.; Kerjaschki, D.; Trzaskos, J.M.; Floege, J. & Ostendorf, T. (2002). In vivo identification of the mitogen-activated protein kinase cascade as a central pathogenic pathway in experimental mesangioproliferative glomerulonephritis. *J Am Soc Nephrol* 13, pp. 1473-1480.

Border, W.A. & Noble, N.A. (1997). TGF-beta in kidney fibrosis: a target for gene therapy. *Kidney Int* 51, pp. 1388-1396.

Boute, N.; Gribouval, O.; Roselli, S.; Benessy, F.; Lee, H.; Fuchshuber, A.; Dahan, K.; Gubler, M.C.; Niaudet, P. & Antignac, C. (2000). NPHS2, encoding the glomerular protein podocin, is mutated in autosomal recessive steroid-resistant nephrotic syndrome. *Nat Genet* 24, pp. 349-354.

Brenner, B.M. (1985). Nephron adaptation to renal injury or ablation. *Am J Physiol* 249, pp. F324-337.

Brunner, H.R. (1992). ACE inhibitors in renal disease. *Kidney Int* 42, pp. 463-479.

Chang, L. & Karin, M. (2001). Mammalian MAP kinase signalling cascades. *Nature* 410, pp. 37-40.

Dhanasekaran, D.N.; Kashef, K.; Lee, C.M.; Xu, H. & Reddy, E.P. (2007). Scaffold proteins of MAP-kinase modules. *Oncogene* 26, pp. 3185-3202.

Dzau, V.J. & Re, R. (1994). Tissue angiotensin system in cardiovascular medicine. A paradigm shift? *Circulation* 89, pp. 493-498.

Ferrell, J.E., Jr. (1996). Tripping the switch fantastic: how a protein kinase cascade can convert graded inputs into switch-like outputs. *Trends Biochem Sci* 21, pp. 460-466.

Giatras, I.; Lau, J. & Levey, A.S. (1997). Effect of angiotensin-converting enzyme inhibitors on the progression of nondiabetic renal disease: a meta-analysis of randomized trials. Angiotensin-Converting-Enzyme Inhibition and Progressive Renal Disease Study Group. *Ann Intern Med* 127, pp. 337-345.

Goldsmith, Z.G. & Dhanasekaran, D.N. (2007). G protein regulation of MAPK networks. *Oncogene* 26, pp. 3122-3142.

Gorin, Y.; Ricono, J.M.; Wagner, B.; Kim, N.H.; Bhandari, B.; Choudhury, G.G. & Abboud, H.E. (2004). Angiotensin II-induced ERK1/ERK2 activation and protein synthesis are redox-dependent in glomerular mesangial cells. *Biochem J* 381, pp. 231-239.

Gruden, G.; Zonca, S.; Hayward, A.; Thomas, S.; Maestrini, S.; Gnudi, L. & Viberti, G.C. (2000). Mechanical stretch-induced fibronectin and transforming growth factor-beta1 production in human mesangial cells is p38 mitogen-activated protein kinase-dependent. *Diabetes* 49, pp. 655-661.

Gupta, S.; Clarkson, M.R.; Duggan, J. & Brady, H.R. (2000). Connective tissue growth factor: potential role in glomerulosclerosis and tubulointerstitial fibrosis. *Kidney Int* 58, pp. 1389-1399.

Habib, R. (1973). Editorial: Focal glomerular sclerosis. *Kidney Int* 4, pp. 355-361.

Haseley, L.A.; Hugo, C.; Reidy, M.A. & Johnson, R.J. (1999). Dissociation of mesangial cell migration and proliferation in experimental glomerulonephritis. *Kidney Int* 56, pp. 964-972.

Hayashi, M.; Kim, S.W.; Imanaka-Yoshida, K.; Yoshida, T.; Abel, E.D.; Eliceiri, B.; Yang, Y.; Ulevitch, R.J. & Lee, J.D. (2004). Targeted deletion of BMK1/ERK5 in adult mice perturbs vascular integrity and leads to endothelial failure. *J Clin Invest* 113, pp. 1138-1148.

Hayashi, M. & Lee, J.D. (2004). Role of the BMK1/ERK5 signaling pathway: lessons from knockout mice. *J Mol Med* 82, pp. 800-808.

Horita, Y.; Tadokoro, M.; Taura, K.; Suyama, N.; Taguchi, T.; Miyazaki, M. & Kohno, S. (2004). Low-dose combination therapy with temocapril and losartan reduces proteinuria in normotensive patients with immunoglobulin a nephropathy. *Hypertens Res* 27, pp. 963-970.

Hugo, C.; Pichler, R.; Gordon, K.; Schmidt, R.; Amieva, M.; Couser, W.G.; Furthmayr, H. & Johnson, R.J. (1996). The cytoskeletal linking proteins, moesin and radixin, are upregulated by platelet-derived growth factor, but not basic fibroblast growth factor in experimental mesangial proliferative glomerulonephritis. *J Clin Invest* 97, pp. 2499-2508.

Jacobs, D.; Glossip, D.; Xing, H.; Muslin, A.J. & Kornfeld, K. (1999). Multiple docking sites on substrate proteins form a modular system that mediates recognition by ERK MAP kinase. *Genes Dev* 13, pp. 163-175.

Johnson, R.J. (1994). The glomerular response to injury: progression or resolution? *Kidney Int* 45, pp. 1769-1782.

Kagami, S.; Border, W.A.; Miller, D.E. & Noble, N.A. (1994). Angiotensin II stimulates extracellular matrix protein synthesis through induction of transforming growth factor-beta expression in rat glomerular mesangial cells. *J Clin Invest* 93, pp. 2431-2437.

Kagami, S.; Urushihara, M.; Kitamura, A.; Kondo, S.; Hisayama, T.; Kitamura, M.; Loster, K.; Reutter, W. & Kuroda, Y. (2004). PDGF-BB enhances alpha1beta1 integrin-mediated activation of the ERK/AP-1 pathway involved in collagen matrix remodeling by rat mesangial cells. *J Cell Physiol* 198, pp. 470-478.

Kagami, S.; Urushihara, M.; Kondo, S.; Loster, K.; Reutter, W.; Tamaki, T.; Yoshizumi, M. & Kuroda, Y. (2001). Requirement for tyrosine kinase-ERK1/2 signaling in alpha 1 beta 1 integrin-mediated collagen matrix remodeling by rat mesangial cells. *Exp Cell Res* 268, pp. 274-283.

Kamakura, S.; Moriguchi, T. & Nishida, E. (1999). Activation of the protein kinase ERK5/BMK1 by receptor tyrosine kinases. Identification and characterization of a signaling pathway to the nucleus. *J Biol Chem* 274, pp. 26563-26571.

Kaplan, J.M.; Kim, S.H.; North, K.N.; Rennke, H.; Correia, L.A.; Tong, H.Q.; Mathis, B.J.; Rodriguez-Perez, J.C.; Allen, P.G.; Beggs, A.H., *et al.* (2000). Mutations in ACTN4, encoding alpha-actinin-4, cause familial focal segmental glomerulosclerosis. *Nat Genet* 24, pp. 251-256.

Kasler, H.G.; Victoria, J.; Duramad, O. & Winoto, A. (2000). ERK5 is a novel type of mitogen-activated protein kinase containing a transcriptional activation domain. *Mol Cell Biol* 20, pp. 8382-8389.

Kato, Y.; Chao, T.H.; Hayashi, M.; Tapping, R.I. & Lee, J.D. (2000). Role of BMK1 in regulation of growth factor-induced cellular responses. *Immunol Res* 21, pp. 233-237.

Kato, Y.; Kravchenko, V.V.; Tapping, R.I.; Han, J.; Ulevitch, R.J. & Lee, J.D. (1997). BMK1/ERK5 regulates serum-induced early gene expression through transcription factor MEF2C. *EMBO J* 16, pp. 7054-7066.

Kohan, D.E. (1998). Angiotensin II and endothelin in chronic glomerulonephritis. *Kidney Int* 54, pp. 646-647.

Krepinsky, J.C.; Ingram, A.J.; Tang, D.; Wu, D.; Liu, L. & Scholey, J.W. (2003). Nitric oxide inhibits stretch-induced MAPK activation in mesangial cells through RhoA inactivation. *J Am Soc Nephrol* 14, pp. 2790-2800.

Kyriakis, J.M. & Avruch, J. (2001). Mammalian mitogen-activated protein kinase signal transduction pathways activated by stress and inflammation. *Physiol Rev* 81, pp. 807-869.

Lafayette, R.A.; Mayer, G.; Park, S.K. & Meyer, T.W. (1992). Angiotensin II receptor blockade limits glomerular injury in rats with reduced renal mass. *J Clin Invest* 90, pp. 766-771.

Ledbetter, S.; Copeland, E.J.; Noonan, D.; Vogeli, G. & Hassell, J.R. (1990). Altered steady-state mRNA levels of basement membrane proteins in diabetic mouse kidneys and thromboxane synthase inhibition. *Diabetes* 39, pp. 196-203.

Lee, J.D.; Ulevitch, R.J. & Han, J. (1995a). Primary structure of BMK1: a new mammalian map kinase. *Biochem Biophys Res Commun* 213, pp. 715-724.

Lee, L.K.; Meyer, T.W.; Pollock, A.S. & Lovett, D.H. (1995b). Endothelial cell injury initiates glomerular sclerosis in the rat remnant kidney. *J Clin Invest* 96, pp. 953-964.

Masaki, T.; Stambe, C.; Hill, P.A.; Dowling, J.; Atkins, R.C. & Nikolic-Paterson, D.J. (2004). Activation of the extracellular-signal regulated protein kinase pathway in human glomerulopathies. *J Am Soc Nephrol* 15, pp. 1835-1843.

McKay, M.M. & Morrison, D.K. (2007). Integrating signals from RTKs to ERK/MAPK. *Oncogene* 26, pp. 3113-3121.

Mezzano, S.A.; Ruiz-Ortega, M. & Egido, J. (2001). Angiotensin II and renal fibrosis. *Hypertension* 38, pp. 635-638.

Morrison, D.K. & Davis, R.J. (2003). Regulation of MAP kinase signaling modules by scaffold proteins in mammals. *Annu Rev Cell Dev Biol* 19, pp. 91-118.

Mulloy, R.; Salinas, S.; Philips, A. & Hipskind, R.A. (2003). Activation of cyclin D1 expression by the ERK5 cascade. *Oncogene* 22, pp. 5387-5398.

Nakamura, T.; Obata, J.; Kimura, H.; Ohno, S.; Yoshida, Y.; Kawachi, H. & Shimizu, F. (1999). Blocking angiotensin II ameliorates proteinuria and glomerular lesions in progressive mesangioproliferative glomerulonephritis. *Kidney Int* 55, pp. 877-889.

Navar, L.G.; Harrison-Bernard, L.M.; Imig, J.D.; Wang, C.T.; Cervenka, L. & Mitchell, K.D. (1999). Intrarenal angiotensin II generation and renal effects of AT1 receptor blockade. *J Am Soc Nephrol* 10 Suppl 12, pp. S266-272.

Nishimoto, S. & Nishida, E. (2006). MAPK signalling: ERK5 versus ERK1/2. *EMBO Rep* 7, pp. 782-786.

Patrakka, J.; Kestila, M.; Wartiovaara, J.; Ruotsalainen, V.; Tissari, P.; Lenkkeri, U.; Mannikko, M.; Visapaa, I.; Holmberg, C.; Rapola, J., *et al.* (2000). Congenital nephrotic syndrome (NPHS1): features resulting from different mutations in Finnish patients. *Kidney Int* 58, pp. 972-980.

Pearson, G.; Robinson, F.; Beers Gibson, T.; Xu, B.E.; Karandikar, M.; Berman, K. & Cobb, M.H. (2001). Mitogen-activated protein (MAP) kinase pathways: regulation and physiological functions. *Endocr Rev* 22, pp. 153-183.

Prols, F.; Hartner, A.; Schocklmann, H.O. & Sterzel, R.B. (1999). Mesangial cells and their adhesive properties. *Exp Nephrol* 7, pp. 137-146.

Raman, M.; Chen, W. & Cobb, M.H. (2007). Differential regulation and properties of MAPKs. *Oncogene* 26, pp. 3100-3112.

Ramos, J.W. (2008). The regulation of extracellular signal-regulated kinase (ERK) in mammalian cells. *Int J Biochem Cell Biol* 40, pp. 2707-2719.

Ravid, M.; Brosh, D.; Levi, Z.; Bar-Dayan, Y.; Ravid, D. & Rachmani, R. (1998). Use of enalapril to attenuate decline in renal function in normotensive, normoalbuminuric patients with type 2 diabetes mellitus. A randomized, controlled trial. *Ann Intern Med* 128, pp. 982-988.

Remenyi, A.; Good, M.C.; Bhattacharyya, R.P. & Lim, W.A. (2005). The role of docking interactions in mediating signaling input, output, and discrimination in the yeast MAPK network. *Mol Cell* 20, pp. 951-962.

Rose, B.A.; Force, T. & Wang, Y. (2010). Mitogen-activated protein kinase signaling in the heart: angels versus demons in a heart-breaking tale. *Physiol Rev* 90, pp. 1507-1546.

Ruiz-Ortega, M. & Egido, J. (1997). Angiotensin II modulates cell growth-related events and synthesis of matrix proteins in renal interstitial fibroblasts. *Kidney Int* 52, pp. 1497-1510.

Rupprecht, H.D.; Schocklmann, H.O. & Sterzel, R.B. (1996). Cell-matrix interactions in the glomerular mesangium. *Kidney Int* 49, pp. 1575-1582.

Schnaper, H.W.; Hayashida, T.; Hubchak, S.C. & Poncelet, A.C. (2003). TGF-beta signal transduction and mesangial cell fibrogenesis. *Am J Physiol Renal Physiol* 284, pp. F243-252.

Schnaper, H.W. & Kopp, J.B. (2003). Renal fibrosis. *Front Biosci* 8, pp. e68-86.

Shih, N.Y.; Li, J.; Karpitskii, V.; Nguyen, A.; Dustin, M.L.; Kanagawa, O.; Miner, J.H. & Shaw, A.S. (1999). Congenital nephrotic syndrome in mice lacking CD2-associated protein. *Science* 286, pp. 312-315.

Shimizu, A.; Kitamura, H.; Masuda, Y.; Ishizaki, M.; Sugisaki, Y. & Yamanaka, N. (1995). Apoptosis in the repair process of experimental proliferative glomerulonephritis. *Kidney Int* 47, pp. 114-121.

Squires, M.S.; Nixon, P.M. & Cook, S.J. (2002). Cell-cycle arrest by PD184352 requires inhibition of extracellular signal-regulated kinases (ERK) 1/2 but not ERK5/BMK1. *Biochem J* 366, pp. 673-680.

Srivastava, T.; Garola, R.E.; Whiting, J.M. & Alon, U.S. (2001). Synaptopodin expression in idiopathic nephrotic syndrome of childhood. *Kidney Int* 59, pp. 118-125.

Suzaki, Y.; Yoshizumi, M.; Kagami, S.; Nishiyama, A.; Ozawa, Y.; Kyaw, M.; Izawa, Y.; Kanematsu, Y.; Tsuchiya, K. & Tamaki, T. (2004). BMK1 is activated in glomeruli of diabetic rats and in mesangial cells by high glucose conditions. *Kidney Int* 65, pp. 1749-1760.

Urushihara, M.; Takamatsu, M.; Shimizu, M.; Kondo, S.; Kinoshita, Y.; Suga, K.; Kitamura, A.; Matsuura, S.; Yoshizumi, M.; Tamaki, T., *et al.* (2010). ERK5 activation enhances mesangial cell viability and collagen matrix accumulation in rat progressive glomerulonephritis. *Am J Physiol Renal Physiol* 298, pp. F167-176.

Wang, X. & Tournier, C. (2006). Regulation of cellular functions by the ERK5 signalling pathway. *Cell Signal* 18, pp. 753-760.

Zhou, G.; Bao, Z.Q. & Dixon, J.E. (1995). Components of a new human protein kinase signal transduction pathway. *J Biol Chem* 270, pp. 12665-12669.

Part 4

Role of Cells and Organelles in Glomerulonephritis

12

Dendritic Cells: Two-Edged Swords in Pathogenesis of Autoimmune Glomerulonephritis

Yahuan Lou
Department of Diagnostic Sciences,
University of Texas Health Science Center at Houston,
USA

1. Introduction

Direct involvement of $CD4^+$ T cells in the pathogenesis of inflammatory glomerulonephritis such as Anti-GBM glomerulonephritis and other glomerular diseases of autoimmune nature, has been well demonstrated. Unlike antibody mediated mechanisms, regulation and/or activation of T cells requires antigen presenting cells (APC) such as dendritic cells (DC). DCs are critical for activation of pathogenic T cells, or for establishing T cell-mediated glomerular inflammation by presenting local self antigens to pathogenic T cells. Thus, recent studies have been focusing on identification of DCs and their functions in various human autoimmune glomerulonephritis or in animal models. Similar to other human autoimmune diseases, DCs involved in glomerulonephritis include diverse subpopulations, which have either pro- or anti-inflammatory functions. Understanding especially their anti-inflammatory function may lead to development of new therapeutic strategies by mimicking those natural mechanisms. Mounting evidence shows the presence of tolerogenic DCs (tDCs) in various kidney diseases, which are involved in inhibition of autoimmunity by elimination or skewing development of self reactive T cells. Several new types of DCs have been characterized in animal models. Among them, one type of tDC may arrest an existing glomerular inflammatory process. This novel tDC specifically infiltrates glomeruli under autoimmune attack and induces apoptosis in auto-reactive T cells, leading to natural recovery in certain strains of animals. Thus, this tDC is an attractive target in cellular immunotherapy for glomerulonephritis by mimicking this natural recovery mechanism.

2. What are dendritic cells (DCs)?

Adaptive immunity, which is unique to vertebrates, is much more efficient than innate immunity, which is common among all types of animals. The high effectiveness of adaptive immunity is due to its specifically defined recognition of any given antigen. Only two types of immune cells in adaptive immunity, B cells and T cells, are capable of such antigen recognition through specified receptors. In T cells, their antigen recognition receptor is the T cell receptor (TcR); in B cells, their receptor is called the B cell receptor (BcR), which in fact is a membrane-bound antibody. Unlike innate immunity, B cells and T cells do not discriminate molecular motifs of microbial antigens from other antigens, and thus, they do not directly recognize microbial antigens, or in a broader meaning, any antigens, by themselves. Rather, they acquire antigen-recognition capacity through "education" by other immune cells. The most important process during "education" is antigen presentation, which is carried out by so-called antigen presenting cells (APCs). In this chapter, we will focus solely on APCs for $CD4^+$ T cells, since $CD4^+$ T cells play a central role in adaptive immunity, inflammatory diseases and autoimmunity including those occurring in glomeruli. A group of phagocytes can present antigens to $CD4^+$ T cells (although B cells can act as APC to $CD4^+$ T cells, it will be excluded in this chapter). We call these phagocytes "professional" APCs since their principal function is to present antigens. These phagocytes, which include monocytes, macrophages and dendritic cells, capture especially microbial antigens through their motif/pattern recognition receptors such as toll like receptors (TLRs). The captured antigens are processed into peptides, which then are presented to $CD4^+$ T cells in a complex of MHC II molecules and antigenic peptides. Thus, these professional APCs function as messengers or connections between innate and adaptive immunity: they capture antigens from microbial pathogens and use these antigens to "educate" T cells and B cells. As a result, a group of T or B cells which solely recognize this antigen would be activated to fight the original pathogens in a more effective way.

The DCs has been recognized as the most potent professional APCs since its discovery three decades ago. So far, immunologists believe that DCs are the only APCs that are able to initiate/direct an adaptive immunity by activation of naïve T cells, because DCs express special signaling molecules called co-stimulatory molecules, such as CD80 and CD86, in addition to their superb capacity in capturing and presenting antigens (1). From this point of view, DCs are also considered a critical immunoregulator. DC was first identified as a population of striking dendritic-shaped cells in the spleen by Ralph Steinman in the 1970s (2). It soon became clear that cells similar to the splenic DCs are present in all lymphoid and non-lymphoid tissues, though in a much smaller number than macrophages. However, soon immunologists realized that DCs in fact are a heterogenic group of phagocytes, which may be generated from different lineages. It seems less arguable that DCs are generated from bone marrow stem cells. As many distinct subtypes of DCs have been described or discovered, it seems difficult to give a simple definition for DCs.

What are DCs? Why did we name certain immune cells DCs? There are several common characteristics shared by the cells, which have been named as DCs (3). *First*, DCs are usually of hematopoietic origin and grow branched projections called dendrites that give the cell its name (δένδρον or déndron in Greek means "tree") at certain development/activation stages. Development of cellular projections greatly increases their cell surface area for contacting/ capturing antigens. *Second*, they are potent professional APCs, and in many cases, they can activate naïve T cells. Their APC function can be reflected by their expression of MHC II, which can be further up-regulated after stimulations, in addition to "dendrite' like cellular projections, which would increase the cell surface area for capturing antigens. In some DCs or at certain activation stages, they also express co-stimulatory molecules for T cells (4). *Third*, they also express multiple "pattern recognition receptors" such as TLRs for recognition of microbial antigens.

Different DCs migrate following a special pattern through circulation, tissue and lymphoid organs (Figure 1) (5). Thus, they express certain sets of chemokine receptors and adhesion molecule. For example, all mouse DCs express an adhesion molecules CD11c. Immature DCs or DC precursors are often found in the peripheral blood before they exit the circulation. As a first line of immune defense, DCs, such as conventional DCs, are present in tissues in contact with the external environment, such as the skin and the mucosal system.

They are actively motile and continuously sample their surroundings. Once activated after encountering invading pathogens or antigens, they migrate to the lymphoid organs where they interact with T cells and B cells to initiate and shape the adaptive immune response. However, this typical migration route may not fit to all types of DCs. For example, plasmocytoid DCs directly enter lymph nodes (6).

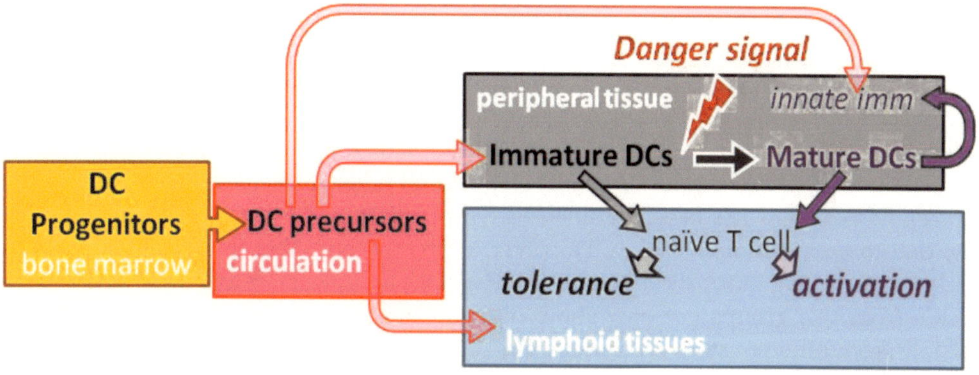

Fig. 1. Schematic diagram shows circulation of DCs, from bone marrow progenitors, precursor in circulation and immature DCs in peripheral tissues and mature DCs in lymphoid organs. This route is representative. Not all DCs migrate or mature as shown.

3. DC classification

Because of the high levels of heterogeneity among identified subsets or types of DCs, their classification is not an easy task for immunologists. DCs have been grouped by their function, lineage, markers, and migration route or residing tissues. *First*, DCs can be grouped by their locations and migration route. DCs and DC precursors can be found in the circulation, and in different anatomic locations, including lymphoid or non-lymphoid tissues. Langerhans cells are a well characterized DC residing in the skin (7). DCs in the interstitial tissue including renal tissue are named IntDC. DCs also populate the entire mucosa system. Those tissue-residing DCs develop from DC precursors in the circulation, and act as "scouts" to detect any invading antigens. Once loaded with antigens, those DCs migrate into afferent lymph, and they are called veiled cells. After migrating through the afferent lymphatic system, they are called interdigitating DCs (IDCs) in T cell areas in the paracortex of lymph nodes. IDCs may activate naïve T cells there. In lymphoid tissue, many DCs are present in the Germinal Center (GC, where B cells differentiate) and are called GC DCs, which function as a strong APC for activating T cells and B cells. In GC, there is a type of cell called follicular DC (fDC). fDC presents antigens to B cells using a totally different mechanism, and thus, is not a typical DC discussed in this chapter. *Second*, DCs have been classified by their lineage (8). For example, the terms "lymphoid DC" and "myeloid or monocyte-related" DC are used for those DCs, which probably differentiate from the same bone marrow stem cells as lymphocytes or monocytes, respectively. However, this classification is largely based on similarity in morphology and surface markers between the cells. Results from *in vitro* differentiation experiments or experiments to identify special differentiation pathways in bone marrow stem cells or DC precursors have provided some evidence to support some DCs' lineage. *Third*, more accurate classifications of DCs that are based on a combination of their lineage, markers and function, and thus, are much more complicated, as well as some times controversial. There are several classification methods for mouse DCs, since various DCs have been well characterized in mice. It seems impossible for this chapter to cover all those classifications for DCs. Furthermore, those classifications may not be able to recover or describe several newly discovered DCs. To avoid confusion, this chapter will mainly introduce one representative classification for mouse DCs which reside in the lymphoid organs, recently summarized by Sato and Fujita (9). Despite the difficulty in comparison of the DC systems between humans and mice, recent work has revealed much common ground (10). We will then compare mouse DCs to their human counterparts.

Mouse DCs are primarily defined by their surface MHC II and CD11c in combination with CD4, CD8αα, CD11b (a myeloid marker) and several other molecules such as CD205 (IDC marker). $CD8\alpha\alpha^+$ DC has been classified as lymphoid DCs, while $CD8\alpha\alpha^-$ DC as myeloid DCs, due to their possible lineage. However, currently, both mouse and human DCs are divided into two big groups: conventional DCs (cDC) and plasmacytoid DCs (pDC) (Figure 2). DCs from two groups not only show different migration routes, but also differentiate probably from different stem cells with quite different functions. In mice, DCs in lymphoid organs have been best characterized. Mouse cDCs in lymphoid tissues can be further divided into five subsets largely based on their CD4 and CD8 expression and their location in different lymphoid tissues. There are three subsets of cDCs in the spleen, which include two of myeloid origin with phenotypes of $CD4^+CD205^-CD11b^+$ and $CD4^-CD8\alpha^-CD205^-CD11b^+$, and one of lymphoid origin with a phenotype of $CD8\alpha\alpha^+CD205^+CD11b^-$ (Figure 2)(11). It needs to be pointed out that "myeloid origin" in this chapter are not equal to "myeloid DC (mDC)", which has been widely used in other classification methods. We will explain the difference later. Each subset shows various functions, which are demonstrated largely by *in vitro* experiments (Figure 2). Both DC subsets of myeloid origin (i.e. $CD11b^+$) in the spleen (some times in lymph nodes as well) express F4/80 (a well known marker for mature macrophages). $F4/80^+$ cDCs are located in the marginal zone between white and red pulp and will migrate to the T-cell area after stimulation. Both splenic $CD8\alpha\alpha^-$ DCs of myeloid origin are able to stimulate $CD4^+$ and $CD8^+$ T cells and to initiate a Th2-type T cell response (12). Splenic DCs of lymphoid origin ($CD8\alpha\alpha^+CD205^+CD11b^-$) are found in the T-cell area; a smaller number of this cDC may also exist in lymph nodes. Interestingly, this DC is a dominant subset among thymic DCs. Several *in vitro* experiments showed that this cDC can function both as a regulator and stimulator of T cells. Although it can stimulate both $CD4^+$ and $CD8^+$ T cells, it subsequently restricts T cell proliferation by either inducing apoptosis in $CD4^+$ T cells, or limiting endogenous cytokine production in $CD8^+$ T cells. Those results suggest that this cDC subset may be responsible for maintenance of T cell tolerance in lymphoid organs in the absence of infection (13). In contrast, other studies suggest this subset cDC to be a potent T cell stimulator. This $CD8\alpha\alpha^+$ lymphoid cDC can activate both $CD4^+$ or, through cross-presentation, $CD8^+$ cytotoxic T cells. More importantly, this DC can trigger the development of a Th1 response *in vivo*, which is in agreement with the fact that activated $CD8\alpha\alpha^+$ lymphoid cDCs are the major source of the Th1-promoting cytokine interleukin-12 (IL-12)(14). In addition to the above three subsets of DCs, there are two extra myeloid DC subsets only found in lymph nodes (Figure 2). In fact, these cDCs are mature DCs which have migrated from peripheral tissues to lymph nodes through the lymphatic system after they are loaded with antigens. The first subset has a $CD4^-CD8\alpha^-CD205^+CD11b^+$ phenotype, which is the mature form of interstitial tissue DCs (IntDCs), and the second subset is $CD8\alpha^{low}CD205^+CD11b^+$, which matures from skin-associated Langerhans cells. Migration of Langerhans cells is restricted to the skin-draining lymph nodes, and thus, $CD8\alpha^{low}CD205^+CD11b^+$ cDCs are found only in skin draining lymph nodes. On the other hand, IntDCs associated $CD4^-CD8\alpha^-CD205^+CD11b^+$ cDC may be found in all lymph nodes. Because of their migration to lymphoid tissues, Langerhans cells and IntDCs are often called "migratory DCs". Mature Langerhans cells (i.e. the $CD8\alpha^{low}CD205^+CD11b^+$ cDC subset) in lymph nodes express characteristic langerin together with high levels of MHC II and co-stimulatory molecules, representing a typical fully activated DC, which can effectively stimulate naïve $CD4^+$ T cells to differentiate into Th1 T cells (15). A constant migration of interstitial tissue immature DC to lymph nodes occurs even in the absence of invading pathogens at steady-state. Since presentation of antigens by immature or semi-mature DCs may lead to unresponsiveness of T cells, the migration of tissue DCs at a steady-state is believed to be critical for the DCs' involvement in the maintenance of peripheral tolerance (16). Before we sum up the classification of cDCs, it is necessary to clarify the terms "myeloid DCs (mDCs)" from DCs with "myeloid origin" described above. The term mDC has been widely used to describe a subset of DCs, which are believed to be from the same lineage of monocytes or macrophages. Some studies revealed that mDCs have at least two subsets: very common mDC-1 and rare mDC-2. However, more recent studies suggest that the mDCs are most likely equivalences of subsets of cDC with myeloid origins in the above classification. For example, mDC is the major source of IL-12. Several recent studies also thought the concept of mDC to be inappropriate (17). Thus, we try to avoid using the term mDC.

pDC is a distinct type of DC, which is characteristically different from cDCs (Figure 2). pDCs are found mainly in the spleen, as well as in bone marrow, thymus and lymph nodes (18). Historically, pDC was first identified in humans, which shared several characteristics with plasma cells (terminally differentiated B cells which secrete antibodies)(19). In fact, freshly isolated pDCs have a morphology which is big and round with only a few dendrites and very different from that of a typical DC. Furthermore, pDCs express B220 (a marker for mouse B cells) and Gr-1, together with CD8α, CD11c, CD205 and MHC II. Recently, additional surface markers, such as mPDCA-1 for mouse pDCs have been identified. While cDC subsets migrate into lymph nodes from tissues, pDCs enter lymph nodes directly from circulation by crossing the high endothelial venule (HEV) using the adhesion molecule CD62L. Freshly isolated pDCs lack expression of co-stimulatory molecules, and show poor capacity to stimulate naïve T cells, suggesting their potential role in the maintenance of peripheral tolerance under steady-state conditions. Although *in vitro* activated pDCs are capable of simulation of T cells by up-regulation of expression of MHC II, CD8α, and co-stimulatory molecules, this capacity is not in the range compatible to that of cDCs. On the other hand, mouse pDCs produce a large quantity of type I interferon (IFN) following a viral infection, suggesting its important role in antiviral responses rather than the APC function in initiation of a T cell response (10, 20). The lineage of mouse pDCs remains controversial. Recent studies showed complicity of pDC lineage, suggesting that its precursor cell may represent a unique hematopoietic lineage with high flexibility in its differentiation. Nevertheless, Flt3L (a cytokine) has been identified to be a major cytokine for the development of pDCs from hematopoietic stem cells (21).

	Tissues	*Subsets*	*Anatomic location*	*Major functions*
Mice		**cDCs**		
		$CD4^-CD8\alpha^{high}$ lymphoid	Spleen T cell area	Th1, cross-presentation
		$CD4^-CD8\alpha^-$ myeloid	Spleen marginal zone	Th2
		$CD4^+CD8\alpha^-$ myeloid	Spleen marginal zone	Th2
	$CD4^-CD8\alpha^-$ LC in skin →	$CD4^-CD8\alpha^{low}$ myeloid	Skin draining LN	Th1
	$CD4^-CD8\alpha^-$ IntDC →	$CD4^-CD8\alpha^-$ IDC myeloid	All LN	Th1/Th2?
		pDCs (IPC)		
		$CD4^{var}CD8\alpha^{var}$ myeloid/ lymphoid	Peripheral lymphoid sheaths	INF-α/β
Humans		**cDCs**		
		DNGR-1$^+$BDCA3$^+$	Spleen	= mouse $CD8\alpha^{high}$ cDC?
	$CD4^+CD1a^+CD11c^{high}$ LC ←	$CD4^+CD1a^+CD11c^{high}$ myeloid	Circulation	Th1 & Th2
	$CD4^+CD1a^-CD11c^{low}$ IntDC ←	$CD4^+CD1a^-CD11c^{low}$ myeloid	Circulation	Th1 & Th2
		pDCs (IPC)		
		$CD4^+CD1a^+CD11c^-$ lymphoid	Peripheral lymphoid sheaths	INF-α/β, Th1/Th2, tolerance

Fig. 2. Simplified classification of DC subsets in humans and mice. Each subset is named by its major markers. Their anatomic locations and major functions are listed for reference. Arrows indicate differentiation direction. *IDC*, interdigitating DC; *IntDC*, interstitial tissue DC; *IPC*, natural IFN-producing cell; *LC*, Langerhans cell; *LN*, lymph node.

Human DCs, especially those residing in the lymphoid organs, have not been characterized as well as those in mice because peripheral blood samples or, in some cases, fetus umbilical cord blood samples, are some times the only readily available source. In rare cases, investigators used human DCs isolated from lymphoid tissues, ranging from the tonsil, thymus, and spleen. Thus, human DCs from peripheral blood will be discussed for their classification. Similar to mouse DCs, human DCs also fall into two distinct groups: human cDC and pDC (9). Although all human cDCs express CD11c, human pDC does not. Thus, unlike for mouse DCs, CD11c is not a common marker for human DCs. In addition, because of a lack of available materials, migration route and maturation of human DCs are less understood. More studies are needed. Nevertheless, for human cDCs, two subsets with myeloid origin have been described in peripheral blood samples thus far, both of which co-express CD11b and CD11c (Figure 2). In addition to common CD11b, CD11c, CD4, and MHC II, the two human cDCs in the blood can be distinguished by other markers: the $CD1a^+$BDCA-1/$CD1c^+$ $CD11c^{high}$ subset and the $CD1a^-$BDCA-3/$CD141^+$ $CD11c^{low}$ subset (22, 23). These two human myeloid cDC subsets show the capacity to stimulate T cells; this capacity will be further augmented in the presence of the cytokine granulocyte-macrophage colony stimulating factor (GM-CSF). *In vitro* experiments showed that under certain culture conditions, these $CD1a^+$BDCA-1/$CD1c^+$ $CD11c^{high}$ subset would differentiate into the cells, which expressed several molecules such as langerin and displayed typical Birbeck granule characteristics of Langerhan cells, suggesting this subset to be the precursor of Langerhans cells. On the other hand, the $CD1a^-$BDCA-3/$CD141^+$ $CD11c^{low}$ subset may be the direct precursors of IntDCs (24). However, this classification is merely based on markers, and may not reflect their lineage but their maturation status. As described above, these two human cDC subsets in the blood, in fact, are precursors of cDCs before their migration into tissue. Therefore, it is difficult to compare human cDCs to mouse cDCs, because of different locations.

Human pDCs share many common features with mouse pDCs. As we mentioned above, pDCs were first identified in humans as a rare type of cells in the paracortical areas in active lymph nodes with a morphology similar to plasma cells. However, this cell also expressed several markers for T cells and monocytes, and thus, it originally was named as plasmacytoid T cell or plasmacytoid monocyte. Recent studies have demonstrated that plasmacytoid monocytes, natural IFN-producing cells (IPCs), and immature DCs in peripheral blood and tonsils turn out to be the same cell known as the pDCs (Figure 2). Similar to mouse pDCs, human pDCs are of lymphoid origin and they poorly stimulate T cells. However, they could differentiate into IDC-like cells and acquire the ability to activate naïve T cells in the presence of IL-3 and CD40L. More studies show that pDCs not only can provoke a Th1 or Th2 responses, but also induce immune tolerance *in vivo* (25). Similar to its mouse counterpart, it can produce large amounts of type I IFN in response to certain viruses (19). Cytokines Flt3L and G-CSF are required for generation and differentiation of pDCs, respectively (26). Administration of Flt3L dramatically increases both myeloid cDCs and pDCs, whereas G-CSF only increases pDCs.

As we described above, all identified human DCs, including cDCs and pDCs, may express CD4, but never CD8. Mouse CD8$\alpha\alpha^+$ DCs have several special functions that other DCs lack in regulation of the T cell response. Hence, they become a promising target for clinical application to manipulate immune responses in autoimmune diseases, organ grafting, and vaccination. Failure of decades-long searching to identify human CD8$\alpha\alpha^+$ DCs has led to question whether CD8$\alpha\alpha^+$ cDCs may exist in humans. However, a recent paper may have made a breakthrough in identifying a human counterpart of mouse CD8$\alpha\alpha^+$ DC; this study identified a population of human DNGR-1$^+$BDCA-3$^+$ leukocytes in the spleen (27). Although this cell lacked expression of CD8, it shares many other markers/molecules, as well as several special functions, with mouse CD8$\alpha\alpha^+$ DCs. It is highly possible that this cell is equivalent to mouse CD8$\alpha\alpha^+$ DCs.

4. Roles of DCs in promoting autoimmunity and immune tolerance

It remains not fully understood how T cells and B cells decide to mount a response to a given antigen. In theory, adaptive immunity is able to mount an immune response to any given antigen, including self antigens, because it does not discriminate self or non-self antigens, or microbial antigens. Yet, our adaptive immune system normally does not respond to self antigens. In other words, the immune system seems to "ignore" the presence of self antigens. However, such unresponsiveness to, or ignorance of, self antigens is neither natural nor inherent. Rather, it is an acquired process. The process for T cells or B cells to actively "ignore" the presence of an antigen is called immune tolerance. If immune tolerance is toward self antigens, it is simply called self tolerance.

The immune system possesses a network of complicated tolerance mechanisms to avoid immune response against all potential self antigens. Self tolerance mechanisms could occur at three levels. The first level is evolutionary. Special molecular patterns of microbes have evolutionally led to the generation of pattern recognition receptors on innate immune cells, which effectively bind to certain microbial molecules. We will not discuss this level of tolerance in this chapter, as it is not related to adaptive immunity. The second level of self tolerance mechanisms occurs prior to or during activation of naïve self reactive T cells. The mechanisms at this level would eliminate pathogenic self reactive T cells, or skew their activation, and thus avoid autoimmunity *de novo*. The majority of known self tolerance mechanisms act at this level. Those mechanisms can be further divided into two categories: central tolerance, which occurs in central lymphoid organs such as the thymus and bone marrow, or peripheral tolerance which occurs mainly in peripheral lymphoid organs. The third level of tolerance mechanisms occurs post activation of pathogenic T cells or after pathogenic T cells have initiated autoimmune tissue damage. This level of tolerance is less explored and thus, remains largely unknown. Failure in tolerance (or a break in self tolerance) to a self antigen at any level is a prerequisite for occurrence of autoimmunity.

With capacities in both promoting and inhibiting autoimmunity, DCs are considered one of the most critical manipulators/regulators in autoimmunity versus immune tolerance. Because DCs are the only APC capable of activating naïve T cells, they first play a pivotal role in breaking self tolerance in T cells as well as supporting autoimmune responses during pathogenesis of autoimmune diseases (28-30). On the other hand, numerous studies have shown that subsets of DCs, or DCs at different maturation stages, function as tolerance inducers by down-regulation of self reactive immune responses, or by skewing activation of a self reactive T cell toward a phenotype related with immune tolerance (29-31). Those DCs are named tolerogenic DCs (tDCs) (Figure 3)(32, 33). A single type of DCs may function as both an activator of an immune response or a tolerance inducer, depending on their maturation/activation status or even their location (33). In other cases, a special subset of DC may act as tDCs and play a sole role in immune tolerance.

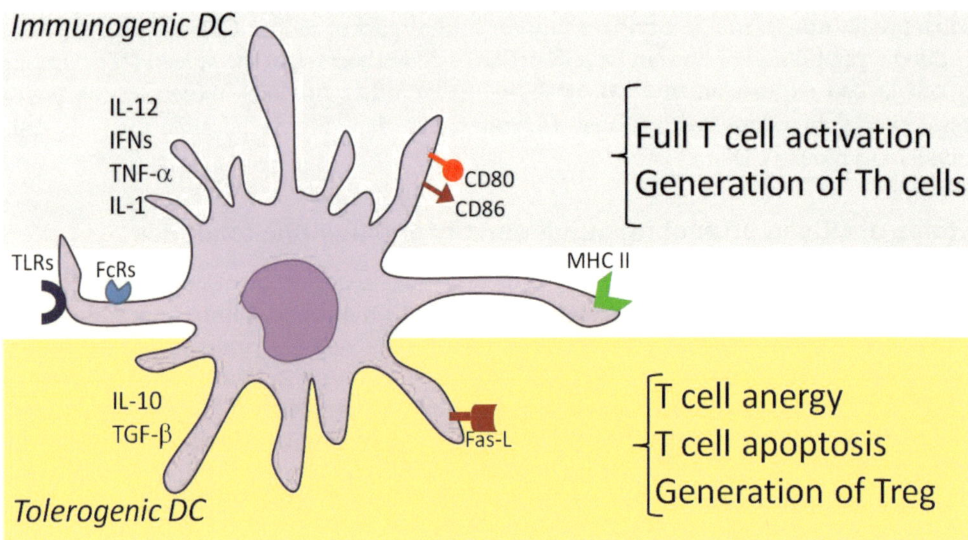

Fig. 3. Comparison of immunogenic DC and tolerogenic DC (tDC). Fates of T cells after their interaction with DCs are shown at the right. Note the differences in expression of co-stimulatory molecules and cytokines. *TLR*, Toll-like receptor; *FcR*, Fc receptor.

Due to their special functions in immunoregulation, DCs have been long investigated for their roles in autoimmune diseases since their discovery. As mentioned in the last paragraph, it is clear that DCs could be pathogenic or protective in autoimmune diseases. From this point of view, DCs can be divided into two groups based on their functions during an autoimmune response: immunogenic DCs, which provoke an autoimmune response to an antigen, and tDCs, which induce tolerance to an antigen. A balance between the two DCs is the key to determine if autoimmunity will occur. Thus, alterations in either DCs due to genetic milieu or environmental factors may lead to unbalance, resulting in autoimmunity.

In the early years after discovery of DCs, investigations mainly focused on DCs' function in promotion or initiation of autoimmunity. It seems there are no arguments that DCs are required to activate naïve self reactive T cells, which is a pivotal player in manifestation of autoimmune diseases. DCs are the only known APCs which are capable of eliciting autoimmune responses and/or autoimmune diseases. In addition, unique functions of DCs in target tissues may further enhance autoimmune inflammation through coordinating recruitment and activation of other immune players. Those early studies have elegantly provided direct evidential support that DCs are a critical player especially in the initiation stage of autoimmunity in animal models such as experimental allergic encephalomyelitis (EAE) models for multiple sclerosis (MS) and non-obese (NOD) model for Type I diabetes. For example, transfer of DCs, which were engineered to constitutively express a T-cell epitope of a model antigen, induced destruction of the β–islet, where this model antigen was expressed (34). In an EAE model, DCs were pulsed *in vitro* with a T cell epitope of well known self antigen for MS called myelin basic protein; transfer of the DCs into untreated mice resulted in MS like symptoms (35). In addition, the role of DCs in autoimmune diseases was indirectly demonstrated, in part, by examination of DCs in tissues of human autoimmune patients. For example, a high number of DCs were detectable in the serum and synovial fluid of patients with various autoimmune diseases such as rheumatoid arthritis, Sjogren's syndrome, multiple sclerosis, thyroiditis and diabetes (36-38). One study further showed a positive association between high levels of circulating DCs secreting pro-inflammatory cytokines with severity of multiple sclerosis (39).

However, unlike in an immune response to invading organisms, the mechanisms for activation of naïve reactive T cells by a DC in an autoimmune response are unique and thus, are a main focus of investigations. Several mechanisms, by which DCs activate pathogenic T cells, have been revealed in the past. *First*, DCs will mature during an infection; the mature DCs may co-present self antigens with those from infectious agents to naïve self reactive T cells. Frequent or persistent viral infections may boost the release of self antigens in the target organ, which in turn would greatly increase the chance for DCs to "accidently" activate naïve self reactive T cells. In addition, overall anti-viral or bacterial immunity may generate cytokine-mediated bystander activation of self reactive lymphocytes. *Second*, DCs present some pathogenic antigens, which mimic certain self antigens, to naïve T cells. Some of those activated T cells may recognize self antigens and cause autoimmunity. Some mimicking peptides may have a low efficiency in stimulating naïve T cells due to a low binding affinity to their TcR. However, increased quantity of microbial antigens during infection could enhance engagement of more mimicking epitopes with TcR, leading to the activation of self reactive T cells. *Third*, certain defects in host tissues may lead to the release of increased amounts of or altered self antigens, which have been previously ignored by the immune system. For example, the defective clearance of apoptotic cell debris due to an impaired uptake may result in an autoimmunity. In this case, DCs may be activated by apoptotic materials such as DNA. A recent study showed that binding of their surface TLR7 and TLR9 to dsDNA from dead cells activates pDCs, which in turn initiate autoimmune skin inflammation in a murine model (40). A common feature for the above three scenarios is that DCs are passively involved in activation of self reactive T cells, and thus, they are "innocent" in those scenarios. In those cases, autoimmunity occurs mainly due to the increase in available self antigens. A "threshold" model has been proposed to summarize the above cases (41). DCs constantly present self antigens, but they fail to activate T cells because antigens are under a "threshold" level. Multiple factors may influence the quantity of presented self antigens to surpass the threshold, resulting in a significant autoimmune response, and subsequently an autoimmune disease. *Fourth,* DCs are also regulated by other immune cells or molecules. DC's maturation and development are controlled by the types of pathogens/antigens as well as cytokines released by the activated T cells. One study suggested that high levels of IFN-α in systemic lupus erythematosus (SLE) may promote differentiation of monocytes to DCs, which in turn initiates an autoimmune response by picking up and further presenting more SLE-specific self antigens to self reactive T cells (42). Generally, regulatory T cells (Tregs) can suppress the maturation, activation and the subsequent production of inflammatory cytokines by recently activated DCs. However, chronically activated DCs, which may be presenting self antigens, could escape this mechanism and provoke an autoimmune response (43). *Fifth,* DCs could initiate autoimmunity because of intrinsic defects in genes controlling the DCs' functions, which results in DCs that behave deviantly. There are numerous genetic defects in DCs, which have been associated with the onset of autoimmune diseases. Unusual differentiation and/or maturation of DCs may lead to an abnormality of DCs either in quantity or quality. Loss of integrin $\alpha_v\beta_8$ on DCs causes autoimmunity and colitis in mice (44). Defects in the apoptosis of immune cells, including DCs, have been blamed for several autoimmune diseases. Abnormal co-stimulatory phenotypes of DCs have been linked to onset of severe murine lupus. By coordinating the recruitment and/or activation of other immune cells, DCs can drive the generation of ectopic lymphoid tissues, as in the case of inflamed synovia in rheumatoid arthritis (RA) and SLE. Thus, more self antigens would be presented more effectively in target organs. Normally, some DCs would be eliminated through apoptosis, because they have the potential to activate naïve self reactive T cells. However, genetic defects in DCs' apoptosis may prolong DCs' life and increase the chances for them to activate self reactive T cells. A transgenic mouse expressing the baculoviral caspase inhibitor, p35, in DCs results in their accumulation and, in turn, chronic lymphocyte activation and systemic autoimmune manifestations (45).

Despite its pivotal role in provoking an autoimmune response as sole APCs that can activate self reactive T cells, many more studies have been devoted to exploring DC's roles in self tolerance and/or autoimmunity prevention/controlling (33). It is clear now that DCs play critical roles in both central and peripheral tolerance. For central tolerance, thymic DCs function similar to but not limited to thymic epithelial cells. Both cells can selectively induce apoptosis in immature potential self reactive T cells. When immature T cells enter the thymus to be "educated", thymic DCs as well as thymic epithelia will present self antigens to immature T cells. If a T cell bears TcR which binds to the self antigens with high affinity, DCs will selectively trigger apoptosis in these potentially self reactive immature T cells. This process is called "negative selection". Unlike thymic epithelial cells, which can only present self antigens within the thymus, thymic DCs also can carry self antigens from outside tissues to eliminate additional self reactive T cells. Furthermore, thymic pDCs or mDCs, which are activated by thymic stromal lymphopoietin, induce generation of natural $CD4^{+}CD25^{+}$ Treg. A significant number of tDC-mediated tolerance mechanisms have been demonstrated in both humans and animals. In general, those tDC-mediated mechanisms are much more complicated and sophisticated than those in central tolerance. Elucidation of the known DC-mediated tolerance mechanisms and discovery of new ones in peripheral tissues remain a big challenge for immunologists, and thus, it is still a hot topic in immunological research today. Known tDC-mediated peripheral tolerance mechanisms, including one from our group, will be summarized in this section. There are two types of tDCs. The first type of tDCs is immature or semi-mature DCs, which are believed to be tolerogenic (33). The second type of tDCs are special types of DCs, or a specially differentiated DC subset, which act solely as an immune tolerance inducer. For the first type of tDCs, in the absence of infection or inflammation, DCs in the tissues will remain in an immature state. Those immature DCs may also capture self antigens from dead cells or accidentally released substances from cells and migrate to lymphoid organs with loaded self antigens due to homeostatic traffic. Unlike a mature DC, the immature or semi-mature DC, which has been loaded with self antigens, actively silence self reactive T cells because they lack co-stimulatory molecules for a full T cell activation. There are several mechanisms for those immature or semi-mature DCs to silence naïve self reactive T cells. Just as they do in central tolerance, some DCs may induce apoptosis in the T cells, which recognize the self antigen presented by DCs (45). Alternatively, the immature DCs induce unresponsiveness in T cells called anergy. It is believed that homeostatic traffic of DCs to silence naïve T cells is critical for maintenance of peripheral tolerance (46). Defect in molecules such as chemokine receptors, which is critical for this homeostatic migration, has been linked to several autoimmune diseases such as rheumatoid arthritis (RA) and MS. Furthermore, it has been reported that immature DCs may stimulate naïve self reactive T cells to differentiate into regulatory T cells (Treg) (47). As one of the most important immunoregulators, Tregs, in turn, actively inhibit pathogenic self reactive T cells. Several studies suggest that Treg can also inhibit maturation of DCs, and thus, more tDCs are generated. On the other hand, the second type of tDCs are specifically differentiated DCs, or from different lineages, which have the sole function of inducing an immune tolerance. Mounting evidence supports the presence of such tDCs. For example, the treatment of DC precursors with certain substances such as glucocorticoid (GC) leads to the generation of a type of DC which was morphologically similar to a mature DC, but was able to induce T cell anergy, suggesting that an anergy-inducing DC could be a special type of DCs (48). 1,25-dihydroxyvitamin D3 (1,25-vitD) has been known to inhibit autoimmune diseases in animal models, as well as in humans. Activation of vitamin D receptor (VDR) by either exogenous or endogenously generated1,25-vitD reprograms DCs to become tolerogenic (49). An experiment showed that systemic administration of *in vitro* generated tDC with TNF-α treatment ameliorates murine inflammatory arthritis, suggesting a critical role of cytokines from a tissue microenvironment in generation of tDC. Obviously, tolerogenicity of those DCs does not depend on its maturation stage but rather on their different maturation pathway. This is probably true for humans as well. A new phenotype of tDC, which induces T cell anergy, can be generated from human monocyte-derived DCs by treatment of proteases from the fungus Aspergillus oryzae (ASP)(50). A long list of substances can induce differentiation of tDCs (32). Dexamethasone-treated DCs are able to induce differentiation of Treg *in vitro* (51). Both immunologists and clinicians expect a potential clinical application from the *in vitro* generated tDCs for inhibition of autoimmunity, and induction of immune tolerance to graft antigens. Some animal models showed encouraging results by transfer of tDC to inhibit autoimmune diseases (52). Vasoactive intestinal peptide induced regulatory dendritic cells showed therapeutic effects on autoimmune disorders (53) On the other hand, investigators are also searching for tDCs with a different lineage from the known cDCs or pDCs. A tDC, which is responsible for inhibition of $CD8^+$ T cell mediated anti-tumor activity, has been described in a murine model (54). This type of tDC has not been characterized well, and further investigation is needed. Our group is currently characterizing a new type of DC, which may be tolerogenic (55).

The common features for the above DC-mediated tolerance mechanisms can be summarized as follows: 1) DCs act on naïve T cells, and 2) DCs induce tolerance in lymphoid tissues but not in peripheral tissues. As a result, those DCs prevent autoimmunity *de novo*, because pathogenic T cells would be eliminated from lymphoid tissues before their activation. However, it is highly possible that naïve autoreactive T cells may escape the above mechanisms and be activated to further differentiate into pathogenic effecter cells through, for example, molecular mimicry or bystander activation during an infection. In fact, the presence of activated self reactive T cells has been widely reported in normal human individuals and animals. Although the tDCs described above have potential clinical applications for treatment of autoimmune diseases, it is worthwhile to emphasize that all those tDCs, either *in vitro* induced tDCs or natural tDCs, may only prevent autoimmunity *de novo*. These tDCs have shown encouraging results with a great promise in animal models. In most cases, the treatment needs to be prior to the onset of the disease. It is, therefore, questionable if these tDCs can be used to treat an existing autoimmune disease, which is common in human patients. It will be equally important to ask if any tolerance mechanisms in target tissues are able to control autoimmune diseases after pathogenic autoreactive T cells have infiltrated the target tissue and caused tissue damage. In other words, are there any tDCs which participate in the third level of immune tolerance? Fortunately, a few studies suggest the existence of tDCs in the third level of tolerance. *In vivo* depletion of pDCs by antibody to mouse pDC antigen-1 (mPDCA-1) after the onset of the disease enhanced T cell activation in target tissue but not in lymphoid organs, which exacerbated CNS inflammation in a mouse EAE model (56). This study suggests the presence of a tissue infiltrating tolerogenic pDCs, which infiltrated inflamed target tissue to inhibit a pathogenic T cell response. However, it remains to be elucidated how this pDC inhibited autoimmune inflammation. A novel DC-mediated mechanism has been recently described in a rat anti-GBM glomerulonephritis model. Unlike many other types of DCs, this DC actively infiltrates inflamed autoimmune target tissues and presents the self antigen locally (55). The DC selectively induces apoptosis in the infiltrating self reactive pathogenic T cells, which recognize the presented self antigen. Subsequently, T cell-mediated autoimmune inflammation is stopped. In contrast to many other tDC-mediated tolerance mechanisms, unique features of the above two are that 1) it contains the autoimmune disease after activation of self reactive T cells/tissue damage rather than prevents it *de novo*, and 2) it occurs in autoimmune target tissue rather than in lymphoid organs. It is conceivable that these tDCs, which are involved in the third level of immune tolerance, could be more effective in treatment of an existing autoimmune disease.

5. Renal DCs in the steady-state

As a first step to studying DCs' role in renal physiology and pathology, many studies have been devoted to identification of DCs in normal renal tissue or related draining lymph nodes in both humans and animals (mainly mice and rats). Historically, as early as 1981, a mononuclear phagocyte with expression of MHC II and a "stellate" morphology was described to reside in the renal interstitium in mice, which probably was the first confirmed DC in renal tissue (57). Since then, various types of DCs have been identified in either steady-state or under pathological conditions mainly in mice, as well as in rats and humans (58-60). Compared to the DCs in other organs or tissues, renal DCs are still poorly understood. However, it has become clear that similar to those in other tissues or organs, renal DCs are comprised of highly heterogeneous subsets (Table 1). Using CX3CR1^{GFP+} transgenic mice, a network composed of a large number of CX3CR1^{+} cells, which are mainly DCs, spanning the entire tubule-interstitium and enclosing all nephrons has been observed (61). Further investigations have suggested that this renal DC network in the steady-state probably is involved in maintenance of renal homeostasis and self tolerance. In addition, several functional subsets of DCs have been identified in the kidney using various markers.
Mouse renal DCs have been best analyzed among all species. Murine renal DCs can be primarily identified using a combination of CD11 and MHC II as markers. With other DC markers, at least three renal DC subsets have been characterized and classified, which have been summarized by Nelson and Kurts, respectively (Table 1)(58, 60). The majority of renal DCs belong to the first subset, which expresses the chemokine Franklin receptor CX3CR1, the macrophage marker F4/80, and the myeloid marker CD11b, but not CD8, suggesting this CX3CR1^{+}F4/80^{+}CD11b^{+}CD8^{-} subset to be the equivalent to the IntDCs (i.e. cDCs of myeloid origin in lymphoid nodes) (refer to Figure 2)(10, 61, 62). This renal DC subset probably is the DCs, which form DC network surrounding renal tubules (61). A small number of the second subset is CD8$\alpha\alpha^{+}$CD11c^{+} CD103^{+}, which seems similar to the CD8$\alpha\alpha^{+}$ cDCs of myeloid origin in the lymph nodes (63). Since this subset is normally observed in skin-associated lymph nodes and is associated with Langerhans cells in the skin, it will be interesting to determine their lineage and function (64). The third subset of renal DCs, which is rare, is similar to the pDCs with a phenotype of CD11c^{+}CD8α^{-}B220^{+}, suggesting that this may be pre-pDCs (61, 65). Human renal DCs in normal kidneys also have been characterized, and several subsets have been described. At least two different HLA-DR^{+} myeloid cDC subtypes have been identified in the cortex of normal kidneys, with phenotypes of BDCA-1^{+}DC-SIGN^{+} and BDCA-1^{+}DC-SIGN^{-} (66). The first subset is probably human cDCs of myeloid origin (see Table). In addition, a subset, which is similar to the pDCs with a phenotype of BDCA-2^{+}DC-SIGN^{-}, is also abundantly present in the renal tissue (66). All of those DC subsets are located in the tubulo-interstitium with a high frequency. These DCs often surround glomeruli, but are rarely observed within glomeruli. Among those subsets, BDCA-1^{+}DC-SIGN^{+} DCs are most abundant and are four times as frequently present as BDCA-2^{+}. Thus, cDCs of myeloid origin are dominant in renal tissues in both humans and mice. In inflamed or injured renal tissue, additional subsets of DCs have been observed in both humans and mice. These pathology-related renal DCs will be discussed in the next section. Several new types of DCs, such as IFN-producing killer DC, inflammatory TNF-α-inducible nitric oxide synthase–producing DCs, and tolerogenic IDO expressing DCs, have been identified (67-69). It remains unclear whether those newly defined DCs are presented in or recruited to renal tissues.

Species	*Subset and phenotype*	*Abundance*	*Note*
Mice	CD8$^-$ cDC myeloid CD11c$^+$CD11b$^+$F4/80$^+$ B220$^-$CX3CR1$^+$	Many	IntDC
	CD8$^+$ cDC myeloid? CD11c$^+$CD11b$^-$CD103$^+$CD205$^-$ Langerin$^+$	Few	= Langerhans cells?
	pDC CD11c$^+$CD11b$^-$CD8$^-$B220$^+$Gr1$^+$	Few	Pre-pDC
	CD8$^-$ Pre-DC (inflammatory) CD11c$^+$CD11b$^+$F4/80$^+$Gr-1$^+$	-	Non-residential?
Humans	cDC BDCA-1$^+$DC-SIGN$^+$	Many	
	cDC BDCA-1$^+$DC-SIGN$^-$	Many	
	pDC BDCA-2$^+$DC-SIGN$^-$	Few	

Table 1. Subsets of DCs in the renal tissue of mice and humans at steady state

Due to the advancement in technologies and the increasing number of DC specific markers, investigators were able to examine renal DCs' function and their lineage in detail by isolation of renal DCs from either animals or humans for *in vitro* experiments, or by using gene manipulated animals or bone marrow chimeras for *in vivo* experiments. Investigations on mice DCs suggest that, like other DCs, renal DCs probably also derive from common bone marrow stem cells for macrophages and DC precursors. Renal DCs may directly derive from circulating pre-DCs (59). Based on the studies on DCs in other non-lymphoid or lymphoid organs, these bone marrow stem cells first differentiate into circulating or patrolling Csf1r$^+$Gr1$^+$ and Csf1r$^+$Gr1$^-$ monocytes in peripheral blood (70, 71). Subsets of Csf1r$^+$Gr1$^-$ or Csf1r$^+$Gr1$^+$ monocytes may become the precursor of different pre-DCs under certain conditions. However, a study suggested the presence of non-monocyte pre-DCs for DCs in other tissues such as the lung (72). On the other hand, some studies showed that diverse renal DC populations probably differentiate from FLT3$^+$ DC precursors for both pDCs and mDCs (73). Microenvironments in renal tissue may determine diversification of renal DCs from this rather flexible common DC precursor. One *in vivo* experiment showed that injection of FLT3 to mice did not alter the proportion of each DC subset in the kidney, although the DCs' number significantly increased (74). Very early studies also suggest a potential of the renal microenvironment in generation of diverse renal DCs from shared progenitors or precursors. Subsets of renal DCs of myeloid origin share several common markers among the mononuclear phagocytes such as F4/80 and CD68. This phenotypic overlap between renal DCs of myeloid origin and macrophages is different in different tissue locations within normal kidneys, suggesting that the environments may affect DCs' phenotypic changes (75). In one experiment, stimulation of the same precursor by different cytokines led to the generation of pro- or anti-inflammatory DCs (70). GM-CFS stimulated DC precursors from bone marrow promotes the generation of DCs with an inflammatory phenotype by both *ex vivo* and *in vivo* experiments (70). On the other hand, FLT3L-derived

DCs are phenotypically similar to DCs at a steady state, which are believed to be mainly anti-inflammatory. Several studies have tried to identify the local factors which determined renal DCs' differentiation. For example, CSF-1 receptor is known to be important for the differentiation and survival of myeloid DCs in general (76). Renal epithelial cells constitutively express CSF-1 (77, 78). It will be interesting to test if epithelium-expressed CFS-1 is involved in shaping renal DCs' repertoire. In summary, the majority of studies on renal DCs of myeloid origin suggest that local inductive factors shape the repertoire of renal DCs.

There are several interesting issues regarding the life cycle of renal DCs at a steady-state. First, how pre-DCs migrate or are recruited into renal tissues. Chemokines and adhesion molecules play a pivotal role in leukocyte trafficking. Thus, renal DCs or their precursors in the circulation are expected to express certain sets of chemokine receptors and adhesion molecules. Several experiments have suggested special chemokines released from renal tissue may be required for recruitment of pre-DCs to the kidney. However, information regarding expression of these two molecules in renal DCs is still lacking or controversial. The second issue is the life span for renal DCs. Using a bone marrow chimera mouse model, the life span of renal DCs in mice has been determined to be 10-14 days in homeostasis (79). On the other hand, BrdU-labeling experiments using normal mice suggest an average half-life of approximately 35 days across all subsets of renal DCs (80). The third issue is whether renal DCs can self renewal or need to be constantly recruited from the circulation. A study observed that a small percent of residential leukocytes were $CX3CR1^{high}GR1^{-}$ but lacked markers for differentiated DCs, suggesting these to be renewal DCs (61). However, more experiments are needed to answer this question.

The subsets of renal DCs, which are constantly present in normal renal tissue and form an immune surveillance network at a steady-state, may have three functions. However, those functions are largely speculated from the results for DCs in other tissues. First, they serve as sentinels in monitoring possible invading pathogens as one part of immune surveillance. Once they are activated by pathogens, mature renal DCs will migrate into renal draining lymph nodes to provoke an adaptive immune response against the pathogens (61, 81). Second, as one part of innate immunity, renal DCs may release cytokines or chemokines upon activation by pathogens to organize an innate immune attack against the pathogens by recruitment or activation of other innate immune cells (82). Third, as an important peripheral tolerance mechanism, immature renal DCs constantly capture self antigens from the tubules and glomeruli, and even some small molecules which are filtered in glomeruli (80, 83-85). Like in other tissue locations, a constant migration of renal DCs into local renal lymph nodes probably also exists (86). Through their APC function, the migrated immature DCs selectively inhibit activation of potential self reactive T cells. It has been reported that additional small self molecules may reach renal lymph nodes, where DCs capture those molecules. If these molecules are not associated with pathogenic antigens, they are used to tolerize harmful T cells by DCs (87, 88).

6. DCs in promotion of autoimmune glomerulonephritis

Like in other peripheral tissues, DCs play a critical role in provoking autoimmunity by breaking self tolerance in renal tissues including glomeruli. We have mentioned earlier that there are no DCs present in normal glomeruli. What type(s) of DCs are responsible for breaking self tolerance and for the maintenance of immune tolerance to glomerular self antigens? It will be interesting to describe a concept called "tubuloglomerular feedback loop" hypothesis (Figure 4). This hypothesis may explain renal DCs' involvement in both self tolerance to tubular/glomerular self antigens, and provoking autoimmune inflammatory kidney diseases including glomerulonephritis (84, 89). In steady-state, this mechanism may prevent autoimmunity in a similar way to that in mucosal tolerance in the intestinal tract, especially for antigens of low molecular mass, although this remains to be formally demonstrated (90). A large population of $CX3CR1^{+}F4/80^{+}$ $CD8^{-}$ DCs, which lines the outer medullary tubules to form a DC network, has been described earlier. There is also a smaller population of renal $CD8\alpha\alpha^{+}$ DCs. Cellular self antigens released from normal apoptotic death or small molecules filtered through glomeruli will reach the lumen of renal tubules; tubular epithelial cells will transfer the self antigens to renal $CD8\alpha\alpha^{-}$ DCs in the renal DC network or $CD8\alpha\alpha^{+}$ DCs directly uptake those antigens (80, 83-85). The self antigens will then be presented to $CD4^{+}$ T cells by renal $CD8\alpha\alpha^{-}$ DCs to induce their unresponsiveness, or cross-presented by renal $CD8\alpha\alpha^{+}$ DCs to $CD8^{+}$ T cells to induce their apoptosis, probably in a similar way to other tissue locations at steady-state (91). Thus, tolerance to normally released self glomerular antigens is induced or maintained. On the other hand, mechanical/chemical, biological renal injury, or autoimmunity would induce cell necrosis, which in turn will release a new set of self antigens called damage-associated molecular patterns (DAMPs), some of which could be ligands for TLRs and serve as a "danger signal". When renal DCs pick up and present these DAMPs as danger antigens under an inflammatory milieu, they may activate self reactive T cells and cause tubulointerstitial inflammation first. The autoimmune response to glomerular antigens will be "feedbacked" to the glomerulus either directly or through a periglomerular infiltration. One recent study showed that renal DCs could become pathogenic during crescentic glomerulonephritis, suggesting that abnormal tissue damages in glomeruli are required for differentiation of pro-inflammatory DCs (92). However, it remains unclear where those pathogenic DCs originate.

Studies, which aimed to demonstrate how and what types of renal or non-renal DCs participate in pathogenesis of glomerulonephritis, remain scarce. However, it is clear that DCs also play a critical role in various renal diseases including autoimmune glomerulonephritis at several levels; these roles are mutually related. *First*, DCs are required to activate pathogenic T cells against renal self antigens. It is not only true for autoimmune glomerulonephritis, but also for other glomerular diseases, as glomerular chronic inflammation may lead to autoimmunity. There is evidence that upon encountering maturation stimuli such as DAMPs or microbial antigens, renal DCs migrate to the renal draining lymph nodes (86) where they activate specific T cells (93). This process is believed to be very similar to the canonical life-cycle of tissue residing DCs extrapolated from the paradigm of Langerhans cells in the skin (73, 91, 94). Activation of self reactive T or B cells in renal draining lymph nodes has been demonstrated in animal models for lupus glomerulonephritis and anti-GBM glomerulonephritis (95, 96). However, renal DCs or renal infiltrating DCs may also activate T cells locally in a lupus model which will be described later. Rodent nephrotoxin nephritis is a model for human crescentic glomerulonephritis. Sheep antibody to mouse GBM will be "embedded" in the host GBM after injection. GBM-"embedded" sheep antigens are taken up by DCs in lymphatic organs, and are used to activate specific Th1 cells and B cells. As a result, glomerular inflammation, characteristic of T cell mediated delayed hypersensitivity, occurs. Although renal DCs show a protective role at early stages (97), later they act as two types of APCs to promote inflammation (60). First, renal DCs migrate to local lymph nodes to cross-present glomerular antigens to CD8+ T cells, which in turn cause glomerular damage. Second, renal DCs present the self antigen from the damage to CD4+ T cells, which in turn orchestrate and maintain glomerular inflammation.

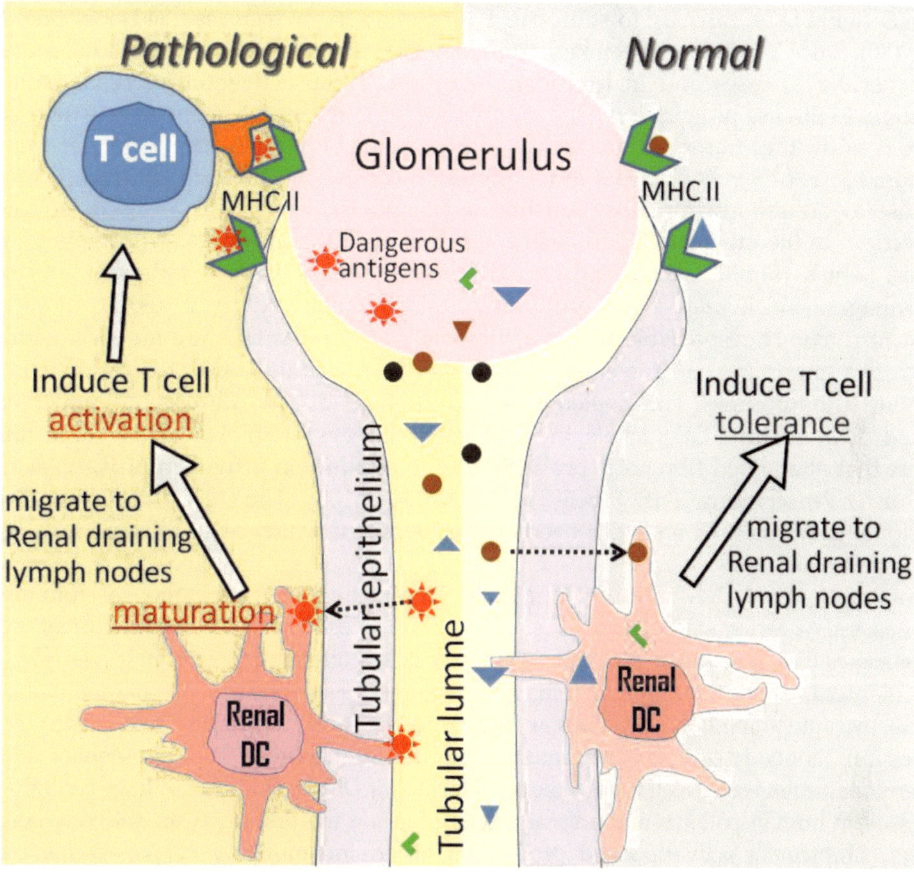

Fig. 4. Diagram shows the tubuloglomerular feedback loop under normal and pathologic conditions in kidneys. In normal kidney, self antigens from glomeruli are released to the lumen of the tubules. The antigens then are up-take by renal DCs, or transferred to renal DCs (arrows) by tubular epithelium. Renal DCs will migrate into renal draining lymph node to induce tolerance toward the glomerular antigens. If renal DCs encounter dangerous antigens from glomeruli, they will mature and induce T cell activation. Activated T cells will in turn attack glomeruli with dangerous pathogens/antigens by recognition of MHC II-antigen complex expressed by Bowman's capsule.

Second, renal DCs also play a role in establishing glomerular inflammation as an innate immune cell. Renal DCs may release a set of pro-inflammatory cytokines and chemokines upon stimulation from injuries, and subsequently orchestrate an acute inflammation. It is important to re-emphasize that such environmental milieu of acute inflammation may in turn provide renal DCs an opportunity to break self tolerance and provoke a pathogenic autoimmunity post acute inflammation. Using two models for renal injury, DCs' roles in establishing acute inflammation post renal injury have been investigated in quite detail.

Ischaemia-reperfusion injury (IRI) is a model to mimic renal transplantation. Renal F4/80+ CD11c+ subset DCs are the earliest source of TNF-α (80), which in turn causes an influx of circulating immune cells including pro-inflammatory DC subsets, monocytes/macrophages and T cells (98). Orchestrated actions of these cells contribute to kidney parenchymal damage. Renal DCs' capacity to stimulate T cells remarkably increased 24 hours post renal injury (80). Since T cells have been known to play critical roles in IRI (99, 100, 101), as well as in glomerular diseases and in transplant rejection, T cell activation by renal DCs may contribute to disease progression. One report showed that renal DCs can be activated under hypoxia with the transcription factor HIF-1a and LPS (102). However, it remains questionable as LPS is not present in the injured renal tissue. Interestingly, renal DCs may also display an anti-inflammatory function in this model, which will be discussed later in this section. In the other model, unilateral urethral obstruction results in progressive renal fibrosis, which mimics human progressive renal diseases (103). Although infiltrating macrophages, which release the profibrotic and pro-inflammatory cytokines TGF-β and TNF-α, are mainly responsible for renal fibrosis, F4/80+ renal DCs are an early source of TNF-α. The importance of this early TNF-α from DCs was demonstrated by depletion of DCs with Clo-liposome. The depletion led to attenuated renal fibrosis, accompanied by reduced TNF-α and TGF-β levels in obstructed kidneys (104). However, some studies suggest that attenuated fibrosis is probably due to a failure in activation of IL-17 secreting Th17 or INF-γ-secreting Th1 T cells by renal DCs (105). Thus, DCs may not directly participate in fibrosis. However, it needs to be identified which renal DCs are involved in the activation of T cells.

In many cases, renal DCs may play dual roles in tandem in the promotion of autoimmune pathogenesis. At earlier stages, renal DCs act as an innate cell to establish an inflammation, and at later stages they function as a potent APC to break self tolerance. This is well exemplified by lupus glomerulonephritis. Lupus is initiated by glomerular deposition of immune complexes formed by autoantibodies and nuclear self antigens, and undergoes two stages during progression: antibody-complex mediated acute lupus nephritis and subsequent chronic glomerulonephritis with T cell involvement. The roles of DCs in this disease have recently been addressed in human patients and animal models. During the first stage, an antibody complex triggers complement activation and production of pro-inflammatory cytokines/chemokines, leading to acute glomerular inflammation. The roles of DCs in this stage can be summarized as 1) a systemic role in breaking T cell tolerance leading to production of autoantibodies, and 2) a local role in establishing glomerular inflammation. Because the systemic role of DCs as a APC in autoantibody generation is less kidney-specific, we will focus on DCs' local role. In addition to renal DCs, DCs have been found to infiltrate glomeruli in lupus glomerulonephritis (95, 106). At least two types of pre-DCs, Gr1+ inflammatory monocyte or Gr1^{low} patrolling monocyte, have been found to infiltrate inflamed glomeruli (107). Those infiltrating DCs are able to produce the Th1-driving cytokine IL-12 within glomeruli, suggesting their ability to provide a pro-inflammatory milieu (104). Blockage of co-stimulatory molecules of DCs together with cyclophosphamide reduced the number of renal CD11c+ cells, as well as T cell infiltration during lupus' chronic stage. This suggests renal DCs themselves function not only as an innate cell population in the promotion/ establishment of renal inflammation but also as APCs to break T cell tolerance. It remains unclear how self reactive T cells are primed. T cell activation and expansion in the renal draining lymph nodes has been reported, suggesting that migration of renal DCs into lymph nodes is necessary (95). Another possibility is that renal DCs may stimulate T cells within glomeruli.

7. DCs in the prevention of autoimmune glomerulonephritis

As we discussed earlier, one of the functions for renal DCs in the steady-state is to maintain peripheral tolerance to renal self antigens. We also mentioned earlier a concept of tubuloglomerular "feedback" loop. This hypothesis may explain how a renal DC network maintains self tolerance to glomerular antigens since no DCs are present in this tissue location. Thus, self tolerance to glomerular self antigens is established indirectly, in a similar way to "oral tolerance". Consequently, non-dangerous self antigens released from glomeruli will be tolerized. This mechanism will prevent glomerular autoimmunity *de novo*. However, recent studies also demonstrated that under acute tissue damage caused by ischemia reperfusion, renal DCs still could control inflammation and probably induce tolerance to the abnormal self antigens leaked from the damage (108), suggesting that this mechanism may also play a role in maintenance of limited self tolerance post acute tissue damages.

In addition to this renal DC network, several subsets of DCs, including residential and infiltrating DCs, also play roles in inhibition of autoimmunity during or post tissue injuries. Those renal DCs induce self tolerance or inhibit glomerular inflammation through several ways. First, the renal DCs may inhibit autoimmune inflammation in glomeruli as APCs to eliminate or anergize pathogenic T cells in glomeruli. In a murine nephrotoxin nephritis model, early depletion of $CD11c^+$ cells aggravated renal damage. Because only DCs in mice express a high level of CD11c, this study suggested a protective role of renal DCs in glomerulonephritis, at least at an early stage of development (97). Mechanistic analysis revealed that renal DCs from nephritic mice stimulated a potent T cell proliferation with the expression of cytokine IL-10. In general, IL-10 is considered an anti-inflammatory. Further study has shown that blockage of IL-10 production aggravated glomerulonephritis. Thus, renal DCs during tissue damage may induce differentiation of T cells into an anti-inflammatory phenotype such as Tregs. A similar phenomenon has been observed in a cisplatin induced nephritis model. In this model, renal tubular cells are first damaged by the toxin and consequently undergo necrotic cell death. Depletion of $CD11c^+$ cells, which are largely murine cDCs but not pDCs, exacerbated renal injury (109). The underlying molecular mechanisms may be similar to that in the lung. An increased expression of inducible costimulatory ligand (ICOS-L) on DCs can suppress T cells (110). In the above two cases, renal cDCs inhibit glomerular inflammation through their APC function to promote generation of anti-inflammatory T cells. Second, renal DCs may also function as anti-inflammatory immune cells to inhibit autoimmune glomerular inflammation. In a murine model, myeloid cells of the kidney, probably renal DCs, have been shown to attenuate ischaemia-reperfusion injury, by production of single Ig IL-1-related receptor (SIGIRR) (111). SIGIRR is a negative regulator of TLR−IL-1 receptor signaling. It inhibits Th17 T cell development, and is an immunosuppressive mediator expressed by DCs and macrophages. The deficiency of this mediator worsened tissue damage. This situation could be reversed by liposome-mediated depletion of phagocytes including renal DCs, suggesting a potential of renal DCs or other renal phagocytes in prevention of further tissue damage by releasing anti-inflammatory molecules such as SIGIRR. However, it needs to be proven if renal DCs expressing SIGIRR actively contain tissue damage. Interestingly, a study by the same group on a murine lupus model also suggested protective roles in renal injury using SIGIRR-deficient mice. Mice that lacked SIGIRR showed aggravated hydrocarbon oil-induced lupus (112).

Despite the above tolerance mechanisms in kidneys, a keen question still remains: why abnormal tissue damage such as an infection in glomeruli usually does not result in autoimmunity, despite the fact that both cell necrosis and microbial antigens provide DAMPs and a danger signal? Thus, other tolerance mechanisms must exist to prevent autoimmunity at the third level (i.e. after self reactive T cells have been activated or autoimmune glomerular damage has been initiated). Indeed, a few studies, including one from our group, suggest the existence of such DC-mediated tolerance mechanisms. As we mentioned before, our group reported a new type of DC with a phenotype of $CD8\alpha\alpha^+CD11b/c^+MHC\text{-}II^+ED1^-OX62^-$ in our rat model for anti-GBM glomerulonephritis (55). This DC is not residential, but rather is selectively recruited into inflamed glomeruli. Both in vivo and in vitro experiments have shown that this DC induces T cell apoptosis in the glomeruli, leading to termination of glomerular inflammation (Figure 5). Further experiments suggest that this DC is responsible for natural recovery from early glomerulonephritis in a disease resistant rat strain by termination of T cell-mediated glomerular inflammation (113, unpublished data, Lou). Importantly, transfer of $CD8\alpha^+$ DCs of a resistant strain cured glomerulonephritis at an early stage in a disease prone strain. This mechanism is very attractive and logical, and could be used for development of a novel cell-based immunotherapeutic strategy for autoimmune glomerulonephritis. DCs have been the target for immunotherapy for treating various diseases including cancer and autoimmune diseases (114). However, more studies are needed to ensure if a similar mechanism also exits in humans (115).

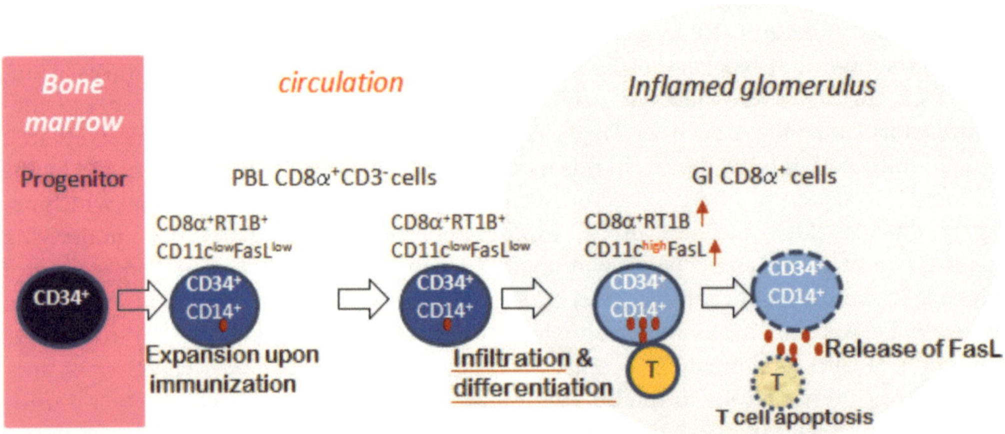

Fig. 5. Diagram for the mechanism, by which a new type of $CD8\alpha^+$ DC terminates glomerular inflammation by active infiltration of inflamed glomeruli and induction of T cell apoptosis through Fas-L. Development of this $CD8\alpha^+$ DC is also shown. *GI CD8α⁺ cells*, glomeruli-infiltrating $CD8\alpha^+$ cells; *RT1B*, rat MHC II molecule. This model used rats as experimental animals.

8. Conclusive remarks

Like in other tissue locations, multiple subsets of both cDCs and pDCs reside in normal renal tissues both in humans and mice. Heterogeneity of residential renal DCs is due to their different precursors and more importantly, renal microenvironmental factors. At a steady-state, these residential renal DCs form an immune surveillance network for detecting pathogens and for maintaining immune tolerance to renal self antigens. Although glomeruli lack residential DCs, those surrounding tubules may monitor antigens from the glomeruli, self or non-self, through the tubuloglomerular feedback loop. During acute glomerular injury, the majority of residential renal DCs play a critical role in controlling tissue damage through their anti-inflammatory function. Under immunological changes in glomeruli, including chronic inflammation and autoimmune attacks, both renal residential DCs and infiltrating DCs are involved in the process. DCs in the renal draining lymph nodes serve as the sole APC to activate naïve self reactive T cells, or those in the renal tissue maintain glomerular inflammation by presenting self antigens locally to pathogenic T cells. However, tolerogenic DCs inhibit autoimmunity in glomeruli by induction of anergy or apoptosis in self reactive T cells, or by inducing differentiation of regulatory T cells (Tregs). It is important to discover new DC subsets, especially tolerogenic DCs, and elucidate their differentiation and function. Using artificially generated tolerogenic DCs, we may be able to develop a novel antigen-specific immunotherapeutic strategy for treatment of glomerular diseases.

9. Acknowledgement

This study was supported by NIH R01-DK60029 (YHL), R01-DK077857 (YHL) and partially by R01-HD049613 (YHL). We thank Miss K. Parker and Mr. T. Bartkowiak for preparing the manuscript. We also thank Ms. J. Wu for her significant contribution to our project on renal dendritic cells. We also apologize to all collegues whose excellent work could not be cited due to space restriction.

10. References

[1] Banchereau J, Steinman RM (1998). Dendritic cells and the control of immunity. *Nature* 392 (6673): 245–52.

[2] Steinman RM, Cohn ZA (1973). Identification of a novel cell type in peripheral lymphoid organs of mice. I. Morphology, quantitation, tissue distribution. *J. Exp. Med.* 137 (5): 1142–62.

[3] Banchereau J, Briere F, Caux C, Davoust J, Lebecque S, Liu Y, Pulendran B, Palucka K. (2000) Immunobiology of dendritic cells. *Ann. Rev. Immunol.* 18: 767-811.

[4] Larsen CP, Kitchie SC, Pearson TC, Linsley PS, Lowry RP. (1992) Functional expression of the costimulatory molecule, B7/BB1, on murine dendritic cell populations. *J. Exp. Med.* 176: 1215-1220.

[5] Alvarez D, Vollmann EH, von Andrian UH. (2008) Mechanisms and consequences of dendritic cell migration. *Immunity* 29(3):325-342.

[6] Penna G, Vulcano M, Sozzani S, Adorini L. (2002) Differential migration behavior and chemokine production by myeloid and plasmacytoid dendritic cells. *Hum. Immunol.* 63(12):1164-1171.

[7] Stoitzner P, Zanella M, Ortner U, Lukas M, Tagwerker A, Janke K, Lutz MB, Schuler G, Echtenacher B, Ryffel B, Koch F, Romani N.(1999) Migration of Langerhans cells and dermal dendritic cells in skin organ cultures: augmentation by TNF-α and IL-1β. *J. Leukoc. Biol.* 66: 462–470.

[8] Steinman RM, Inaba K. (1999) Myeloid dendritic cells. *J. Leukoc. Biol.* 66(2):205-208.

[9] Sato K, Fujita S. (2007) Dendritic cells: nature and classification. *Allergol Int.* 56(3):183-191.

[10] Shortmann K, Liu Y.(2002) Mouse and human dendrictic cell subtypes. *Nat. Rev. Immunol.* 2: 151-161.

[11] Vremec D, Pooley J, Hochrein H, Wu L, Shortman K.(2000) CD4 and CD8 expression by dendritic cell subtypes inmouse thymus and spleen. *J. Immunol.* 12164:2978-2986.

[12] Yasumi T, Katamura K, Yoshioka T *et al.* (2004) Differential requirement for the CD40-CD154 costimulatory pathway during Th cell priming by CD8α+ and CD8α− murine dendritic cell subsets. *J. Immunol.* 172:4826-4833.

[13] Liu K, Iyoda T, Saternus M, Kimura Y, Inaba K, Steinman RM. (2002) Immune tolerance after delivery of dying cells to dendritic cells *in situ*. *J. Exp. Med.* 196:1091-1097.

[14] Maldonado-Lopez R, De Smedt T, Michel P *et al.* (1999) CD8α+ and CD8α− subclasses of dendritic cells direct the development of distinct T helper cells *in vivo*. *J. Exp. Med.* 189:587-592.

[15] Merad M, Fong L, Bogenberger J, Engleman EG.(2000) Differentiation of myeloid dendritic cells into CD8α-positive dendritic cells *in vivo*. *Blood* 24:1865-1872.

[16] Lutz MB, Schuler G.(2000) Immature, semi-mature and fully mature dendritic cells: which signals induce tolerance or immunity? *Trends Immunol.* 23:445-449.

[17] Wu L, D'Amico A, Hochrein H, O'Keeffe M, Shortman K, Lucas K. (2001) Development of thymic and splenic dendritic cell populations from different hemopoietic precursors. *Blood* 98:3376-3382.

[18] Asselin-Paturel C, Boonstra A, Dalod M *et al.* (2001) Mouse type I IFN-producing cells are immature APCs with plasmacytoid morphology. *Nat. Immunol.* 2:1144-1150.

[19] Trinchieri G, Santoli D, Dee RR, Knowles BB. (1978) Anti-viral activity induced by culturing lymphocytes with tumor-derived or virus transformed cells: identification of the anti-viral activity as interferon and characterization of the human effector lymphocyte subpopulation. *J. Exp. Med.* 147:1299–313.

[20] Schuster P, Boscheinen JB, Tennert K, Schmidt B. (2011) The Role of Plasmacytoid dendritic cells in innate and adaptive immune responses against α herpes virus infections. *Adv Virol.* 2011 Article ID 679271, 12 pages

[21] Brawand P, Fitzpatrick DR, Greenfield BW, Brasel K, Maliszewski CR, De Smedt T.(2000) Murine plasmacytoid predendritic cells generated from Flt3ligand-supplemented bone marrow cultures are immature APCs. *J. Immunol.* 169:6711-6719.

[22] Ito T, Inaba M, Inaba K *et al.* (1999) A $CD1a^{+}/CD11c^{+}$ subset of human blood dendritic cells is a direct precursor of Langerhans cells. *J. Immunol.* 163:1409-1419.

[23] Dzionek A, Fuchs A, Schmidt P *et al.* (2000) BDCA-2, BDCA-3, and BDCA-4: three markers for distinct subsets of dendritic cells in human peripheral blood. *J. Immunol.* 165:6037-6046.

[24] Ito T, Amakawa R, Inaba M *et al.* (2004) Plasmacytoid dendritic cells regulate Th cell responses through OX40 ligand and type I IFNs. *J. Immunol.* 2004;172:4253-4259.

[25] Colonna M, Trinchieri G, Liu Y. (2004) Plasmacytoid dendritic cells in immunity. *Nat Immunol.* 5(12):1219-26.

[26] Ito T, Amakawa R, Inaba M, Ikehara S, Inaba K, FukuharaS. (2001) Differential regulation of human blood dendritic cell subsets by IFNs. *J. Immunol.* 166:2961-2969.

[27] Poulin LF, Salio M, Griessinger E, Anjos-Afonso F, et al.(2010) Characterization of human DNGR-1+ BDCA3+ leukocytes as putative equivalents of mouse CD8α+ dendritic cells *J. Exp. Med.* 207(6):1261-1271.

[28] Drakesmith H, Chain B, Beverley P. (2000) How can dendritic cells cause autoimmune disease? *Trends in Immunol.*21:214-217.

[29] Bayry J, Thirion M, Delignat S, Misra N, Lacroix-Desmazes S, Kazatchkine MD, Kaveri SV.(2004) Dendritic cells and autoimmunity. ***Autoimmunity Rev.*** 3(3):183-187.

[30] Gonzalez B, Guerra C, Morris D, Gray D, Venketaraman V. (2010) Dendritic cells in infectious disease, hypersensitivity, and autoimmunity. ***Int. J. Interferon, Cytokine Mediator Res.*** 2:137 - 147.

[31] Thomson AW, Robbins PD. (2008) Tolerogenic dendritic cells for autoimmune disease and transplantation. *Ann Rheum Dis* 67:iii90-iii96

[32] Torres-Aguilar H, Blank M, Jara L, Shoenfeld Y. (2010) Tolerogenic dendritic cells in autoimmune diseases crucial players in induction and prevention of autoimmunity. *Autoimmunity Rev.* 2010 doi:10.1016/j.

[33] Steinman RM, Hawiger D, Nussenzweig. (2003) Tolerogenic dendritic cells. *Ann. Rev. Immunol.* 21:685-711.

[34] Ludewig B, Odermatt B, Landmann S, Hengartner H, Zinkernagel RM. (1998) Dendritic cells induce autoimmune diabetes and maintain disease via *de novo* formation of local lymphoid tissue. *J. Exp. Med.* 188:1493 –501.

[35] Dittel BN, Visintin I, Merchant RM, Janeway CA jr. (1999) Presentation of the self antigen myelin basic protein by dendritic cells leads to experimental autoimmune encephalomyelitis. *J. Immunol.* 163:32 –39.

[36] Thomas R, Lipsky PE. (1996) Presentation of self peptides by dendritic cells: possible implications for the pathogenesis of rheumatoid arthritis. *Arthritis. Rheum.* 39:183 –90.

[37] Serafini B, Columba-Cabezas S, Di Rosa F, Aloisi F. (2000) Intracerebralr ecruitment and maturation of dendritic cells in the onset and progression of experimental autoimmune encephalomyelitis. *Am. J. Pathol.* 157:1991–2002.

[38] Quadbeck B, Eckstein AK, Tews S, Walz M, Hoermann R, Mann K, et al. (2000) Maturation of thyroidal dendritic cells in Graves' disease. *Scand. J. Immunol.* 55:612–620.

[39] Huang YM, Xiao BG, Ozenci V, Kouwenhoven M, Teleshova N, Fredrikson S, et al. (1999) Multiple sclerosis is associated with high levels of circulating dendritic cells secreting pro-inflammatory cytokines. *J. Neuroimmunol.* 99:82 –90.

[40] Guiducci C, Tripodo C, Gong M, Sangaletti S, Colombo MP, Coffman RL, Barrat FJ. (2010) Autoimmune skin inflammation is dependent on plasmacytoid dendritic cell activation by nucleic acids via TLR7 and TLR9 . J. Exp. Med. 2010 doi:10.1084/jem.20101048

[41] Ludewig B, Junt T, Hengartner H, Zinkernagel RM. (2001) Dendritic cells in autoimmune diseases. *Curr. Opin. Immunol.* 13(6):657-662.

[42] Blanco P, Palucka AK, Gill M, Pascual V, Banchereau J. (2001) Induction of dendritic cell differentiation by IFN-α in systemic lupus erythematosus. *Science* 294:1540 –1543.

[43] Barchet W, Price JD, Cella M, Colonna M, MacMillan SK, Cobb JP, Thompson PA, Murphy KM, Atkinson JP, Kemper K. (2006) Complement-induced regulatory T cells suppress T-cell responses but allow for dendritic-cell maturation. *Blood* 107: 1497-1504

[44] Travis MA, Reizis B, Melton AC, Masteller E, Tang Q, Proctor JM, Wang Y, Bernstein X, Huang X, Reichardt LF, Bluestone JA, Sheppard D. (2007) Loss of integrin $\alpha_v\beta_8$ on dendritic cells causes autoimmunity and colitis in mice. *Nature* 449:361-365.

[45] Chen M, Wang YH, Wang Y, Huang L, Sandoval H, Liu YJ, Wang J. (2006) Dendritic cell apoptosis in the maintenance of immune tolerance. *Science* 24(5764):1160-1164.

[46] Mahnke K, Schmitt E, Bonifaz L, Enk AH, Jonuleit H. (2002) Immature, but not inactive: the tolerogenic function of immature dendritic cells. *Immunol Cell Biol.* 80:477–483.

[47] Belkaid Y, Oldenhove G. (2008) Tuning Microenvironments: induction of regulatory T cells by dendritic Cells. *Immunity* 29(3): 362-371.

[48] Piemonti L, Monti P, Allavena P, Sironi P, Soldini M, Leone L, et al.(1999) Glucocorticoids affect human dendritic cell differentiation and maturation. *J. Immunol.* 162:6473–6481.

[49] Penna G, Adorini L. (2000) 1α, 25-dihydroxyvitamin D3 inhibits differentiation, maturation, activation, and survival of dendritic cells leading to impaired alloreactive T cell activation. *J. Immunol.* 164:2405–2411.

[50] Zimmer A, Luce S, Gaignier F, Nony E, Naveau M, Biola-Vidamment A, Pallardy M, Van Overtvelt L, Mascarell L, Moingeon P. (2011) Identification of a New Phenotype of Tolerogenic Human Dendritic Cells Induced by Fungal Proteases from Aspergillus oryzae. *J. Immunol.* 186(7):3966-3976.

[51] Unger WW, Laban S, Kleijwegt FS, van der Slik AR, Roep BO.(2009) Induction of Treg by monocyte-derived DC modulated by vitamin D3 or dexamethasone: differential role for PD. Eur. *J. Immunol.* 39(11):3147-3159.

[52] Healy LJ, Collins HL, Thompson SJ. (2008) Systemic administration of tolerogenic dendritic cells ameliorates murine inflammatory arthritis. *Open Rheumatol. J.* 2:71-80.

[53] Chorny A, Gonzalez-Rey E, Fernandez-Martin A, Pozo D, Ganea D, Delgado M. (2005) Vasoactive intestinal peptide induces regulatory dendritic cells with therapeutic effects on autoimmune disorders. *Proc. Natl. Acad. Sci. USA* 102, 13562-13567.

[54] Kusmartsev S, Nagaraj S, Garbrilovich DI. (2005) Tumor-associated $CD8^+$ T cell tolerance induced by bone marrow-derived immature myeloid cells. *J. Immunol.* 175, 4853-4592.

[55] Wu J, Zhou C, Robertson J, Weng CY, Meistrich ML, Tailor RC, Lou YH.(2010) Identification of a bone marrow derived $CD8\alpha\alpha^+$ dendritic cell like population in inflamed autoimmune target tissue with capability of inducing T cell apoptosis. *J. Leukoc. Biol.* 88: 839-848.

[56] Bailey-Bucktrout SL, Caulkins CS, Goings G, Fischer JAA, Dzionek A, Miller SD.(2008) Central nervous system plasmacytoid dendritic cells regulate the severity of relapsing experimental autoimmune encephalomyelitis. *J. Immunol.* 180:6457 -6461.

[57] Schreiner GF, Kiely JM, Cotran RS, Unanue ER. (1981) Characterization of resident glomerular cells in the rat expressing Ia determinants and manifesting genetically restricted interactions with lymphocytes. *J. Clin. Invest.* 68: 920–931.

[58] John R, Nelson PJ. (2006) Dendritic cells in the kidney. *J. Am. Soc. Nephrol.* 18:2628-2635.

[59] Velazquez P, Dustin ML, Nelson PJ. (2009) Renal dendritic cells: an update. *Nephron Exp. Nephrol.* 111:e67-71.

[60] Hochheiser K, Tittel A, Kurts C. (2010) Kidney dendritic cells in acute and chronic disease. *Int. J. Exp. Pathol.* Doi: 10.1111

[61] Soos TJ, Sims TN, Barisoni L, Lin K, Littman DR, Dustin ML, Nelson PJ. (2006) CX3CR1_ interstitial dendritic cells form a contiguous network throughout the entire kidney. *Kidney Int.* 70: 591–596.

[62] Kruger T, Benke D, Eitner F. et al. (2004) Identification and functional characterization of dendritic cells in the healthy murine kidney and in experimental glomerulonephritis. *J. Am. Soc. Nephrol.* 15:613–621.

[63] Ginhoux F., Liu K., Helft J. et al. (2009) The origin and development of nonlymphoid tissue $CD103^+$ DCs. *J. Exp. Med.* 206:3115–3130.

[64] Hildner K., Edelson B.T., Purtha W.E. et al. (2008) Batf3 deficiency reveals a critical role for $CD8\alpha^+$ dendritic cells in cytotoxic T cell immunity. *Science* 322:1097–1100.

[65] Coates PT, Duncan FJ, Colvin BL, Wang Z, Zahorchak AF, Shufesky WJ, Morelli AE, Thomson AW. (2004) In vivo-mobilized kidney dendritic cells are functionally immature, subvert alloreactive T-cell responses, and prolong organ allograft survival. *Transplantation* 77: 1080–1089.

[66] Woltman A, de Fijter J, Zuidwijk K, Vlug A, Bajema I, van der Kooij S, van Ham V, van Kooten C. (2007) Quantitation of dendritic cell subsets in human renal tissues under normaland pathologic conditions. *Kidney Int.* 71: 1001–1008.

[67] Chan CW, Crafton E, Fan HN, Flook J, Yoshimura K, Skarica M, Brockstedt D, Dubensky TW, Stins MF, Lanier LL, Pardoll DM, Housseau F. (2006) Interferon-producing killer dendritic cells provide a link between innate and adaptive immunity. *Nat. Med.* 12: 207–213.

[68] Taieb J, Chaput N, Menard C, Apetoh L, Serbina NV, Salazar-Mather TP, Biron CA, Kuziel WA, Pamer EG.(2003) TNF/iNOS-producing dendritic cells mediate innate immune defense against bacterial infection. *Immunity* 19: 59–70.

[69] Munn DH, Sharma MD, Lee JR, Jhaver KG, Johnson TS, Keskin DB, Marshall B, Chandler P, Antonia SJ, Burgess R, Slingluff CL Jr, Mellor AL. (2002) Potential regulatory function of human dendritic cells expressing indoleamine 2,3-dioxygenase. *Science* 297:1867–1870.

[70] Naik SH. (2008) Demystifying the development of dendritic cell subtypes, a little. *Immunol. Cell Biol.* 86: 439–452.

[71] Geissmann F, Auffray C, Palframan R, Wirrig C, Ciocca A, Campisi L, Narni-Mancinelli E, Lauvau G. (2008) Blood monocytes: distinct subsets, how they relate to dendritic cells, and their possible roles in the regulation of T-cell responses. *Immunol. Cell Biol.* 86:398–408.

[72] Landsman L, Varol C, Jung S.(2007) Distinct differentiation potential of blood monocyte subsets in the lung. *J. Immunol.* 178:2000–2007.

[73] Shortman K, Naik SH.(2007) Steady-state and inflammatory dendritic-cell development. *Nat. Rev. Immunol.* 7:19–30.

[74] Maraskovsky E, Brasel K, Teepe M, Roux ER, Lyman SD, Shortman K, McKenna HJ. (1996) Dramatic increase in the numbers of functionally mature dendritic cells in Flt3 ligand-treated mice: Multiple dendritic cell subpopulations identified. *J. Exp. Med.* 184:1953–1962.

[75] Hume DA, Gordon S. (1983) Mononuclear phagocyte system of the mouse defined by immunohistochemical localization of antigen F4/80: identification of resident macrophages in renal medullary and cortical interstitium and the juxtaglomerular complex. *J. Exp. Med.* 157: 1704–1709.

[76] MacDonald KP, Rowe V, Bofinger HM, Thomas R, Sasmono T, Hume DA, Hill GR.(2005) The colony-stimulating factor 1 receptor is expressed on dendritic cells during differentiation and regulates their expansion. *J. Immunol.* 175: 1399–1405.

[77] Isbel NM, Hill PA, Foti R, Mu W, Hurst LA, Stambe C, Lan HY, Atkins RC, Nikolic-Paterson DJ. (2001) Tubules are the major site of M-CSF production in experimental kidneydisease: Correlation with local macrophage proliferation. *Kidney Int.* 60: 614–625.

[78] Jang MH, Herber DM, Jiang X, Nandi S, Dai XM, Zeller G, Stanley ER, Kelley VR.(2006) Distinct in vivo roles of colony-stimulating factor-1 isoforms in renal inflammation. *J. Immunol.* 177: 4055–4063.

[79] Leszczynski D, Renkonen R, Hayry P. (1985) Localization and turnover rate of rat renal "dendritic' cells. *J. Scan. Immunol.* 21:355-360.

[80] Dong X, Swaminathan S, Bachman LA, Croatt AJ, Nath KA, Griffin MD. (2005) Antigen presentation by dendritic cells in renal lymph nodes is linked to systemic and local injury to the kidney. *Kidney Int.* 68: 1096–1108.

[81] Foti M, Granucci F, Ricciardi-Castagnoli P. (2004) A central role for tissue-resident dendritic cells in innate responses. *Trends Immunol.* 25: 650–654.

[82] Munz C, Steinman RM, Fujii S.(2005) Dendritic cell maturation by innate lymphocytes: Coordinated stimulation of innate and adaptive immunity. *J. Exp. Med.* 202: 203–207.

[83] Kurts C, Kosaka H, Carbone FR, Miller JF, Heath WR. (1997) Class I-restricted cross-presentation of exogenous self-antigens leads to deletion of autoreactive CD8(+) T cells. *J. Exp. Med.* 186: 239–245.

[84] Heymann F, Meyer-Schwesinger C, Hamilton-Williams EE et al. (2009) Kidney dendritic cell activation is required for progression of renal disease in a mouse model of glomerular injury. *J. Clin.Invest.* 119: 1286–1297.

[85] Lukacs-Kornek V., Burgdorf S., Diehl L., Specht S., Kornek M., Kurts C. (2008) The kidney-renal lymph node-system contributes to cross-tolerance against innocuous circulating antigen. *J. Immunol.* 180: 706–715.

[86] Roake JA, Rao AS, Morris PJ, Larsen CP, Hankins DF, Austyn JM. (1995) Dendritic cell loss from nonlymphoid tissues after systemic administration of lipopoly saccharide, tumor necrosis factor, and interleukin 1. *J. Exp. Med.* 181: 2237–2247.

[87] Kelly CJ, Korngold R, Mann R, Clayman M, Haverty T, Neilson EG.(1986): Spontaneous interstitial nephritis in kdkd mice. II. Characterization of a tubular antigen-specific, H-2Krestricted Lyt-2^{+} effector T cell that mediates destructive tubulointerstitial injury. *J. Immunol.* 136: 526–531,

[88] Hancock WW, Tsai TL, Madaio MP, Gasser DL.(2003) Multiple autoimmune pathways in kd/kd mice. *J. Immunol.* 171:2778–2781.

[89] Sung, SS, Bolton WK. (2010) T cells and dendritic cells in glomerular disease: the new glomerulotubular feedback loop. *Kidney Int.* 77:393-399.

[90] Faria AM, Weiner HL. (2005) oral tolerance. *Immunol. Rev.* 206:232-259.

[91] Steinman RM, Hawiger D, Liu K et al. (2003) Dendritic cell function in vivo during the steady state: a role in peripheral tolerance. *Ann. N Y Acad. Sci.* 987: 15–25.

[92] Hochheiser K, Engel DR, Hammerich L, Heymann F, Knolle PA, Panzer U, Kurts C. (2011) Kidney dendritic cells become pathogenic during crescentic glomerulonephritis with proteinuria. *J. Am. Soc. Nephrol.* 22(2):306-316.

[93] Edgtton KL, Kausman JY, Li M et al. (2008) Intrarenal antigens activate CD4+ cells via co-stimulatory signals from dendritic cells. *J. Am. Soc. Nephrol.* 19: 515–526.

[94] Geissmann F., Manz MG., Jung S, Sieweke MH, Merad M, Ley K. (2010) Development of monocytes, macrophages, and dendritic cells. *Science* 327: 656–661.

[95] Bagavant H, Deshmukh US, Wang H, Ly T, Fu SM. (2006) Role for nephritogenic T cells in lupus glomerulonephritis: progression to renal failure is accompanied by T cell activation and expansion in regional lymph nodes. *J. Immunol.* 177: 8258–8265.

[96] Robertson J, Wu J, Arends J, Zhou C, McMahon J, Torres L, Lou YH.(2005) Activation of GBM-specific B cells in the renal draining lymph node following T cell mediated glomerular injury. *J. Am. Soc. Nephrol.* 16: 3256-3263.

[97] Scholz J, Lukacs-Kornek V, Engel DR et al. (2008) Renal dendritic cells stimulate IL-10 production and attenuate nephrotoxic nephritis. *J. Am. Soc. Nephrol.* 19: 527–537.

[98] Ysebaert DK, De Greef KE, Vercauteren SR et al. (2000) Identification and kinetics of leukocytes after severe ischaemia / reperfusion renal injury. *Nephrol. Dial. Transplant.* 15: 1562–1574.

[99] Yokota N, Daniels F, Crosson J, Rabb H. (2002) Protective effect of T cell depletion in murine renal ischemia-reperfusion injury. *Transplantation* 74:759–763.

[100] Ysebaert DK, De Greef KE, De Beuf A et al. (2004) T cells as mediators in renal ischemia / reperfusion injury. *Kidney Int.* 66:491–496.

[101] Burne-Taney MJ, Kofler J, Yokota N, Weisfeldt M, Traystman RJ, Rabb H (2003) Acute renal failure after whole body ischemia is characterized by inflammation and T cell-mediated injury. *Am. J. Physiol. Renal. Physiol.* 285: F87–94.

[102] Jantsch J, Chakravortty D, Turza N et al. (2008) Hypoxia and hypoxia-inducible factor-1 alpha modulate lipopolysaccharideinduced dendritic cell activation and function. *J. Immunol.* 180: 4697–4705.

[103] Nagler W. (1973) Vertebral artery obstruction by hyperextension of the neck: report of three cases. *Arch. Phys. Med. Rehabil.* 54: 237–240.

[104] Kitamoto K, Machida Y, Uchida J et al. (2009) Effects of liposome clodronate on renal leukocyte populations and renal fibrosis in murine obstructive nephropathy. *J. Pharmacol. Sci.* 111: 285–292.

[105] Machida Y, Uchida J, Kitamoto K, Nishikawa N, Morimoto K, Maeda S, Kamata R, Iwai T, Naganuma T, Nakatani T, Miura K. (2010) Role of renal dendritic cells and macrophages on renal fibrosis in obstructive nephropathy. *Transplantation* 90: 476-

[106] Tucci M, Ciavarella S, Strippoli S, Dammacco F, Silvestris F. (2009) Oversecretion of cytokines and chemokines in lupus nephritis is regulated by intraparenchymal dendritic cells: a review. *Ann. N Y Acad. Sci.* 1173:449–457.

[107] Li L, Huang L, Sung SS et al. (2008) The chemokine receptors CCR2 and CX3CR1 mediate monocyte / macrophage trafficking in kidney ischemia–reperfusion injury. *Kidney Int.* 74:1526–1537.

[108] Lassen S, Lech M, Römmele C, Mittruecker HW, Mak TW, Anders HJ. (2010) Ischemia reperfusion induces IFN Regulatory Factor 4 in renal dendritic cells, which suppresses postischemic inflammation and prevents acute renal failure. *J. Immunol.* 185(3): 1976-1983.

[109] Tadagavadi RK, Reeves WB. (2010) Renal dendritic cells ameliorate nephrotoxic acute kidney injury. *J. Am. Soc. Nephrol.* 21: 53–63.

[110] Akbari O, Freeman GJ, Meyer EH et al. (2002) Antigen-specific regulatory T cells develop via the ICOS-ICOS-ligand pathway and inhibit allergen-induced airway hyperreactivity. *Nat. Med.* 8:1024–1032.

[111] Lech M, Avila-Ferrufino A, Allam R et al. (2009) Resident dendritic cells prevent postischemic acute renal failure by help of single Ig IL-1 receptor-related protein. *J. Immunol.* 183: 4109–4118.

[112] Lech M, Kulkarni OP, Pfeiffer S et al. (2008) Tir8 / Sigirr prevents murine lupus by suppressing the immunostimulatory effects of lupus autoantigens. *J. Exp. Med.* 205: 1879–1888.Robertson J, Wu J, Arends J, Zhou C, Adrogue H, Chan J, Lou YH. (2008) Spontaneous recovery from early glomerular inflammation is associated with resistance to anti-GBM glomerulonephritis: tolerance and autoimmune tissue injury. *J. Autoimmunity* 30: 246-256. Overes IM, Fredrix H, Kester MG, *et al.* (2009). Efficient activation of LRH-1-specific CD8+ T-cell responses from transplanted leukemia patients by stimulation with P2X5 mRNA-electroporated dendritic Cells. *J. Immunotherapy* 32 (6): 539

[115] SJ Sung, WK Bolton. (2010) Are men rats? dendritic cells in autoimmune glomerulonephritis. *J. Leukoc. Biol.* 88:831-835.

13

Endoplasmic Reticulum: The Master Regulator of Stress Responses in Glomerular Diseases

Reiko Inagi
Division of Nephrology and Endocrinology, University of Tokyo School of Medicine, Hongo Bunkyo-ku, Tokyo, Japan

1. Introduction

The glomerulus is composed of glomerular resident cells, which include podocytes, mesangial cells, and glomerular endothelial cells, and is response for glomerular filtration. A range of pathogenic conditions can cause structural and functional damage to these glomerular cells, including hypertension, diabetes, and inflammation; these induce glomerulonephritis, which in turn leads to end-stage renal failure. Extensive investigations have uncovered the molecular mechanisms by which glomerulonephritis progresses, including the contribution of cellular stress signals induced by oxidative stress, hypoxia, or inflammation.

The endoplasmic reticulum (ER) is an organelle that maintains protein homeostasis, which includes regulation of the concentration, conformation, folding, and trafficking of client proteins. ER dysfunction causes an imbalance between protein-folding capacity and protein-folding load, a condition referred to as ER stress. This stress triggers the accumulation of unfolded proteins in the ER and subsequent activation of an intracellular stress signal, the unfolded protein response (UPR). ER stress and the UPR can result from various disturbances, such as hypoxia, glucose deprivation, and oxidative stress. The UPR, which initially serves as an adaptive response to maintain the homeostasis of the ER, induces ER resident chaperones, which act to enhance protein-folding capacity, the activation of pathways that degrade unfolded proteins accumulated in the ER (ERAD), and the attenuation of translation. The physiological level of the UPR transformes to a pathogenic response when ER stress is overwhelming or prolonged. At its pathogenic level, the UPR produces an apoptotic response, namely the activation of UPR-related proapoptotic molecules and inhibition of anti-apoptotic molecules. Accumulating evidence demonstrates that ER stress contributes not only to protein conformational diseases, but also to the progression of various diseases, including cardiac disease, diabetes, cancer, and kidney disease. Given the linkage of ER stress with oxidative stress or hypoxia, both of which are pathogenic, it is hardly surprising that the potential pathophysiological significance of ER stress is evoked across a wide range of diseases.

Recent evidence demonstrates that ER stress is a significant contributor to glomerulonephritis. Podocytes play an important role in the glomerular filtration barrier that is maintained by filtration slits (slit diaphragm), and express various proteins associated with the slit diaphragm. Congenital nephrotic syndrome is caused by genetic mutation of slit diaphragm-associated molecules, such as nephrin and α-actinin-4. These mutated proteins are malfolded and accumulated in the ER of podocytes, and thereby induce the UPR, namely ER chaperone expression and proapoptotic gene induction. Mesangial cells are responsible for the structural and functional maintenance of glomerular tufts and mesangial cell damage in glomerulonephritis is associated with induction of the UPR, which involves ER chaperone expression and the attenuation of protein translation. The induction level of the UPR increases in parallel with disease progression. These data suggest that the UPR maintains ER homeostasis in glomerular cells and ensures cell survival under pathogenic conditions. ER stress pathophysiologically contributes to tubulointerstitial damage not only in glomeruli, but also tubules. Tubular damage, such as tubular cell death caused by proteinuria, ischemia-reperfusion, or nephrotoxin, predominantly enhances the UPR, especially UPR-induced apoptosis and autophagy.

These findings emphasize not only the importance of ER stress as a new progression factor but also the interesting future possibility of renoprotective strategies which target ER stress. In experimental glomerular and tubular injury model animals, overexpression of GRP78 (glucose-regulated protein 78), a master regulator of UPR, or administration of the chemical compounds that regulate UPR activation shows renoprotective effects. Preconditioning of ER stress with non-nephrotoxic dose of ER stress inducers protects against the podocyte and mesangial cell damage they induced. Interestingly, some oxidative stress inhibitors and advanced glycation inhibitors also act as UPR inhibitors, suggesting a link between oxidative stress, hypoxia, and ER stress. Therapeutic approaches which target ER stress may act by breaking the vicious cycle of this stress signal crosstalk in kidney disease.

Here, I summarize the role of ER stress as the master regulator of the stress response in glomerular disease and the therapeutic possibility of targeting UPR molecules.

2. ER stress and the unfolded protein response (UPR)

The ER plays an important role in the quality control of proteins by the regulating their synthesis, folding and trafficking. ER homeostasis depends on a balance in capacity between protein synthesis and folding. Various disturbances; decrease folding capacity, including folding mutations, hypoxia, or starvation, and thereby induce the accumulation of malfolded protein in the ER, which in turn leads to ER stress. This enforces the cellular stress signal, called the unfolded protein response (UPR) (Ron & Walter, 2007) (Figure 1).

The UPR pathway is regulated by three ER resident transducers (ER stress sensors), namely inositol-requiring protein-1 (IRE1), protein kinase RNA (PKR)-like ER kinase (PERK), and activating transcription factor 6 (ATF6). Under normal conditions, they are inactivated by binding with an ER chaperone, glucose-regulated protein 78 (GRP78 or BiP). When unfolded proteins accumulate in the ER lumen, however, they are dissociated from GRP78, activated by dimerization, phosphorylation, or translocation to the Golgi, and then induce signals to attenuate translation or upregulate adaptive UPR target gene expression. The three ER resident transducers induce the ER chaperones to enhance folding capacity and activate the pathway for ER-associated protein degradation (ERAD) to reduce the accumulation of malfolded proteins. The UPR pathway maintains ER homeostasis to ensure cell survival.

When severe ER stress results in excessive or prolonged UPR activation, cells are unable to resolve the protein-folding defect or restore ER homeostasis via the adaptive UPR pathway.

In these circumstances, the proapoptotic UPR mediated by CHOP (CCAAT/enhancer-binding protein homologous protein) or caspase 12 is induced to ensure cell death (Tabas & Ron, 2011). The UPR pathway is thus a double-edged sword for cells under ER stress, and the final outcome represents the sum of the effects of the various possible UPR branches.

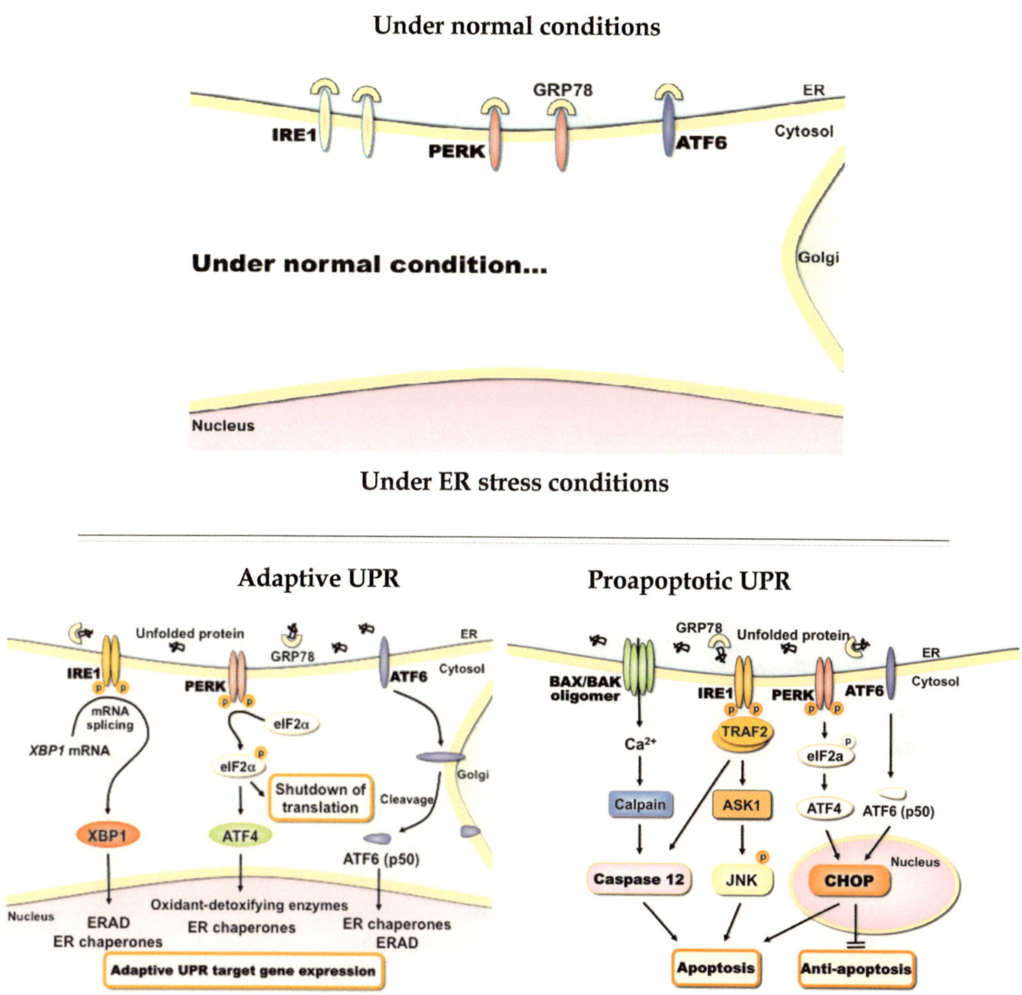

Fig. 1. Unfolded protein response (UPR)

Under normal conditions (upper panel), the ER stress sensors IRE1, PERK, and ATF6 are inactivated by binding with ER chaperone GRP78. When an imbalance between protein synthesis and folding capacity under ER stress causes the accumulation of unfolded proteins in the ER, however, these sensors are dissociated from GRP78 and activated by dimerization and phosphorylation (IRE1 and PERK) or translocation and cleavage (ATF6), thereby inducing the adaptive UPR for cell survival (lower left panel). The adaptive UPR consists of 1) translation attenuation to ensure a balance of protein synthesis and folding, 2) induction of ER chaperone expression to enhance folding capacity, and 3) activation of the ER-associated protein degradation (ERAD) system to reduce unfolded protein accumulation. In stark contrast, prolonged or severe UPR activation leads to induction of the proapoptotic UPR, which is mediated by CHOP and caspase 12 for cell death (lower right panel). The balance of UPR states contributes to the consequence of ER stress. IRE1, inositol-requiring protein-1; PERK, protein kinase RNA (PKR)-like ER kinase; ATF6, activating transcription factor 6; GRP78, glucose-regulated protein 78; CHOP, CCAAT/enhancer-binding protein homologous protein. (modified from Reiko Inagi, Curr Opin Pharmacol, 2009 with permission)

2.1 Adaptive UPR: IRE-XBP, PERK-eIF2α, and ATF6 pathways

The IRE1 pathway is initiated by the RNAase activity of IRE1, which induces mRNA splicing in X-box-binding protein 1 (XBP1), thereby creating a potent transcriptional activator (XBP1s) of genes which encode ERAD components and ER chaperones such as GRP78, GRP94, and calreticulin. The IRE1-XBP1 pathway serves mainly as an ER homeostatic response to ER stress by degrading or refolding misfolded proteins accumulated in the ER lumen. Recent publication of the crystal structure and autophosphorylation mechanism of IRE1 protein has provided new insights into the regulation mechanism of IRE1-XBP1 axis and subsequently the entire UPR (Lee et at, 2008; Ali et al, 2011).

The PERK pathway alleviates the ER burden by reducing the frequency of initiation of mRNA translation, thereby decreasing the influx of new proteins into the ER. PERK is a Ser/Thr protein kinase whose active homodimer phosphorylates and inactivates eukaryotic initiation factor 2α (eIF2α), thereby shutting off protein translation globally and reducing protein load on the ER. In addition to this function, the PERK-eIF2α pathway activates in parallel activating transcription factor 4 (ATF4), and thereby selectively induces UPR-inducible gene expression, including ER chaperones, as well as antioxidant enzymes, such as glutathione S-transferase and hemoxygenase 1 (HO-1), to protect cells from both oxidative as well as ER stresses (Bardag-Gorce et al, 2010). Although PERK and IRE1 share functionally similar ER-luminal sensing domains and are both simultaneously activated in cellular paradigms of ER stress in vitro, they are selectively engaged in vivo by the physiological stress of unfolded proteins.

The ATF6 pathway is activated by its transloation to the Golgi where it is cleaved by S1P and S2P (site-1 and site-2 proteases). The cytosolic fragment of cleaved ATP6 (p50) further translocates to the nucleus, where it subsequently activates the transcription of its target genes, which encode ER chaperones and ERAD components.

2.2 Proapoptotic UPR: CHOP and IRE1-TRAF2 pathways

ER stress-induced apoptosis is mainly mediated by CHOP, also referred to as GADD153 (growth arrest and DNA damage 153). CHOP, a transcription factor which induces several proapoptotic factors, occurs downstream of the PERK (PERK-ATF4 pathway) and ATF6 pathways in the proapoptotic UPR axis. The CHOP pathway also down-regulates anti-apoptotic Bcl-2, leading to enhanced oxidant injury and apoptosis. These findings are consistent with the previous observation that overexpression of Bcl-2 specifically in the ER protects renal tubular cells against ER stress-induced apoptosis (Bhatt et al, 2008).

The IRE1-TRAF2 pathway is another proapoptotic UPR branch. The cytoplasmic domain of activated IRE1 interacts with the adaptor factor TRAF2 (tumor necrosis factor receptor-associated factor 2), leading to activation of both the caspase 12-dependent and JNK-mediated apoptotic pathways. Several components of the caspase cascade are reported to be involved in ER stress-induced apoptosis. In particular, caspase 12, which is associated with the ER membrane, is a proximal regulator of ER stress-induced caspase activation followed by apoptosis. Caspase 12 is expressed in rodents but not primates, and caspase 4 is instead thought to contribute to ER stress-induced apoptosis in human cells.

ER stress-induced dysfunction of ER Ca^{+} homeostasis also contributes to apoptosis through multiple pathways. Ca^{+} leaked from the ER lumen enters the mitochondria, depolarizes the inner mitochondrial membrane, and generates mitochondrial ROS. This enhanced ROS production is associated with a vicious cycle of oxidative stress in both the ER and mitochondria, where it activates several apoptotic pathways, including the caspase 9-mediated or BAX/BAK-mediated pathways. This dispensation with dysfunctional cells represents a last resort on the part of multicellular organisms.

3. Pathophysiology of ER stress in kidney disease

It was recently established that ER stress is induced in various kidney diseases (Inagi, 2010). This is not entirely unexpected given that ER function is easily influenced by various cellular stresses. Further, ER stress contributes to disease progression in cardiac, vascular, and metabolic diseases, all of which are linked to the development of kidney disease. ER stress and consequent imbalance of UPR is one of the potent pathogenic mechanisms of kidney disease.

The initial filtrating component of functional nephrons are the glomeruli, which are capillary tufts that receive their blood supply from afferent arterioles of the renal circulation. The specialized capillary bed in each glomerulus consists of a network of interconnected loops surrounded by Bowman's capsule. Podocytes, which play an important role in the filtration barrier, have foot processes that extend over the glomerular basement membrane. These foot processes are bridged by slit diaphragms (filtration barrier) which connect adjacent foot process and thereby act to prevent larger molecules filtering into Bowman's capsule. Mesangial cells, some of which have phagocytic properties, are located between the capillary loops, and form the central stalk of the glomerulus. These form part of the functional nephron unit and interact closely with endothelial cells and indirectly with podocytes. Recent evidence increasingly emphasizes the link between ER stress and both glomerular cell damage and tubulointerstitial injury.

3.1 Podocytes and ER stress

Mutation of components of the slit diaphragms, including nephrin and alpha-actinin-4, leads to congenital nephrotic syndromes. These mutations are mostly associated with conformational abnormalities. Thus, they induce defects in the related protein trafficking and retention of mutant proteins in the ER, and thereby lead to ER stress in podocytes. Indeed, Cybulsky and collegues have demonstrated that mice overexpressing human mutated alpha-actini-4 develop the pathological and functional features of congenital nephrotic syndrome, including podocyte injury and proteinuria. They also show associated ER stress, namely an increase in ER chaperones and adaptive and proapoptotic UPR molecules (Cybulsky et al, 2009), suggesting that ER stress in podocytes contributes to congenital nephrotic syndrome. We have also demonstrated that ER stress is induced by malfolded protein accumulation in podocytes, and that this leads to proteinuria. We previously established a transgenic rat in which the protein encoded by the transgene (megsin, a kidney specific serine protease inhibitor) is consistently malfolded and polymerized under overexpression conditions and accumulated in the ER lumen of podocytes (Inagi et al, 2005a). Pathological changes in these podocytes, such as ER dilation, were associated with severe proteinuria. Importantly, these transgenic rats showed an increase in ER chaperone expressions in damaged podocytes, including GRP78 or oxygen-regulated protein 150 (ORP150) (Inagi et al, 2005b). Collectively, these data suggest that the decline in protein-folding capacity in podocytes triggers cellular dysfunction which in turn results in derangement of the structure of slit diaphragms and thereby causes proteinuria.

We have also established an advanced diabetic nephropathy model mouse, which develops severe albuminuria and renal damage with all of the characteristics of human advanced diabetic nephropathy, such as acellular nodule-like lesions (Inagi et al, 2006). Immunohistochemistry for the detection of GRP78 revealed that these changes were associated with ER stress mainly in podocytes. (Inagi R, unpublished data)

ER stress induction in podocytes was further confirmed by studies utilizing the XBP1-venus fusion Tg mouse, which is an ER stress monitoring mouse (Iwawaki et al, 2004). These mice produce XBP1-GFP fusion protein only when XBP1 is activated by alternative splicing under ER stress conditions, and not under normal conditions. On treatment with anti-GBM antibody, a model of rapidly progressive glomerulonephritis, untreated mice showed the basal level of GFP expression in podocytes. In contrast, this expression was significantly increased in the diseased mice in association with proteinuria. This finding suggests that the XBP-1 axis is activated in damaged podocytes.

Taken together, our and previous findings demonstrating UPR activation in other podocyte-injury disease models (e.g., membranous nephropathy and minimal change nephrotic syndrome) highlight the link between ER stress and podocyte homeostasis, and that the ER stress state in podocytes might be changed by these various factors.

3.2 Mesangial cells and ER stress

Mesangioproliferative glomerulonephritis, which is caused by mesangial cell damage, is one of the major glomerulonephritises. We previously demonstrated that ER chaperone expression was significantly increased in the damaged mesangial area in anti-Thy1 nephritis rats, a representative mesangioproliferative glomerulonephritis model (Inagi et al, 2008). For example, immunohistochemistry for the detection of GRP78 and ORP150 followed by quantitative morphometry confirmed that the UPR for the induction of ER chaperone expression was markedly enhanced as the disease progressed. Similar results were observed by Western blot analysis followed by densitometry utilizing isolated glomeruli in experimental rats. Further, another adaptive UPR axis for translation attenuation was also significantly increased, as estimated by the phosphorylation of PERK and eIF2α. These data emphasize the association between mesangial cell damage and ER stress, and that significant activation of the adaptive UPR axis contributes to the progression of glomerulonephritis. Given that oxidative stress is also induced in anti-Thy1 nephritis rats, mesangial cell damage may be orchestrated by the link between ER stress and oxidative stress as pathogenic mediators.

This evidence from a rat disease model might be consistent with evidence that ER stress estimated by GRP78 and CHOP expression is higher in patients with proliferative glomerulonephritis than in those with other glomerular diseases (Markan et al, 2009).

Trigger	Disease state	References
Folding mutant proteins		
	Congenital nephrotic syndrome	
		Cybulsky AV et al., Am J Physiol-Renal 2009
ATP depletion		
	Puromycin nephrosis	Nakajo A et al., J Am Soc Nephrol 2007
Complement (C5b-9)		
	Heymann nephritis	Cybulsky AV et al., J Biol Chem 2002
Oxidative stress (ROS), fatty acid		
	Diabetic nephropathy	Morse E et al., Am J Physiol-Renal 2010
Lowering of folding capacity		
	Proteinuria	Inagi R et al., Kidney Int 2005

Table 1. Triggers for ER stress in podocytes

Various pathogenic factors trigger ER stress in podocytes. Heymann nephritis and puromycin nephrosis are representative experimental animal disease models which mimic human membranous nephropathy and minimal change nephrotic syndrome, respectively.

3.3 Tubular cells and ER stress

Several disturbances have been shown to induce ER stress in tubules as cellular damage progresses. (Table 2) Among them, we showed that the proapoptotic UPR axis, which is predominantly mediated by caspase 12, is induced by proteinuria and contributes to tubular cell death in a minimal change nephrotic syndrome model rats (puromycin nephropathy) (Ohse et al, 2006). In chronic kidney disease, we further showed that uremic toxin might act as an ER stress inducer. In particular, in chronic kidney disease model rats (5/6-nephrectomized rats), CHOP-positive tubular cells were significantly increased in parallel with the accumulation of a representative uremic toxin, indoxyl sulfate, in the serum (Kawakami et al, 2010). These changes were ameliorated by the administration of a uremic toxin absorbent, AST-120, clearly suggesting the causal effect of indoxyl sulfate in ER stress induction in tubular cells.

Not only in experimental animals but also in humans, mRNA levels of ER chaperons (GRP78 and ORP150) and URP transcription factors (XBP1 and CHOP) in tubules is increased in patients with both advanced diabetic nephropathy and minimal change nephrotic syndrome as compared with healthy individuals (Lindenmeyer et al, 2008).

Disease site (trigger)	Consequence(s)	Reference
Ischemia-reperfusion		
(hypoxia)	ORP150 ↑	Bando Y, et al, FASEB J 2004
Minimal change nephrotic syndrome		
(proteinuria)	GRP78 ↑ , ORP150 ↑ , CHOP ↑ , caspase 12 ↑	Ohse T, et al, Kidney Int 2006
	GRP78 ↑ , ORP150 ↑ , XBP1 ↑ , CHOP ↑	Lindernmeyer MT, et al., J Am Soc Nephrol 2008
Diabetic nephropathy		
(hyperglycemia)	GRP78 ↑ , ORP150 ↑ , XBP1 ↑ , CHOP ↑	Lindernmeyer MT, et al., J Am Soc Nephrol 2008
Tubular injury		
(nephrotoxin, cyclosporine)	GRP78 ↑ , CHOP ↑	Pallet N, et al., Autophagy 2009
Chronic kidney disease		
(uremic toxin, indoxyl sulfate)	GRP78 ↑ , CHOP ↑	Kawakami T, et al., Am J Physiol-Renal 2010

Table 2. Triggers for ER stress in tubular cells.

3.4 Other kidney cells and ER stress

While ER stress is induced in retinal endothelial cells and pericytes in diabetic retinopathy, the role of ER stress in glomerular endothelial or tubulointerstitial cells is still unclear. Tubulointerstitial cells are heterogeneous, and a certain subpopulation of these cells includes pericyte-like cells producing erythropoietin (EPO). The role of ER stress in tubulointerstitial cells is an interesting issue, particularly its contribution to the regulation of EPO expression.

Recently, it was demonstrated that renal anemia is not due to loss of EPO-producing cells but rather derangement of the oxygen-sensing mechanism which regulates EPO expression (Bernhardt et al, 2010). We investigated the effect of ER stress on EPO production in an EPO-producing hepatic cell line, HepG2. Hypoxia-induced EPO mRNA expression was significantly blunted by ER stress in HepG2 when the cells were treated with the ER stress inducer tunicamycin under low oxygen tension (Chiang CK, et al., unpublished data). Our observations suggest that renal pathogens, which can trigger ER stress, derange renal EPO production capacity and may thereby enhance the development of renal anemia. Further studies of the suppressive mechanism of this finding are under way.

4. ER stress and other stress signals

It is known that ER stress is initiated by hypoxia or oxidative stress and vice versa. Hypoxia and oxidative stress induce the cellular stress signals, namely the hypoxia-inducible factor (HIF) and NF-E2-related factor 2 (Nrf2) pathways, respectively. Imbalance of these stress signals contributes to the pathological features of various kidney diseases (e.g., diabetic nephropathy, ischemia-reperfusion injury, glomerulonephritis) (Nangaku, 2006), which are also associated with ER stress. This suggests that the UPR, HIF, and Nrf2 pathways are linked, and that stress signal crosstalk might orchestrate the disease progression.

4.1 UPR and HIF pathway

Hypoxia, leading to the loss of energy, initiates a defect in protein-folding capacity, and thereby induces UPR activation. In tumor cells, for example, the hypoxic microenvironment brought on by poor vascularization brings about ER stress due to the loss of energy for protein folding. It has now been established that not only the HIF pathway but also the UPR is crucial to the survival of tumor cells against their hypoxic microenvironment: increased expression of ER chaperones, which enhances protein-folding capacity, is observed in a wide range of human cancers, and expression level correlates with tumor progression, metastasis, and drug resistance (Lee, 2007).

Further, it has also been demonstrated that the HIF pathway upragulates the expression of the UPR molecules, indicating the presence of molecular crosstalk between the HIF and URP pathways. Cultured endothelial cells under hypoxia showed an increased in GRP78, GRP94 and caspase 12 expressions. A chemical stabilizer of HIF, $CoCl_2$, also increased the expression of both GRP78 and GRP94, revealing that HIF activation alters UPR state (Ostergaard et al, 2009). Conversely, ER stress by tunicamycin and brefeldin A triggered HIF-1α mRNA expression in the human hepatocyte cell line HepG2 under hypoxia (Werno et al, 2008). These findings suggest the presence of positive feedback between the HIF pathway and the UPR under hypoxic conditions and the possibility of indirect regulation of the HIF pathway by the UPR. In addition, one study demonstrated that certain UPR molecule expression is translationally regulated by an HIF regulator: ATF4, a UPR transcription factor, alters its protein stability through interaction of the zipper II domain of ATF4 with the oxygen sensor prolyl-4-hydroxylase domain 3 (PHD3) (Koditz et al, 2007). PHDs are well-known regulators of HIF, and treatment with the PHD inhibitor increased ATF4 protein levels. These data demonstrate that PHD-dependent oxygen-sensing recruits both the HIF and ATF4 systems in parallel. To further emphasize the biological significance of interaction between the HIF and ER stress pathways, studies utilizing *C. elegans* showed that HIF-1 deficiency extended lifespan in a UPR transducer IRE-1-dependent manner (Chen et al, 2009)

4.2 UPR and oxidative stress

Oxidative stress as well as hypoxia initiates ER stress (Malhorta & Kaufman, 2007). Nitric oxide (NO), produced in excessive levels following ischemia, contributes to ER stress. Ischemia-reperfusion-induced activation of the PERK-eIF2α axis for translation attenuation is blocked in endothelial or neuronal NO synthase (NOS) knockout mice with bilateral carotid artery occlusion (DeGracia & Montie, 2004). Consistent with this, the NO-releasing reagent SNAP activates the PERK pathway, indicating that NO plays a role in the ischemia-reperfusion-induced UPR. Pretreatment with neuroprotective levels of an NOS inhibitor recovered the proapoptotic UPR state induced by a ischemia-induced defect in ER Ca^{2+} homeostasis, which occurs due to Ca^{2+} leakage into the cytosol and subsequent uptake into mitochondria, resulting in mitochondrial ROS generation. The aberrant NO production seen in hypoxia, which alters calcium homeostasis in both the ER and mitochondria, may initiate a vicious cycle of ER stress, oxidative stress, and apoptosis.

Under oxidative stress, reactive oxygen species (ROS) interfere with not only cellular redox-dependent reactions but also protein-folding capacity, including protein disulfide bonding, ultimately resulting in protein misfolding in the ER. Studies utilizing the overexpression of anti-oxidant enzymes have emphasized the linkage of oxidative stress to the ER stress response. The ischemia-induced ER stress response was markedly less pronounced in animals overexpressing copper/zinc superoxide dismutase (Cu/Zn-SOD), suggesting that superoxide radicals play a role in this pathological process (Hayashi et al, 2003). Further, cadmium caused the generation of ROS with subsequent induction of ER stress in a cultured renal proximal tubular cell line, which in turn led to apoptosis; this cadmium-induced ER stress and apoptosis were significantly attenuated by manganese SOD overexpression (Yokouchi et al, 2008). Paradoxically, ER stress also increases intracellular ROS production: increased protein disulfide bonding enhances ROS production in the ER lumen, and alteration of ER Ca+ homeostasis increases cytosolic Ca+, thereby stimulating mitochondrial ROS production. Of particular note, recent studies have demonstrated that the accumulation of intracellular ROS is attenuated by the adaptive UPR through PERK activation, which simultaneously activates an anti-oxidative stress signal, the Nrf2 pathway, and maintains redox homeostasis, thereby ensuring cell survival. The antioxidant effects of the PERK axis of the UPR are supported by the finding that PERK-deficient cells exposed to tunicamycin, an ER stress inducer, showed a toxic accumulation of intracellular ROS compared to wild-type cells (Cullinan & Diehl, 2006). Translation attenuation through the PERK-eIF2α pathway effectively prevents the misfolded protein-inducible oxidative stress and maintains the cell (Back et al, 2009).

4.3 UPR and advanced glycation

Under oxidative stress conditions with hyperglycemia, proteins and DNA are non-enzymatically modified by oxidative glycation, which occurs mainly due to increased ROS generation, and converted to advanced glycation endproducts (AGEs). Advanced glycation is one of the major pathophysiological posttranslational modifications and induces the derangement of protein functions or apoptosis. Functional abnormalities of glycated proteins perturb cellular homeostasis and increase mitochondrial ROS generation, accelerating the vicious cycle of oxidative stress and thereby enhancing subsequent glycation modification. From the viewpoint that ER stress is predominantly induced by hypoxic or oxidative stress, it is reasonable to speculate the presence of a link between advanced glycation and ER stress on the disease development and progression caused by these disturbances.

It has been reported that AGEs induce ER stress directly. Among findings, it is reported that glycated serum albumin (AGE-bovine serum albumin) induces ER stress, as estimated by GRP78 expression, and apoptosis in a dose- and time-dependent manner in mouse podocytes via an increase in intracellular Ca^{2+} concentration. ER stress inhibitor taurine-conjugated ursodeoxycholic acid (TUDCA), which acts as a chaperone that promotes the folding and trafficking of unfolded or malfolded proteins, prevents AGE-induced apoptosis, suggesting that this apoptosis is mediated by the apoptotic UPR pathway (Chen et al., 2008). Like glycated albumin, extracellular matrix is frequently modified by advanced glycation in the skin of diabetic patients. The advanced-glycated type I collagen also causes proapoptotic UPR-mediated apoptosis via CHOP activation in dermal fibroblasts, suggesting a pathophysiological role for the link between advanced glycation and ER stress in diabetic wounds (Loughlin & Artlett, 2010).

5. Therapeutic approach targeting ER stress in kidney disease

Accumulating evidence, including ours, has recently indicated the therapeutic benefits of targeting ER stress in various diseases, including cardiac, vascular, and metabolic diseases as well as kidney disease. Therapeutic modalities which targeting ER stress are summarized in Table 3. While artificial modulation of ER stress may provide protection to various kinds of cells (Kim et al, 2008), this chapter focuses on the beneficial effects on kidney disease.

Modality	Function(s)
ER chaperone overexpression	
GRP78	Translation shutdown ↑
ORP150	Protein folding ↑
Chemical chaperones	
4-PBA	Protein folding ↑ , ERAD ↑ , caspase 12 ↓
TUDCA	Adaptive UPR ↑ , proapoptotic UPR ↓
Chemical compounds	
DTTox	GRP78 ↑
BIX	GRP78 ↑
Salubrinal	Adaptive UPR (PERK-eIF2α) ↑
Benzodiazepinones	IRE1/TRAF2/ASK1 ↓
Methoxyflavone	GRP78 ↑
ER stress preconditioning	
ER stress inducers	Basal adaptive UPR ↑
Others	
Anti-oxidative stress compounds	
TM2002	Oxidative stress ↓
Butylated hydroxyanisole	Protein-folding capacity ↑
Anti-hypoxia compound (HIF stabilizer)	
Dimethyloxalylglycine	proapoptotic UPR (CHOP) ↓ , GRP78 ↑ , ATF4 ↑
Anti-inflammatory drug	
Mizoribine	Intracellular energy for protein folding ↑
Anti-hypertensive drug	
Angiotensin II type 1 receptor blocker	proapoptotic UPR (CHOP) ↓

Table 3. Therapeutic modalities targeting ER stress.
Abberant UPR state, which contributes to the progression of various diseases, is suppressed by ER chaperone overexpression, the chemical chaperones themselves, or chemical compounds which selectively activate the adaptive UPR axis or suppress the apoptotic UPR axis. ER stress preconditioning upregulates the basal UPR state and protects cells from variuos pathogenic stresses.

5.1 ER chaperones and chemical chaperones

ER chaperone overexpression (e.g., GRP78 and ORP150) and chemical or pharmaceutical chaperones (e.g., 4-phenyl butyric acid (PBA), TUDCA, and dimethyl sulfoxide) stabilize protein conformation, enhance ER protein-folding capacity to normalize the imbalance of protein synthesis and folding, and thereby maintain ER homeostasis. In particular, protein folding augmentation therapies utilizing these UPR modulators or chemical chaperones may improve conditions associated with protein malfolding, such as congenital nephrotic syndromes, which are caused by a defect in the retention and accumulation of mutant proteins in the ER of podocytes.

As the evidences for the effectiveness of ER chaperone enhancement in the kidney, ORP150 transgenic mice showed resistance to renal ischemia-reperfusion injury (Bando et at, 2004). 4-Phenylbutyric acid (4-PBA), a chemical chaperone, rescues mutated nephrin, which is associated with misfolding and mislocalization, from the ER to the cell surface, suggesting the beneficial effect of protein folding augmentation therapy in congenital nephrotic syndrome (Liu et al, 2004). 4-PBA also exerts a marked renoprotective effect possibly by modulating ER stress and the related inflammatory cascade in diabetic nephropathy (Qi et al, 2011). Endogenous bile acids and derivatives such as ursodeoxycholic acid and its taurine-conjugated derivative (TUDCA) can also modulate ER function, restore glucose homeostasis in type 2 diabetic mice, and thereby ameliorate the development of diabetic complications, including diabetic nephropathy in these animals (Xie et al, 2002; Ozcan et al, 2006; Ozcan et al, 2009). In studies of TUDCA therapy for obese men and women, TUDCA has consistently shown promise as an effective pharmacological approach to the treatment of insulin resistance and obesity-related disease including chronic kidney disease (Kars et al, 2010). Unlike 4-PBA, however, TUDCA has not been shown to act as a chaperone that promotes the folding and trafficking of malfolded proteins; instead, it is likely to increase folding capacity, possibly by enhancing the ERAD pathway (ER-associated malfolded protein degradation system). Murine podocytes suffered from ER stress-induced apoptosis on exposure to advanced glycation end product (AGE)-modified bovine serum albumin, but TUDCA prevented this apoptosis by suppressing the apoptotic UPR activation (Chen et al, 2008).

Aberrant UPR state, which contributes to the progression of various diseases, is suppressed by ER chaperone overexpression, the chemical chaperones themselves, or chemical compounds which selectively activate the adaptive UPR axis or suppress the apoptotic UPR axis. ER stress preconditioning upregulates the basal UPR state and protects cells from various pathogenic stresses.

5.2 Chemical UPR modulators

Chemical compounds which selectively activate the adaptive UPR branches act as enhancers of translation attenuation as well as of ER chaperone expression. Other chemical compounds which suppress the proapoptotic UPR branches protect cells from ER stress-induced cell death. The UPR pathway is a double-edged sword for cells suffering from ER stress; normalization of the balance between the adaptive and proapoptotic UPR branches by these chemical compounds might thus be effective in promoting ER homeostasis.

Several chemical compounds have demonstrated renal protective effects against ER stress suggesting the therapeutic possibility of targeting the UPR. Trans-4,5-dihydroxy-1,2-dithiane (DTTox) protected the proximal tubular epithelium against a nephrotoxic chemical via stimulation of GRP78 (Asmellash et al, 2005), while BIX (BiP inducer X, 1-(3,4-dihydroxyphenyl)-2-thiocyanato-ethanone) ameliorated disease manifestations of renal ischemia-reperfusion injury in mice by activating the ATF6 axis with subsequent induction of GRP78 (Prachasilchai et al, 2009). Salubrinal suppresses the protein phosphatases responsible for the dephosphorylation of eIF2α, and significantly reduces tubular injury in a rat cyclosporine nephropathy model by increasing the amounts of phosphorylated eIF2α (Pallet et al, 2008). Methoxyflavone, a group of flavonoids, is also identified as a strong ER stress modulator. Pretreatment of mice with tangeretin, a methoxyflavone, enhanced the expression of GRP78 and HO-1 in renal tubular epithelium and prevented tunicamycin-induced cell death (Takano et al, 2007).

5.3 Others

The previous evidences regarding the crosstalk of oxidative stress, hypoxia, and ER stress emphasize that anti-oxidative stress or anti-hypoxia drugs may also hold promising in reducing pathogenic ER stress. In fact, effective attenuation of the ER stress response has also been observed in compounds which suppress oxidative stress. TM2002, an inhibitor of oxidative protein glycation, shows renoprotective effects against glomerular and tubular interstitial damage in association with a decrease in ER stress in anti-Thy1 nephritis and renal ischemic-reperfusion rats (Izuhara et al, 2008). Further, a chemical HIF stabilizer, prolyl hydroxylase inhibitor (Dimethyloxalylglycine) which attenuates ischemic cardiac injury by HIF pathway activation, selectively activates the adaptive UPR (GRP78 and ATF4 inductions), and weakens the proapoptotic UPR, suggesting that HIF stabilizer has the renoprotective effects as a UPR modulator (Natarajan et al, 2009).

One study demonstrated that treatment with mizoribine, an immunosuppressant used clinically, reduced ER stress and rescued the mislocalization of nephrin from the ER to the cytoplasm in podocytes with glucose starvation. Mizoribine is known to inhibit purine nucleotide biosynthesis, and might thereby restore the intracellular energy balance under ER stress by salvaging ATP levels. These data suggest that the effect of mizorbine in inducing the remission of proteinuria in human nephrotic syndrome might be mediated by a reduction in ER stress (Nakajo et al, 2007).

Further, similar inhibitory effects to those of mizoribine on ER stress were seen with another clinically used anti-hypertensive drugs, namely angiotensin converting enzyme (ACE) inhibitors and angiotensin II type 1 receptor blockers. The angiotensin II type 1 receptor is thought to be an ER stress inducer, albeit that the molecular mechanisms by which angiotensin II induces ER stress remain unclear. It is therefore reasonable to consider that the increased tubular apoptosis in experimental diabetic rats is attenuated by ACE inhibitors in association with a reduction in aberrant apoptotic UPR activation and subsequent maintenance of the physiological UPR state in the tubulointerstitium (Sun et al, 2009)

5.4 ER stress preconditioning

The effects of ER stress preconditioning highlight the possibility of therapy based on ER stress. The concept of preconditioning was originally identified in ischemic diseases. Brief ischemic treatment for preconditioning prior to the subsequent insult induces a state of resistance to the loss of blood supply by initiating cellular protective responses in the tissue. These findings suggest that ER stress preconditioning may initiate the adaptive UPR and attenuate the subsequent insult. An increasing number of reports have demonstrated the beneficial effects of preconditioning in ER stress-related diseases, such as cardiac and neuronal diseases and retinopathy.

To evaluate the beneficial effect of ER stress preconditioning in kidney disease, we investigated whether a non-nephrotoxic dose of the ER stress inducers tunicamycin or thapsigargin for preconditioning ameliorate the development of anti-Thy1 nephritis, a mesangioproliferative glomerulonephritis model. As we expected, disease progression was dramatically improved by preconditioning, in association with a decrease in microaneurysm formation, adhesion of Bowman's capsule to the tuft, and proteinuria (Inagi et al, 2008). Importantly, the protective effect of preconditioning against glomerular damage was associated with modulation of the adaptive UPR. While the expression of ER chaperones (GRP78 and ORP150) was significantly increased as the disease progressed, the preconditioning slightly enhanced the basal level of this expression and significantly suppressed the aberrant ER chaperone expression after disease induction. Similarly, preconditioning slightly enhanced the basal level of the PERK-eIF2α axis in translation attenuation and suppressed its augmentation by disease induction. These findings demonstrate that ER preconditioning induces a robust basal (physiological) UPR state and maintains a stable UPR level in the kidney.

Other reports have also emphasized the effectiveness of ER stress preconditioning in the kidney. Preconditioning with tunicamycin or doxorubicin mitigates experimental membranous nephropathy via ER chaperone enhancement (Cybulsky et al, 2002). Kitamura and colleagues extensively investigated the role of ER stress in inflammation, and clearly showed that inflammatory cytokine-induced NF-κB activation in mesangial cells was suppressed by preconditioning via the IRE1-XBP1 axis (Hayakawa et al, 2010).

Modality	Site (disease) and enhanced UPR	Reference
Tunicamycin or Doxorubicin		
	Podocytes (Heymann nephritis) GRP78 ↑, PERK-eIF2α axis	
		Cybursky AV, et al, J Biol Chem 2002
Tunicamycin or thapsigargin		
	Mesangial cells (anti-Thy1 nephritis) GRP78 ↑, PERK-eIF2α axis	
		Inagi R, et al, Am J Soc Nephrol 2008
	(NF-kB-related Inflammation) IRE1, PERK-eIF2α axis	
		Hayakawa K, et al, Am J Soc Nephrol 2010
Tunicamycin, thapsigargin, or trans-4,5-dihydroxy-1,2-dithiane,		
	Tubular epithelial cells (oxidative stress) GRP78 ↑	
		Hung CC, et al, J Biol Chem 2003
BIX (GRP78 inducer)		
	Tubular epithelial cells (ischemia-reperfusion) ATF6 axis	
		Prachasilchai W et al., J Pharmacal Sci, 2009

Table 4. ER stress preconditioning in kidney disease

Preconditioning with an ER stress inducer such as tunicamycin and thapsigargin confers a protective effect against kidney disease. BIX is a GRP78 inducer, 1-(3,4-dihydroxyohenyl)-2-thiocyanate-ethanone which markedly induces GRP78 production and is preferentially mediated by the ATF6 pathway.

6. Conclusion

The physiological state of the UPR pathway is important to the maintenance of ER homeostasis. Under pathogenic conditions, however, ER stress and the subsequent overwhelming UPR activation are significantly induced in various kidney cells and

contribute to kidney disease progression rather than regulating ER homeostasis. Enhancement of the basal level of the UPR, particularly the adaptive UPR axis, might support appropriate ER homeostasis and a robust cell state. Cells might accordingly become resistant to pathogenic factors, and an aberrant UPR might be suppressed (Fig. 2).
It is now established that ER stress is involved in cardiac, vascular, and metabolic diseases, which in turn affect kidney disease development. UPR is intricately linked to two other important stress pathways, HIF and Nrf2, which also contribute to disease progression. Keeping intact the balance of these stress signal networks via regulation of the UPR will allow us to maintain cellular homeostasis and disease prevention.

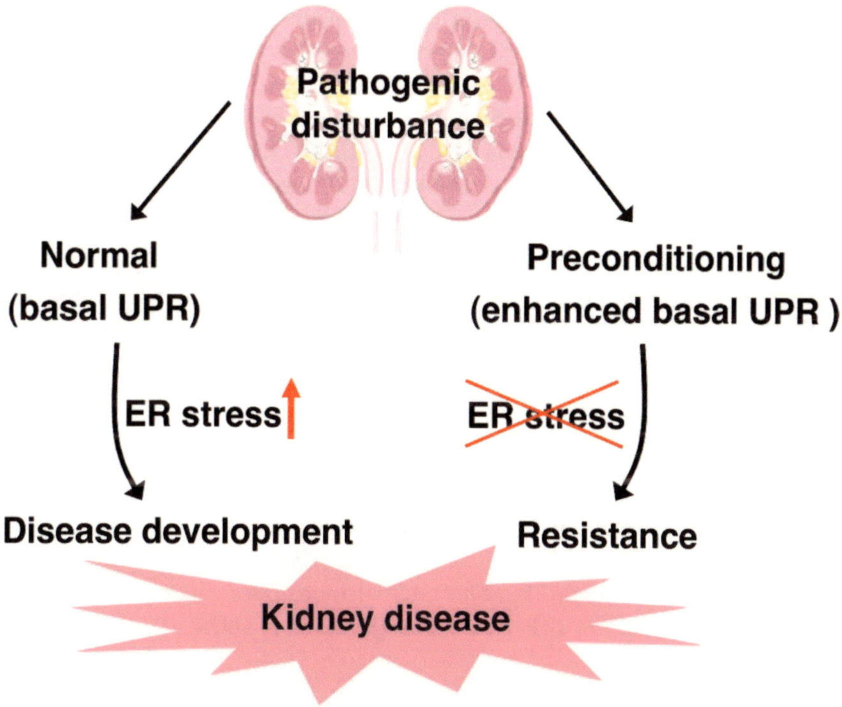

Fig. 2. ER stress preconditioning in the kidney.

Under pathogenic conditions, the basal UPR for ER homeostasis transformed to the pathogenic state, and thereby leads to the features of ER stress-related kidney diseases. In contrast, preconditioning with ER stress enhances the basal UPR level and induces kidney cells to develop resistance to pathogens.

7. Acknowledgments

I am grateful to Masaomi Nangaku, MD, PhD, of the Tokyo University School of Medicine, for critically reviewing the manuscript. Our studies regarding ER stress and kidney disease were supported by Grants-in-Aid for Scientific Research from the Japan Society for the Promotion of Science (22590880), and grants from The Kidney Foundation, Japan (JKFB09-2), Nakayama Foundation for Human Science, Japan, and the Japanese Association of Dialysis Physician (22051) to RI.

8. References

Ali, MM.; Bagratuni, T.; Davenport, EL.; Nowak, PR.; Silva-Santisteban, MC.; Hardcastle, A.; McAndrews, C.; Rowlands, MG.; Morgan, GJ.; Aherne, W.; Collins, I.; Davies, FE. & Pearl, LH. (2011). Structure of the Ire1 autophosphorylation complex and implications for the unfolded protein response. *EMBO J*, Vol.30, No.5, pp. 894-905.

Asmellash, S.; Stevens, JL. & Ichimura, T (2005). Modulating the endoplasmic reticulum stress response with trans-4,5-dihydroxy-1,2-dithiane prevents chemically induced renal injury in vivo. *Toxicol Sci,* Vol.88, No.2, pp. 576-584.

Back, SH.; Scheuner, D.; Han, J.; Song, B.; Ribick, M.; Wang, J.; Gildersleeve, RD.; Pennathur, S. & Kaufman, RJ. (2009). Translation attenuation through eIF2alpha phosphorylation prevents oxidative stress and maintains the differentiated state in beta cells. *Cell Metab*, Vol.10, No.1, pp.13-26.

Bando, Y.; Tsukamoto, Y.; Katayama, T.; Ozawa, K.; Kitao, Y.; Hori, O.; Stern, DM.; Yamauchi, A. & Ogawa, S. (2004). ORP150/HSP12A protects renal tubular epithelium from ischemia-induced cell death. *FASEB J*, Vol.18, No.12, pp. 1401-1403.

Bardag-Gorce, F.; Oliva, J.; Lin, A.; Li, J.; French, BA. & French, SW. (2010). Proteasome inhibitor up regulates liver antioxidative enzymes in rat model of alcoholic liver disease. *Exp Mol Pathol*, Vol.90, No.1, pp. 123-130.

Bernhardt, WM.; Wiesener, MS.; Scigalla, P.; Chou, J.; Schmieder, RE.; Günzler, V. & Eckardt, KU. (2010). Inhibition of prolyl hydroxylases increases erythropoietin production in ESRD. *J Am Soc Nephrol,* Vol.21, No.12, pp. 2151-2156.

Bhatt, K,; Feng, L.; Pabla, N.; Liu, K.; Smith, S. & Dong, Z. (2008). Effects of targeted Bcl-2 expression in mitochondria or endoplasmic reticulum on renal tubular cell apoptosis. *Am J Physiol Renal Physiol*, Vol.294, No. 3, pp. F499-507.

Chen, D.; Thomas, EL. & Kapahi, P. (2009). HIF-1 modulates dietary restriction-mediated lifespan extension via IRE-1 in Caenorhabditis elegans. *PLoS Genet,* Vol.5, No.5, pp. e1000486.

Chen, Y.; Liu, CP.; Xu, KF.; Mao, XD.; Lu, YB.; Fang, L.; Yang, JW. & Liu, C. (2008). Effect of taurine-conjugated ursodeoxycholic acid on endoplasmic reticulum stress and apoptosis induced by advanced glycation end products in cultured mouse podocytes. *Am J Nephrol*, Vol.28, No.6, pp. 1014-1022.

Cullinan, SB. & Diehl, JA. (2006). Coordination of ER and oxidative stress signaling: the PERK/Nrf2 signaling pathway. *Int J Biochem Cell Biol*, Vol.38, No.3, 317-332.

Cybulsky, AV.; Takano, T.; Papillon, J.; Khadir, A.; Liu, J. & Peng, H. (2002). Complement C5b-9 membrane attack complex increases expression of endoplasmic reticulum stress proteins in glomerular epithelial cells. *J Biol Chem,* Vol.277, No.44, pp. 41342-41351.

Cybulsky, AV.; Takano, T.; Papillon, J.; Bijian, K,; Guillemette, J. & Kennedy, CR. (2009). Glomerular epithelial cell injury associated with mutant alpha-actinin-4. *Am J Physiol Renal Physiol*, Vol.297, No.4, pp. F987-95.

DeGracia, DJ. & Montie, HL. (2004). Cerebral ischemia and the unfolded protein response. *J Neurochem*, Vol.91, No.1, pp. 1-8.

Hayakawa, K.; Nakajima, S.; Hiramatsu, N.; Okamura, M.; Huang, T.; Saito, Y.; Tagawa, Y.; Tamai, M.; Takahashi, S.; Yao, J. & Kitamura, M. (2010). ER stress depresses NF-kappaB activation in mesangial cells through preferential induction of C/EBP beta. *J Am Soc Nephrol,* Vol.21, No.1, pp. 73-81.

Hayashi, T.; Saito, A.; Okuno, S.; Ferrand-Drake, M.; Dodd, RL.; Nishi, T.; Maier, CM.; Kinouchi, H. & Chan, PH. (2003). Oxidative damage to the endoplasmic reticulum is implicated in ischemic neuronal death. *J Cereb Blood Flow Metabol,* Vol.23, No.10, pp.1117-1128.

Hung, CC.; Ichimura, T.; Stevens, JL. & Bonventre, JV. (2003). Protection of renal epithelial cells against oxidative injury by endoplasmic reticulum stress preconditioning is mediated by ERK1/2 activation. *J Biol Chem,* Vol.278, No.31, pp. 29317-29326.

Inagi, R.; Nangaku, M.; Usuda, N.; Shimizu, A.; Onogi, H.; Izuhara, Y.; Nakazato, K.; Ueda, Y.; Oishi, H.; Takahashi, S.; Yamamoto, M.; Suzuki, D.; Kurokawa, K.; van Ypersele de Strihou, C. & Miyata, T. (2005a). Novel serpinopathy in rat kidney and pancreas induced by overexpression of megsin. *J Am Soc Nephrol,* Vol.16, No.5, pp. 1339-1349.

Inagi, R.; Nangaku, M.; Onogi, H.; Ueyama, H.; Kitao, Y.; Nakazato, K.; Ogawa, S.; Kurokawa, K.; Couser, WG. & Miyata, T. (2005b). Involvement of endoplasmic reticulum (ER) stress in podocyte injury induced by excessive protein accumulation. *Kidney Int,* Vol.68, No.6, pp. 2639-2650.

Inagi, R.; Yamamoto, Y.; Nangaku, M.; Usuda, N.; Okamato, H.; Kurokawa, K.; van Ypersele de Strihou, C.; Yamamoto, H. & Miyata, T. (2006). A severe diabetic nephropathy model with early development of nodule-like lesions induced by megsin overexpression in RAGE/iNOS transgenic mice. *Diabetes,* Vol.55, No.2, pp. 356-366.

Inagi, R.; Kumagai, T.; Nishi, H.; Kawakami, T.; Miyata, T.; Fujita, T. & Nangaku, M. (2008). Preconditioning with endoplasmic reticulum stress ameliorates mesangioproliferative glomerulonephritis. *J Am Soc Nephro,* Vol.19, No.5, pp. 915-922.

Inagi, R. (2010). Endoplasmic reticulum stress as a progression factor for kidney injury. *Curr Opin Pharmacol.* Vol.10, No.2, pp. 156-165. Review.

Iwawaki, T.; Akai, R.; Kohno, K. & Miura, M. (2004). A transgenic mouse model for monitoring endoplasmic reticulum stress. *Nat Med,* Vol.10, No.1, pp. 98-102.

Izuhara, Y.; Nangaku, M.; Takizawa, S.; Takahashi, S.; Shao, J.; Oishi, H.; Kobayashi, H.; van Ypersele de Strihou, C. & Miyata, T. (2008). A novel class of advanced glycation inhibitors ameliorates renal and cardiovascular damage in experimental rat models. *Nephrol Dial Transplant,* Vol.23, No.2, pp. 497-509.

Kawakami, T.; Inagi, R.; Wada, T.; Tanaka, T.; Fujita, T. & Nangaku, M. (2010). Indoxyl sulfate inhibits proliferation of human proximal tubular cells via endoplasmic reticulum stress. *Am J Physiol Renal Physio,* Vol.299, No.3, pp. F568-576.

Kars, M.; Yang, L.; Gregor, MF.; Mohammed, BS.; Pietka, TA.; Finck, BN.; Patterson, BW.; Horton, JD.; Mittendorfer, B.; Hotamisligil, GS. & Klein, S. (2010). Tauroursodeoxycholic Acid may improve liver and muscle but not adipose tissue insulin sensitivity in obese men and women. *Diabetes,* Vol.59, No.8, pp. 1899-905.

Kim, I.; Xu, W. & Reed, JC. (2008). Cell death and endoplasmic reticulum stress: disease relevance and therapeutic opportunities. *Nat Rev Drug Discov*, Vol.7, No.12, pp. 1013-1030. Review.

Koditz, J.; Nesper, J.; Wottawa, M.; Stiehl, DP.; Camenisch, G.; Franke, C.; Myllyharju, J.; Wenger, RH. & Katschinski, DM. (2007). Oxygen-dependent ATF-4 stability is mediated by the PHD3 oxygen sensor. *Blood*, Vol.110, No.10, pp. 3610-3617.

Lee AS. (2007). GRP78 induction in cancer: therapeutic and prognostic implications. *Cancer Res*, Vol.67, No.8, pp. 3496-3499.

Lee, KP.; Dey, M.; Neculai, D.; Cao, C.; Dever, TE. & Sicheri, F. (2008). Structure of the dual enzyme Ire1 reveals the basis for catalysis and regulation in nonconventional RNA splicing. *Cel,l* Vol.132, No.1, pp. 89-100.

Liu, XL.; Doné, SC.; Yan, K.; Kilpeläinen, P.; Pikkarainen, T. & Tryggvason, K. (2004). Defective trafficking of nephrin missense mutants rescued by a chemical chaperone. *J Am Soc Nephrol*, Vol.15, No.7, pp. 1731-1738.

Lindenmeyer, MT.; Rastaldi, MP.; Ikehata, M.; Neusser, MA.; Kretzler, M.; Cohen, CD. & Schlöndorff, D. (2008). Proteinuria and hyperglycemia induce endoplasmic reticulum stress. *J Am Soc Nephrol*, Vol.19, No.11, pp. 2225-2236.

Loughlin, DT. & Artlett, CM. (2010). Precursor of advanced glycation end products mediates ER-stress-induced caspase-3 activation of human dermal fibroblasts through NAD(P)H oxidase 4. *PLoS One*, Vol.5, No.6, pp. e11093.

Malhotra, JD. & Kaufman RJ. (2007). Endoplasmic reticulum stress and oxidative stress: a vicious cycle or a double-edged sword? *Antioxid Redox Signal*, Vol.9, No.12, pp. 2277-93.

Markan, S.; Kohli, HS.; Joshi, K.; Minz, RW.; Sud, K.; Ahuja, M.; Anand, S. & Khullar, M. (2009). Up regulation of the GRP-78 and GADD-153 and down regulation of Bcl-2 proteins in primary glomerular diseases: a possible involvement of the ER stress pathway in glomerulonephritis. *Mol Cell Biochem*, Vol.324, No.1-2, pp. 131-138.

Morse, E.; Schroth, J.; You, YH.; Pizzo, DP.; Okada, S.; Ramachandrarao, S.; Vallon, V.; Sharma, K. & Cunard, R. (2010). TRB3 is stimulated in diabetic kidneys, regulated by the ER stress marker CHOP, and is a suppressor of podocyte MCP-1. *Am J Physiol Renal Physiol*, Vol.299, No.5, pp. F965-72.

Nakajo, A.; Khoshnoodi, J.; Takenaka, H.; Hagiwara, E.; Watanabe, T.; Kawakami, H.; Kurayama, R.; Sekine, Y.; Bessho, F.; Takahashi, S.; Swiatecka-Urban, A.; Tryggvason, K. & Yan, K. (2007). Mizoribine corrects defective nephrin biogenesis by restoring intracellular energy balance. *J Am Soc Nephrol*, Vol.18, No.9, pp. 2554-2564.

Nangaku, M. (2006). Chronic hypoxia and tubulointerstitial injury: a final common pathway to end-stage renal failure. *J Am Soc Nephrol*, Vol.17, No.1, pp. 17-25.

Natarajan, R.; Salloum, FN.; Fisher, BJ.; Smithson, L.; Almenara, J. & Fowler, AA 3rd. (2009). Prolyl hydroxylase inhibition attenuates post-ischemic cardiac injury via induction of endoplasmic reticulum stress genes. *Vascul Pharmacol*, Vol.51, No.2-3, pp.110-118.

Ohse, T.; Inagi, R.; Tanaka, T.; Ota, T.; Miyata, T.; Kojima, I.; Ingelfinger, JR.; Ogawa, S.; Fujita, T. & Nangaku, M. (2006). Albumin induces endoplasmic reticulum stress and apoptosis in renal proximal tubular cells. *Kidney Int,* Vol.70, No.8, pp. 1447-1455.

Ostergaard, L.; Simonsen, U.; Eskildsen-Helmond, Y.; Vorum, H.; Uldbjerg, N.; Honoré, B. & Mulvany, MJ. (2009). Proteomics Reveals Lowering Oxygen Alters Cytoskeletal and Endoplasmatic Stress Proteins in Human Endothelial Cells. *Proteomics,* Vol.9, No.19, pp. 4457-4467.

Ozcan, L.; Ergin, AS.; Lu, A.; Chung, J.; Sarkar, S.; Nie, D.; Myers, MG Jr. & Ozcan, U. (2009). Endoplasmic reticulum stress plays a central role in development of leptin resistance. *Cell Metab,* Vol.9, No.1, pp. 35-51.

Ozcan, U.; Yilmaz, E.; Ozcan, L.; Furuhashi, M.; Vaillancourt, E.; Smith, RO.; Gorgun, CZ. & Hotamisligil, GS. (2006). Chemical chaperones reduce ER stress and restore glucose homeostasis in a mouse model of type 2 diabetes. *Science,* Vol.313, No.5790, pp. 1137-1140.

Pallet, N.; Bouvier, N.; Bendjallabah, A.; Rabant, M.; Flinois, JP.; Hertig, A.; Legendre, C.; Beaune, P.; Thervet, E. & Anglicheau, D. (2008). Cyclosporine-induced endoplasmic reticulum stress triggers tubular phenotypic changes and death. *Am J Transplant,* Vol.8, No.11, pp. 2283-2296.

Prachasilchai, W.; Sonoda, H.; Yokota-Ikeda, N.; Ito, K.; Kudo, T.; Imaizumi, K. & Ikeda, M. (2009). The protective effect of a newly developed molecular chaperone-inducer against mouse ischemic acute kidney injury. *J Pharmacol Sci,* Vol.109, No.2, pp. 311-3114.

Qi, W.; Mu, J.; Luo, ZF.; Zeng, W.; Guo, YH.; Pang, Q.; Ye, ZL.; Liu, L.; Yuan, FH. & Feng, B. (2011). Attenuation of diabetic nephropathy in diabetes rats induced by streptozotocin by regulating the endoplasmic reticulum stress inflammatory response. *Metabolism,* Vol.60, No.5, pp.594-603.

Ron, D. & Walter, P. (2007). Signal integration in the endoplasmic reticulum unfolded protein response. *Nat Rev Mol Cell Biol,* Vol.8, No.7, pp. 519-529. Review. Sun, HL.;

Sun, L.; Li, YY.; Shao, MM.; Cheng, XY.; Ge, N.; Lu, JD. & Li, SM. (2009). ACE-inhibitor suppresses the apoptosis induced by endoplasmic reticulum stress in renal tubular in experimental diabetic rats. *Exp Clin Endocrinol Diabetes,* Vol.117, No.7, pp. 336-344.

Tabas, I. & Ron, D. (2011). Integrating the mechanisms of apoptosis induced by endoplasmic reticulum stress. *Nat Cell Biol,* Vol.13, No.3, pp. 184-190. Review.

Takano, K.; Tabata, Y.; Kitao, Y.; Murakami, R.; Suzuki, H.; Yamada, M.; Iinuma, M.; Yoneda, Y.; Ogawa, S. & Hori, O. (2007). Methoxyflavones protect cells against endoplasmic reticulum stress and neurotoxin. *Am J Physiol Cell Physiol,* Vol.292, No.1, pp. C353-61.

Werno, C.; Zhou, J. & Brüne, B. (2008). A23187, ionomycin and thapsigargin upregulate mRNA of HIF-1alpha via endoplasmic reticulum stress rather than a rise in intracellular calcium. *J Cell Physiol,* Vol.215, No.3, pp. 708-714.

Xie, Q.; Khaoustov, VI.; Chung, CC.; Sohn, J.; Krishnan, B.; Lewis, DE. & Yoffe, B. (2002). Effect of tauroursodeoxycholic acid on endoplasmic reticulum stress-induced caspase-12 activation. *Hepatology*, Vol.36, No.3, pp. 592-601.

Yokouchi, M.; Hiramatsu, N.; Hayakawa, K.; Okamura, M.; Du, S.; Kasai, A.; Takano, Y.; Shitamura, A.; Shimada, T.; Yao, J. & Kitamura, M. (2008). Involvement of selective reactive oxygen species upstream of proapoptotic branches of unfolded protein response. *J Biol Chem,* Vo.283, No.7, pp. 4252-4260.

Part 5

Miscellaneous

14

Urinary Biomarkers in Glomerulonephritis

Sophie Ohlsson
Lund University
Sweden

1. Introduction

A biomarker refers to a biologic, biochemical or molecular event that can be assayed qualitatively and quantitatively by laboratory techniques. The level of biomarkers should correlate with disease pathogenesis or activity. Biomarker discovery for kidney diseases is currently an active area of investigation. Today golden standard for diagnosis and for evaluation of treatment results is kidney biopsy - an invasive test with considerable risks.
Biomarkers have the potential to be useful tools for non invasive evaluation and management of patients suffering from glomerulonephritis. Biomarkers that predict impending disease activity could be used to initiate treatment early, which could minimize the initial insult, allow a reduction in duration and intensity of therapy, improve outcomes and lessen chronic renal injury. Biomarkers that predict response to therapy could be used to choose the most appropriate regimen for an individual patient and biomarkers that reflect disease severity could be used to adjust the intensity of therapy.
Profiles as well as individual markers, with the potential to reduce the use of renal biopsy, improve therapeutic efficacy, and limit toxicity are emerging and this chapter will describe some examples in the context of IgA nephropathy, lupus nephritis, ANCA-associated small vessel vasculitis (ASVV) with renal involvement and focal segmental glomerulosclerosis (FSGS).

2. Proteomics – biomarker patterns

Renal and urinary proteomics are among the most rapidly growing sub disciplines of proteomics applied to biomedical research. There is much interest of nephrologists and renal physiologists in applying proteomics to address clinical and basic questions. Urinary proteome analysis offers opportunities for pattern recognition as well as single biomarker discovery. Urine as a body fluid for clinical analysis is relatively stable, presumably due to the fact that its "stored" for some time in the bladder, hence proteolytic degradation by endogenous proteases may be essentially complete by the time of voiding. Urinary proteins and peptides originate not only from glomerular filtration, but also from tubular secretion, epithelial cells shed from the kidney and urinary tract, secreted exosomes and seminal secretions. Urine is thus a rich source of biomarkers for a wide range of diseases, due to specific changes in its proteome. Commonly used methods for urinary proteome analyses include two-dimensional polyacrylamide gel electrophoresis (2-D PAGE), different types of mass spectrometry, capillary electrophoresis and protein microarrays [Fliser D, Novak J et al 2007; Muller GA, Muller CA & Dihazi 2007].

2.1 Possible clinical applications in glomerulonephrits

2.1.1 Immunoglobulin A (IgA) nephropathy

There are several proteomics studies on IgA nephropathy, showing promising results. A specific urinary polypeptide pattern can distinguish IgA nephropathy from healthy controls with a sensitivity of 100% and specificity of 90%, and from membranous nephropathy with a sensitivity of 77% and a specificity of 100%. In addition, compared with patterns established earlier in minimal change disease, focal segmental glomerulosclerosis and diabetic nephropathy, the pattern of IgA nephropathy had both sensitivity and specificity of 100%. Even most patients in clinical remission with normal clinical testing (dipstick urinalysis and quantitative proteinuria) were correctly classified by the pattern of polypeptides identified. Sequencing of three of the discriminatory polypeptides identified three different fragments of serum albumin. [Haubitz M, Wittke S et al, 2005].

2.1.2 Lupus nephritis

Urinary proteomic profiling was described in lupus nephritis by Mosley et al, 2006. The authors reported that two protein ions had been detected, which could distinguish between active and inactive lupus nephritis with 92% sensitivity and specificity each. The two biomarkers could predict early relapse and remission, but were not further isolated and identified. Zhang et al, 2008, identified three potential low-molecular-weight biomarkers, namely hepcidin, alpha 1 antitrypsin and an N-terminal fragment of albumin. There were two isoforms of hepcidin, 20 and 25 amino acid (aa) long. Hepcidin 20 increased 4 months pre-flare and then slowly returned to baseline by 4 months post-flare. Hepcidin 25 decreased at flare and returned to baseline by 4 months post-flare. There was no correlation between the 20 and 25 aa isoforms. Hepcidin is a LMW peptide hormone that has antimicrobial activity, regulates iron homeostasis, and has been implicated in the pathogenesis of the anemia of chronic inflammation, including that of chronic kidney Disease [Deicher R, Horl W H 2004]. Urine hepcidin has been shown to increase during inflammation and decline as inflammation resolved. The expression is induced by interleukin-6 (IL-6) and is suppressed by TNF-alpha, cytokines that are implicated in the pathogenesis of SLE [Aringer M, Smolen J S 2005].

2.1.3 ANCA associated small vessel vasculitis

Haubitz et al recently presented one of the first urinary proteomics studies on ANCA associated small vessel vasculitis (ASVV) with renal involvement. Urinary proteome analysis with CE-MS was shown to permit differentiation of patients with active AAV *versus* healthy individuals and patients with other chronic renal diseases. A panel of biomarkers also permits distinguishing between patients with active AAV and patients in remission. Initiation of immunosuppressive treatment results in a change of the pattern from active to inactive disease, correlating with clinically decreasing vasculitis activity and the achievement of remission. The most frequently observed peptides were proteolytic products of hemoglobin. The existence of these fragments is to be expected as microhematuria is a characteristic finding in vasculitis. Remarkably only C- and N-terminal fragments could be defined as biomarkers, whereas fragments from the core of the molecules, although present in urine, showed no significant value as biomarkers. The existence of specific fragments may be a result of the specifically released proteases in ANCA-associated vasculitis after activation of neutrophils by ANCA [Haubitz M, Good D M et al 2009].

2.1.4 Focal segmental glomerulosclerosis

Candiano et al published a proteomics study on idiopathic nephrotic syndrome in 2006, comprising patients suffering from minimal change disease, membranous glomerulonephritis or focal segmental glomerulosclerosis (FSGS). Albumin and alpha 1AT fragments represent the major proteins in urine of patients with nephrotic syndrome, where at least 50 isoforms of these proteins were characterized by proteomics analysis. Most of these isoforms derive from plasma, but a few were formed *in situ* by specific proteolysis. Albumin adducts that harbor both the COOH and NH2 terminal parts of the protein also were detected, suggesting the formation of covalent chemical adducts [Candiano G, Musante L et al 2006]. Two years earlier, Weissinger et al described urinary proteome patterns in healthy subjects, compared to different primary renal diseases. One-hundred seventy-three polypeptides were present in more than 90% of the urine samples obtained from healthy individuals, while 690 polypeptides were present with more than 50% probability. These data permitted the establishment of a "normal" polypeptide pattern in healthy individuals. Polypeptides found in the urine of patients differed significantly from the normal controls. These differences allowed the distinction of specific protein spectra in patients with minimal change disease (MCD), membranous glomerulonephritis (MGN), and focal segmental glomerulosclerosis (FSGS). Abnormal pattern of proteins were found even in urine from patients in clinical remission [Weissinger E M, Wittke S et al 2004].

3. Individual biomarkers

3.1 Immunoglobulin A (IgA) nephropathy

Urinary concentration of several cytokines involved in proliferation and repair has been evaluated as potential biomarkers of histopathological changes and as predictors of long-term prognosis in IgA nephropathy. Urinary IL-6 has been shown to predict long term renal outcome in IgA nephropathy [Harada K, Akai Y et al 2002]. The excretion of IL-6 and epidermal growth factor (EGF) has been correlated with degree of tubulointerstitial damage, with the urinary IL-6/EGF ratio proposed as a marker for progression of the renal damage [Ranieri E, Gesualdo L et al 1996]. Other potential markers that have been evaluated include urinary alpha 1 antitrypsin and heparan sulfate [Mitsuhashi H, Tsukada Y et al 1993]. Urine N-acetyl-alpha-D-glucosaminidase (NAG) levels are measured in some clinics. NAG is a lysosomal enzyme abundant in lesions of proximal tubular damage in patients with nephrotic syndrome, glomerulonephritis and diabetic nephropathy. Nonetheless, the sensitivity and specificity of this biomarker for IgAN is not ideal. In patients characterized with tubulointerstitial lesion, urinary NAG levels correlated well with the extent of tubulointerstitial changes. In patients characterized with primary glomerular lesion and accompanied tubulointerstitial changes such as IgAN, the elevated urinary NAG levels often lag the morphologic changes due to tubulointerstitial injury [Bazzi C, Petoni V et al 2002]. Ding et al presented a study in 2007, claiming that urinary NGAL level holds promise as a noninvasive marker, more sensitive and specific than NAG, for early detection of sub-microscopic tubulointerstitial injury of IgAN [Ding H, Yani H et al 2007]. Urinary IgG and IgA correlated with glomerular filtration rate and grading of histological features and was significantly elevated compared to healthy controls [Halling S F E, Söderberg M P & Berg U B 2005]. Despite these promising reports of differential presence of proteins and protein complexes, none of the tests has so far been developed into a clinically useful assay. Very recently, Peters et al published a study demonstrating high urinary levels of kidney injury molecule 1 (KIM-1) as an independent predictor of end stage renal disease in patients with IgA nephropathy [Peters H P, Waanders F et al 2011].

3.2 Lupus nephritis

Current laboratory markers, such as proteinuria, urine protein-to-creatinine ratio, creatinine clearance, anti-dsDNA and complement levels are unsatisfactory. They lack sensitivity and specificity for differentiating renal activity and damage in lupus nephritis. There are many candidate biomarkers in lupus nephritis. In this chapter, we have chosen to describe some of the most promising ones.

3.2.1 Monocyte chemoattractant protein 1

Monocyte chemoattractant protein 1 (MCP-1) is a leukocyte chemotactic factor, involved in mediating inflammation and injury in lupus nephritis. MCP-1 drives fibrosis both indirectly via macrophages, but also through direct induction of a fibrotic response in glomerular mesangial cells [Tesch G H 2008]. The urinary MCP-1 level is elevated in active lupus nephritis, compared to inactive disease and healthy controls, and reduced after immunosuppressive treatment [Wada T, Segawa C et al 1996]. In a longitudinal follow up, urinary MCP-1 increased 2-4 months before renal flares and remained high for at least 4 months after treatment of flares. In patients who improved clinically, MCP-1 levels fell to control levels, whereas in treatment refractory patients, the levels remained high [Rovin B H, Song D J et al 2005]. Thus MCP-1 is a very promising biomarker in lupus nephritis and possibly also a future therapeutic target.

3.2.2 Neutrophil gelatinase-associated lipocalin

Neutrophil gelatinase-associated lipocalin (NGAL) is constitutively expressed at low levels in the kidneys, but up regulated following acute renal injury and various insults such as inflammation, ischemia and infection and considered as a good biomarker for acute kidney injury, with high sensitivity and specificity [Bolignano D, Donato V et al 2008]. NGAL In lupus nephritis, urinary levels of NGAL has been found to differentiate between patients with or without active renal disease. NGAL correlates more strongly with histological activity scores than chronicity scores on renal biopsies. Significant correlation has been seen with urine protein-to-creatinine ratios but not with proteinuria, serum creatinine level or conventional markers such as anti-dsDNA and complement levels. In longitudinal studies, NGAL was found to increase up to 3 months before renal flare and is considered to be a very promising biomarker in lupus nephritis [Hinze C H, Suzuki M et al 2008].

3.2.3 Tumor Necrosis Factor-Like Inducer of Apoptosis

Tumor necrosis factor-like inducer of apoptosis (TWEAK) is a multifunctional cytokine, involved in up regulation of pro inflammatory mediators and induction of cell death and apoptosis. TWEAK expression is dramatically increased in the context of inflammation and injury and its expression is found to be dysregulated in chronic inflammatory states [Winkles J A 2008]. Stimulation of kidney cells with TWEAK induces expression of chemokines and inflammatory mediators, such as MCP-1, RANTES, IP-10, VCAM-1 and ICAM-1 - which have all been suggested as biomarkers in SLE. Urinary TWEAK levels were significantly higher in patients with active nephritis, compared to inactive. Urinary TWEAK also correlated with renal SLE activity scores, anti-dsDNA and complement levels, but there was on the other hand no correlation with proteinuria - suggesting that the increased levels in urine was not merely due to glomerular damage. The urinary TWEAK levels peaked at the time of flare, with an increasing trend before and a decreasing trend after flares. Unfortunately, the small rise in uTWEAK prior to the disease flare does not appear to have any predictive value [Gaipl U S, Voll R E et al 2005]. Urinary TWEAK did not discriminate between different LN histological classes. This is a common problem in LN biomarker studies. The problem probably relates to the small number of subjects studied who are then sub grouped into a number of histological classes, the inherent sampling error associated with renal biopsy, and the lack of a clear system to assess inflammatory disease activity at the tissue level.

3.3 ANCA associated small vessel vasculitis

Previous studies have shown that the renal function at diagnosis is a strong predictor not only for renal survival but also for patient survival in ASVV. Other factors have also been reported to predict outcome in ASVV, such as severity of the disease at diagnosis, treatment related infections, alpha 1 antitrypsin deficiency, high levels of PR3-ANCA measured by capture ELISA and low levels of thrombocytes. However these findings have usually not been confirmed in repeated investigations. Proteinuria, severe interstitial fibrosis and glomerulosclerosis, which are known to predict outcome in chronic proteinuric glomerulonephritides have also been found to be important risk factors for development of renal failure in ASVV [Pallan L, Savage CO & Harper L 2009]. The need of better non invasive prognostic markers is significant.

3.3.1 Monocyte chemoattractant protein 1

Indirectly, by macrophage recruitment, and also via direct induction of a fibrotic response in glomerular mesangial cells - MCP-1 has the potential to drive the process of renal fibrosis [Tesch G H 2008]. Urinary excretion of MCP-1 is increased in patients with ASVV. The degree of excretion correlates significantly with patient outcome, considering critical damage or death. The association with poor prognosis was stronger for U-MCP-1 than for conventional prognostic markers like CRP, BVAS (Birmingham vasculitis activity score), and ANCA, as well as compared to candidate markers like U- IgM and U-IL-8 [Ohlsson S, Bakoush O et al 2009]. Urinary MCP-1 is considered very promising biomarker in ASVV. A longitudinal study for validation of these results is ongoing.

3.3.2 IgM

In other glomerulonephritides, not associated with vasculitis, elevated urine excretion of high molecular weight proteins, e. g. IgM, has been found to be a better predictor of renal outcome than the degree of albuminuria. In ASVV, urinary levels of IgM was found to be a better independent predictor of renal survival than serum creatinine at diagnosis and, in addition to age, it was an important predictor for patient survival. Patients with low urinary IgM excretion maintained their kidney function despite a high degree of albuminuria, and patients with high urine IgM excretion were more likely to develop ESRD [Bakoush O, Segelmark M et al 2006]. The authors of this study recommend routine measurement of urine IgM concentrations at diagnosis in patients with ANCA-associated small vessel vasculitis, as a relatively cheap, non-invasive and early prognostic marker.

3.3.3 FSGS

The glomerular microenvironment is influenced by circulating growth factors that are filtered from the blood stream and pass the glomerular filtration barrier. The role of IGF-binding proteins (IGFBPs) has been studied in two diseases that concern podocytes. The glomerular expression and urinary excretion of IGFBP-1, -2, and -3 were studied in patients with focal segmental glomerulosclerosis (FSGS) or minimal change disease (MCD). It was found that patients with active FSGS excrete high amounts of IGFBP-1 and -3. In human podocytes, we can induce mRNA expression of IGFBP-3 in response to TGF-β and in human microvascular endothelial cells expression of IGFBP-1 and -3 in response to TGF-β and Bradykinin. The conclusion was that the local expression of IGFBPs in podocytes and endothelial cells might contribute to the pathogenesis of glomerular disease and that IGFBP-1 and -3 are potential non-invasive markers of FSGS, differentiating against MCD [Worthmann K, Peters I et al 2010].

4. Summary

Urinary proteomics has great potential in biomarker discovery in kidney diseases. So far we have partially achieved the goals to better understand the biology and physiology of the kidney, and to unravel pathogenic mechanisms and /or pathophysiology of kidney disorders.

Biomarker	**Diagnosis/Reference**
Hepcidin	Lupus/Zhang et al 2008
Alpha-1-antitrypsin	Lupus/Zhang et al 2008 IgAN/Mitsuhashi et al 1993
Albumin, N-terminal	Lupus/Zhang et al 2008
Albumin fragments	IgAN/Haubitz et al 2005
Hemoglobulin, N- and C-terminal parts	ASVV/Haubitz et al 2005
IL-6	IgAN/Harada et al 2002
EGF	IgAN/Raniere et al 1996
Heparansulfate	IgAN/Mitsuhashi et al 1993
NAG	IgAN/Bazzi et al 2002
NGAL	IgAN/Ding et al 2007 Lupus/Hinze et al 2008
IgG	IgAN/Halling et al 2005
IgA	IgAN/Halling et al 2005
IgM	ASVV/Bakoush et al 2006
KIM-1	IgAN/Peters et al 2011
MCP-1	Lupus/Wada et al 1996, Rovin et al 2005 ASVV/Ohlsson et al 2009
TWEAK	Lupus/Gaipl et al 2005
IGFBP-1, -3	FSGS/Worthmann et al 2010

Table I. Urinary biomarkers in glomerulonephritis. IgAN: IgA-nephritis, IL-6: interleukin 6, EGF: epidermal growth factor, NAG: N-acetyl-alpha-D-glucosaminidase, NGAL: neutrophil gelatinase associated lipocalin, KIM-1: kidney injury molecule, MCP-1: monocyte chemoattactant protein 1, TWEAK: Tumor necrosis factor-like inducer of apoptosis, IGFBP: insulin-like growth factor binding protein

For biomarker discovery, although a large number of biomarker candidates have been identified, they are neither fully validated in a large cohort, nor ready for routine clinical practice at present. NGAL and MCP-1 are both extremely promising urinary biomarkers. Whereas NGAL seems to be more of a marker of acute kidney injury, the prognostic value of MCP-1 most likely comes from this protein's role in driving the process of fibrosis and scarring. In experimental glomerulonephritis, there is increased glomerular synthesis of MCP-1, and systemic administration of an anti-MCP-1 antibody has been demonstrated to reduce the severity of acute glomerulonephritis as well as subsequent scarring, implying that MCP-1 could be a possible therapeutic target also in man [Wada T, Yokoyama H et al 1996].

5. References

Aringer M, Smolen J S (2005). Cytokine expression in lupus kidneys. *Lupus*, Vol14, pp. 13-18

Bakoush O, Segelmark M et al (2006). Urine IgM excretion predicts outcome in ANCA-associated renal vasculitis. *Nephrol Dial Transplant*, Vol.21, pp. 1263-1269

Bazzi C, Petoni V et al (2002). Urinary N-acetyl-beta-glucosaminidase excretion is a marker of tubular cell dysfunction and a predictor of outcome in primary glomerulonephritis. *Nephrol Dial Transplant*, Vol.17, pp. 1890-1896

Bolignano D, Donato V et al (2008). Neutrophil gelatinase-associated lipocalin (NGAL) as a marker of kidney damage. *Am J Kidney Dis*, Vol.52, pp. 595-605

Candiano G, Musante L et al (2006). Repetitive fragmentation products of albumin and alpha 1 antitrypsin in glomerular disease associated with nephrotic syndrome. *J Am Soc Nephrol*, Vol.17, pp. 139-148

Deicher R, Horl W H (2004). Hepcidin: a molecular link between inflammation and anemia. *Nephrol Dial Transplant*, Vol.12, pp. 521-524

Ding H, Yani H et al (2007). Urinary neutrophil gelatinase-associated lipocalin (NGAL) is an early biomarker for renal tubulointerstitial injury in IgA nephropathy. *Clin Immunol*, Vol.123, pp. 227-234

Fliser D, Novak J et al. (2007). Advances in urinary proteome analysis and biomarker discovery. *J Am Soc Nephrol*, Vol.18, pp. 1057-1071

Gaipl U S, Voll R E et al (2005). Impaired clearance of dying cells in systemic lupus erythematosus. *Autoimm Rev*, Vol.4, pp. 189-194

Halling S F E, Söderberg M P & Berg U B (2005). Henoch-Schönlein nephritis: clinical findings related to renal function and morphology. *Pediatr Nephrol*, Vol.20, pp. 46-51

Harada K, Akai Y et al. (2002). Prognostic value of urinary interleukin 6 in patients with IgA nephropathy: an 8-year follow-up study. *Nephron*, Vol.92, pp. 824-826

Haubitz M, Good D M et al. (2009). Identification and validation of urinary biomarkers for differential diagnosis and evaluation of therapeutic intervention in anti-neutrophil cytoplasmic antibody associated vasculitis. *Mol Cell Proteomics*, Vol.8, pp. 2296-2307

Haubitz M, Wittke S et al. (2005). Urine protein patterns can serve as diagnostic Tools in patients with IgA nephropathy. *Kidney Int*, Vol.67, pp. 2313-2320

Hinze C H, Suzuki M et al (2008). Neutrophil gelatinase-associated lipocalin is a predictor of the course of global and renal childhood-onset systemic lupus erythematosus disease activity. *Arthritis and Rheumatism*, Vol.60, pp. 2772-2781

Mitsuhashi H, Tsukada Y et al (1993). Urine glycosaminoglycans and heparan sulfate excretions in adult patients with gomerular diseases. *ClinNephrol*, Vol.39, pp. 231-38

Mosley K, Tam F W et al. (2006). Urinary proteomic profiles distinguish between active and inactive lupus nephritis. *Rheumatology (Oxford)*, Vol.45, pp. 1497-1504

Muller GA, Muller CA & Dihazi H. (2007). Clinical proteomics - on the long way from bench to bedside? *Nephrol Dial Transplant*, Vol.22, pp. 1297-1300

Ohlsson S, Bakoush O et al (2009). Monocyte Chemoattractant Protein 1 (MCP-1) is a prognostic marker in ANCA-associated Small Vessel Vasculitis. *Mediators Inflamm*, Vol.2009, 7 pp

Pallan L, Savage C O & Harper L (2009). ANCA-associated vasculitis: from bench research to novel treatments. *Nat Rev Nephrol*, Vol.5, pp. 278-286

Peters HP, Waanders F et al (2011). High urinary excretion of kidney injury molecule 1 is an independent predictor of endstage renal disease in patients with IgA nephropathy. *Nephrol Dial Transplant*, Vol 2011, pp.

Ranieri E, Gesualdo L et al (1996). Urinary IL-6/EGF ratio: a useful prognostic marker for the progression of renal damage in IgA nephropathy. *Kidney Int*, Vol.50, pp. 1990-2001

Rovin B H, Song D J et al (2005). Urine chemokines as biomarkers of human systemic lupus erythematosus activity. *J Am Soc Nephrol*, Vol.16, pp. 467-473

Tesh G H (2008). MCP-1/CCL2: a new diagnostic marker and therapeutic target for progressive renal injury in diabetic nephropathy. *Am J Physiol Renal Physiol*, Vol.294, pp. 697-701

Wada T, Segawa C et al (1996). Monitoring urinary levels of monocyte chemotactic and activating factor reflects disease activity of lupus nephritis. *Kidney Int*, Vol.49, pp. 761-767

Wada T, Yokoyama H et al (1996). Intervention of crescentic glomerulonephritis by antibodies to monocyte chemotactic and activating factor (MCAF/MCP-1). *FASEB Journal*, Vol.10, pp. 1418-1425

Weisinger E M, Wittke S et al (2004). Proteomic patterns established with capillary electrophoresis and mass spectrometry for diagnostic purposes. *Kidney Int*, Vol.65, pp. 2426-2434

Winkles J A (2008). The TWEAK-Fn14 cytokine-receptor axis: discovery, biology and therapeutic targeting. *Nature Rev Drug Discov*, Vol.7, pp. 411-425

Worthmann K, Peters I et al (2010). Urinary excretion of IGFBP-1 and 3 correlate with disease activity and differentiate focal segmental glomerulosclerosis and minimal change disease. *Growth factors*, Vol.28, pp. 129-138

Zhang X, Jin M et al. (2008). Biomarkers of lupus nephritis determined by serial urine proteomics. *Kidney Int*. Vol.74, pp. 799-807